T0263239

Non-Invasive Ventilation

Editors

BRADLEY A. YODER
HARESH KIRPALANI

CLINICS IN PERINATOLOGY

www.perinatology.theclinics.com

Consulting Editor
LUCKY JAIN

December 2016 • Volume 43 • Number 4

ELSEVIER

1600 John F. Kennedy Boulevard ● Suite 1800 ● Philadelphia, Pennsylvania, 19103-2899

http://www.theclinics.com

CLINICS IN PERINATOLOGY Volume 43, Number 4
December 2016 ISSN 0095-5108, ISBN-13: 978-0-323-47748-2

Editor: Kerry Holland
Developmental Editor: Casey Jackson

© **2016 Elsevier Inc. All rights reserved.**

This periodical and the individual contributions contained in it are protected under copyright by Elsevier, and the following terms and conditions apply to their use:

Photocopying

Single photocopies of single articles may be made for personal use as allowed by national copyright laws. Permission of the Publisher and payment of a fee is required for all other photocopying, including multiple or systematic copying, copying for advertising or promotional purposes, resale, and all forms of document delivery. Special rates are available for educational institutions that wish to make photocopies for non-profit educational classroom use. For information on how to seek permission visit www.elsevier.com/permissions or call: (+44) 1865 843830 (UK)/(+1) 215 239 3804 (USA).

Derivative Works

Subscribers may reproduce tables of contents or prepare lists of articles including abstracts for internal circulation within their institutions. Permission of the Publisher is required for resale or distribution outside the institution. Permission of the Publisher is required for all other derivative works, including compilations and translations (please consult www.elsevier.com/permissions).

Electronic Storage or Usage

Permission of the Publisher is required to store or use electronically any material contained in this periodical, including any article or part of an article (please consult www.elsevier.com/permissions). Except as outlined above, no part of this publication may be reproduced, stored in a retrieval system or transmitted in any form or by any means, electronic, mechanical, photocopying, recording or otherwise, without prior written permission of the Publisher.

Notice

No responsibility is assumed by the Publisher for any injury and/or damage to persons or property as a matter of products liability, negligence or otherwise, or from any use or operation of any methods, products, instructions or ideas contained in the material herein. Because of rapid advances in the medical sciences, in particular, independent verification of diagnoses and drug dosages should be made. Although all advertising material is expected to conform to ethical (medical) standards, inclusion in this publication does not constitute a guarantee or endorsement of the quality or value of such product or of the claims made of it by its manufacturer.

Clinics in Perinatology (ISSN 0095-5108) is published quarterly by Elsevier Inc., 360 Park Avenue South, New York, NY 10010-1710. Months of issue are March, June, September, and December. Business and Editorial Offices: 1600 John F. Kennedy Blvd., Ste. 1800, Philadelphia, PA 19103-2899. Customer Service Office: 3251 Riverport Lane, Maryland Heights, MO 63043. Periodicals postage paid at New York, NY and additional mailing offices. Subscription prices are $290.00 per year (US individuals), $502.00 per year (US institutions), $340.00 per year (Canadian individuals), $614.00 per year (Canadian institutions), $420.00 per year (international individuals), $614.00 per year (international institutions), $100.00 per year (US students), and $195.00 per year (Canadian and international students). International air speed delivery is included in all Clinics subscription prices. All prices are subject to change without notice. **POSTMASTER:** Send address changes to *Clinics in Perinatology*, Elsevier Health Sciences Division, Subscription Customer Service, 3251 Riverport Lane, Maryland Heights, MO 63043. **Customer Service: Telephone: 1-800-654-2452** (U.S. and Canada); **1-314-447-8871** (outside U.S. and Canada). **Fax: 1-314-447-8029. E-mail: journalscustomerservice-usa@elsevier.com** (for print support); **journalsonlinesupport-usa@elsevier.com** (for online support).

Reprints. For copies of 100 or more, of articles in this publication, please contact the Commercial Reprints Department, Elsevier Inc., 360 Park Avenue South, New York, NY 10010-1710. Tel. 212-633-3874; Fax: 212-633-3820; E-mail: reprints@elsevier.com.

Clinics in Perinatology is also pubilshed in Spanish by McGraw-Hill Interamericana Editores S.A., P.O. Box 5-237, 06500 Mexico D.F., Mexico.

Clinics in Perinatology is covered in *MEDLINE/PubMed (Index Medicus) Current Contents, Excepta Medica, BIOSIS* and *ISI/BIOMED.*

Contributors

CONSULTING EDITOR

LUCKY JAIN, MD, MBA
Richard W. Blumberg Professor and Interim Chair, Emory University School of Medicine, Department of Pediatrics, Executive Medical Director and Interim Chief Academic Officer, Children's Healthcare of Atlanta, Atlanta, Georgia

EDITORS

BRADLEY A. YODER, MD
Professor, Division of Neonatology, Department of Pediatrics, University of Utah School of Medicine, Salt Lake City, Utah

HARESH KIRPALANI, BM, MSc, FRCPC
Professor of Pediatrics, Division of Neonatology, Children's Hospital of Philadelphia, University of Pennsylvania, Philadelphia, Pennsylvania; Emeritus Professor, Department of Clinical Epidemiology and Biostatistics, McMaster University, Hamilton, Ontario, Canada

AUTHORS

JENNIFER BECK, PhD
Department of Pediatrics, Keenan Research Centre for Biomedical Science, St. Michael's Hospital, University of Toronto; Department of Chemistry and Biology, Institute for Biomedical Engineering and Science Technology (iBEST), Ryerson University and St. Michael's Hospital, Toronto, Ontario, Canada

TAMARA BLEAK, BSN, RN, MBA
Manager, Intermountain Life Flight Children's Services, Salt Lake City, Utah

KEVIN CREZEE, BS, RRT-NPS
Clinical Specialist, Department of Medical Affairs, Mallinckrodt Pharmaceuticals, Hampton, New Jersey

PETER G. DAVIS, MD
Neonatal Research, The Royal Women's Hospital, Parkville, Victoria, Australia

NICOLE R. DOBSON, MD
Department of Pediatrics, Uniformed Services University of Health Sciences, Bethesda, Maryland

STEVEN M. DONN, MD, FAAP
Professor of Pediatrics, Division of Neonatal-Perinatal Medicine, C.S. Mott Children's Hospital, University of Michigan Health System, Ann Arbor, Michigan

MICHAEL DUNN, MD, FRCP(C)
Department of Pediatrics, University of Toronto; Department of Newborn and
Developmental Pediatrics, Sunnybrook Health Sciences Centre, Toronto, Ontario,
Canada

KEVIN C. DYSART, MD
Associate Professor of Clinical Pediatrics, Perelman School of Medicine, University of
Pennsylvania, Philadelphia, Pennsylvania

KIMBERLY S. FIRESTONE, MSc, RRT
Neonatology Department, Neonatal Respiratory Outreach Clinical Liaison, Neonatal
Intensive Care Unit, Akron Children's Hospital, Akron, Ohio

ELIZABETH E. FOGLIA, MD, MSCE
Division of Neonatology, The Children's Hospital of Philadelphia, The Hospital of the
University of Pennsylvania, The University of Pennsylvania Perelman School of Medicine,
Philadelphia, Pennsylvania

SAMIR GUPTA, MD, DM, FRCPCH, FRCPI
Professor of Neonatology, Durham University; Director, Research & Development;
Consultant Neonatologist, Department of Paediatrics, University Hospital of North Tees,
Stockton-on-Tees, United Kingdom

KEVIN IVES, MD
Newborn Services, John Radcliffe Hospital, Oxford University Hospitals, NHS Foundation
Trust, Oxford, United Kingdom

HARESH KIRPALANI, BM, MSc, FRCPC
Professor of Pediatrics, Division of Neonatology, Children's Hospital of Philadelphia,
University of Pennsylvania, Philadelphia, Pennsylvania; Emeritus Professor, Department
of Clinical Epidemiology and Biostatistics, McMaster University, Hamilton, Ontario,
Canada

ANGELA KRIBS, MD
Department of Neonatology and Pediatric Intensive Care, Children's Hospital, University
of Cologne, Cologne, Germany

BRIGITTE LEMYRE, MD, FRCPC
Department of Pediatrics, University of Ottawa, Ottawa, Ontario, Canada

BRETT J. MANLEY, MB BS (Hons), PhD
Neonatal Services, Newborn Research Centre, The Royal Women's Hospital;
The Department of Obstetrics and Gynaecology, The University of Melbourne, Parkville,
Victoria, Australia

LARS MENSE, MD
Department of Pediatrics, University of Ottawa, Ottawa, Ontario, Canada

AMIT MUKERJI, MD, FRCP(C)
Division of Neonatology, Department of Pediatrics, McMaster Children's Hospital,
McMaster University, Hamilton, Ontario, Canada

DONALD NULL Jr, MD, FAAP
Professor of Pediatrics, Division of Neonatology; Director, Newborn ICU; Director,
Neonatal Transport, UC Davis Children's Hospital, Sacramento, California

RAVI MANGAL PATEL, MD, MSc
Division of Neonatal-Perinatal Medicine, Department of Pediatrics, Children's Healthcare of Atlanta, Emory University School of Medicine, Atlanta, Georgia

RICHARD A. POLIN, MD
William T Speck Professor of Pediatrics, College of Physicians and Surgeons, Columbia University, New York, New York

CHARLES C. ROEHR, MD, PhD
Newborn Services, John Radcliffe Hospital, Oxford University Hospitals, NHS Foundation Trust, Oxford, United Kingdom; Department of Neonatology, Charitè University Medical School, Berlin, Germany

HOWARD STEIN, MD
Medical Director, Neonatal Intensive Care Unit, Promedica Toledo Children's Hospital; Clinical Professor of Pediatrics, University of Toledo-Health Science Campus, Toledo, Ohio

ARJAN B. TE PAS, MD, PhD
Division of Neonatology, Department of Pediatrics, Leiden University Medical Center, Leiden, Netherlands

MARKUS WAITZ, MD
Department of Pediatrics, University of Ottawa, Ottawa, Ontario, Canada

STEPHEN E. WELTY, MD
Professor of Pediatrics and Translational Biology and Molecular Medicine, Department of Pediatrics, Baylor College of Medicine, Houston, Texas

CLYDE J. WRIGHT, MD
Assistant Professor, Section of Neonatology, Department of Pediatrics, Perinatal Research Center, Children's Hospital Colorado, University of Colorado School of Medicine, Aurora, Colorado

BRADLEY A. YODER, MD
Professor, Division of Neonatology, Department of Pediatrics, University of Utah School of Medicine, Salt Lake City, Utah

Contents

Noninvasive support modalities have become ever more present in the care of newborns with a wide variety of disease processes. As clinicians have continued to avoid intubation and mechanical ventilation in preterm and term infants, the technologies available to support these groups have grown. Despite this rapid growth they can be broken down into 3 large categories of support, all attempting to deliver both flow and pressure to the nasopharynx supporting both phases of spontaneous breathing. The goal of all of the therapies is to stabilize a heterogeneous group of disorders with some common pathologies and avoid invasive support modalities.

Lung aeration is the most critical task newborns must accomplish after birth. Almost all extremely preterm infants require respiratory support during this process, but the best method to promote lung aeration in preterm infants is unknown. The current standard practice is intermittent positive pressure ventilation with positive end-expiratory pressure. Sustained inflation is a promising alternative strategy for lung liquid clearance and aeration. Here we review the physiologic rationale for sustained inflation and the available clinical evidence for sustained inflation in preterm infants.

Continuous positive airway pressure (CPAP) systems can be broadly grouped into continuous flow or variable flow devices. Bubble CPAP (bCPAP) is a continuous flow device and has physiologic properties that could facilitate gas exchange. Its efficacy has been reported to be similar to variable flow CPAP systems when used as a primary mode of respiratory support. Post-extubation bCPAP is reported to significantly reduce extubation failure rates among preterm infants ventilated for less than 2 week when compared to Infant flow driver CPAP (variable flow). bCPAP has been successfully used in resource-poor settings. The success on

CPAP is however dependant on good nursing care and clear management protocols for weaning and escalation of care.

Premature neonates are predisposed to complications, including bronchopulmonary dysplasia (BPD). BPD is associated with long-term pulmonary and neurodevelopmental consequences. Noninvasive respiratory support with nasal continuous positive airway pressure (CPAP) has been recommended strongly by the American Academy of Pediatrics. However, CPAP implementation has shown at least a 50% failure rate. Enhancing nasal CPAP effectiveness may decrease the need for mechanical ventilation and reduce the incidence of BPD. Bubble nasal CPAP is better than nasal CPAP using mechanical devices and the bubbling provides air exchange in distal respiratory units. The Seattle PAP system reduces parameters that assess work of breathing.

Heated, humidified, nasal high-flow (HF) therapy is a promising treatment for preterm infants, and almost certainly has a place in the clinical care of this population. It is only in the last few years that data have become available from randomized trials comparing HF with other noninvasive respiratory support modes, particularly nasal continuous positive airway pressure. This article discusses the evidence for HF use from randomized clinical trials in preterm infants and proposes recommendations for evidence-based practice.

Nasal high-flow therapy (nHFT) has become a popular form of noninvasive respiratory support in neonatal intensive care units. A meeting held in Oxford, UK, in June 2015 examined the evidence base and proposed a consensus statement. In summary, nHFT is effective for support of preterm infants following extubation. There is growing evidence evaluating its use in the primary treatment of respiratory distress. Further study is needed to assess which clinical conditions are most amenable to nHFT support, the most effective flow rates, and escalation and weaning strategies. Its suitability as first-line treatment needs to be further evaluated.

Noninvasive ventilation (NIV) is frequently used in the NICU to avoid intubation or as postextubation support for spontaneously breathing infants experiencing respiratory distress. Neurally adjusted ventilatory assist (NAVA) is used as a mode of noninvasive support in which both the timing and degree of ventilatory assist are controlled by the patient. NIV-NAVA has been successfully used clinically in neonates as a mode of ventilation to prevent intubation, allow early extubation, and as a novel way to deliver nasal continuous positive airway pressure.

High-frequency ventilation (HFV) as a mode of noninvasive respiratory support (NRS) in preterm neonates is gaining popularity. Benefits may accrue from combining the ventilatory efficiency of HFV delivered through a noninvasive interface, enhancing respiratory support while potentially limiting lung injury. Current evidence suggests that noninvasive HFV (NIHFV) may be superior to other NRS modes in eliminating carbon dioxide and preventing endotracheal ventilation after failure of other NRS modes. Animal data suggest NIHFV may promote improved alveolar development compared to endotracheal ventilation. However, adequately powered large-scale controlled trials are required to evaluate efficacy and safety prior to widespread use of NIHFV.

To minimize ventilator-associated lung injury in neonates, use of noninvasive (NIV) respiratory support has markedly increased over the past decade, especially in neonates younger than 28-weeks gestational age and 1250 g. Previously, neonates with respiratory failure who required anything greater than an oxyhood or low-flow nasal cannula were intubated for transport. This increased use has required transport teams to develop or incorporate a new set of support tools to minimize lung injury. This article reviews the various modes of NIV used during neonatal transport, important patient selection criteria, appropriate assessment, and the associated risks and benefits.

Respiratory distress syndrome (RDS) caused by surfactant deficiency is major cause for neonatal mortality and short- and long-term morbidity of preterm infants. Continuous positive airway pressure and other modes of noninvasive respiratory support and intubation and positive pressure ventilation with surfactant therapy are efficient therapies for RDS. Because continuous positive airway pressure can fail in severe surfactant deficiency, and because traditional surfactant therapy requires intubation and positive pressure ventilation, this entails a risk of lung injury. Several strategies to combine noninvasive respiratory therapy with minimally invasive surfactant therapy have been described. Available data suggest that those strategies may improve outcome of premature infants with RDS.

Caffeine is one of the most commonly prescribed medications in preterm neonates and is widely used to treat or prevent apnea of prematurity.

Caffeine therapy is safe, effectively decreases apnea, and improves short- and long-term outcomes in preterm infants. In this review, the authors summarize the role of caffeine therapy for preterm infants receiving noninvasive respiratory support. As caffeine is already widely used, recent data are summarized that may guide clinicians in optimizing the use of caffeine therapy, with a review of the timing of initiation, dose, and duration of therapy.

Noninvasive support of preterm infants with respiratory distress is an evidenced-based strategy to decrease the incidence of bronchopulmonary dysplasia. Continuous positive airway pressure (CPAP) is the only noninvasive strategy with sufficient evidence to support its use in acute respiratory distress syndrome. It is unclear if one method for delivering CPAP is superior to another. Future research will focus on strategies (eg, sustained lung inflation, and administration of surfactant using a thin plastic catheter) that increase the likelihood of success with CPAP, especially in infants with a gestational age of less than 26 weeks.

Although continuous positive airway pressure (CPAP) is an effective strategy to prevent invasive ventilation, failure rates are high and many babies require endotracheal intubation. Prolonged exposure to mechanical ventilation is linked with bronchopulmonary dysplasia and other morbidities. Different techniques of nasal intermittent positive pressure ventilation (NIPPV) have been proposed as an alternative to CPAP. Bilevel NIPPV and conventional mechanical ventilator-driven NIPPV are used in clinical practice. Both methods differ substantially in pressures and cycling times, potentially affecting their mechanism of action. This review focuses on noninvasive ventilation strategies, their physiologic effects, impact on clinical outcome parameters, and effects of synchronization.

PROGRAM OBJECTIVE

The goal of *Clinics in Perinatology* is to keep practicing perinatologists, neonatologists, obstetricians, practicing physicians and residents up to date with current clinical practice in perinatology by providing timely articles reviewing the state of the art in patient care.

TARGET AUDIENCE

Perinatologists, neonatologists, obstetricians, practicing physicians, residents and healthcare professionals who provide patient care utilizing findings from *Clinics in Perinatology*.

LEARNING OBJECTIVES

Upon completion of this activity, participants will be able to:
1. Review the physiologic basis for non-invasive ventilating devices.
2. Discuss evidence for various methods of non-invasive respiratory support options.
3. Recognize research trends in the use of non-invasive respiratory support methods in neonates.

ACCREDITATION

The Elsevier Office of Continuing Medical Education (EOCME) is accredited by the Accreditation Council for Continuing Medical Education (ACCME) to provide continuing medical education for physicians.

The EOCME designates this enduring material for a maximum of 15 *AMA PRA Category 1 Credit*(s)™. Physicians should claim only the credit commensurate with the extent of their participation in the activity.

All other health care professionals requesting continuing education credit for this enduring material will be issued a certificate of participation.

DISCLOSURE OF CONFLICTS OF INTEREST

The EOCME assesses conflict of interest with its instructors, faculty, planners, and other individuals who are in a position to control the content of CME activities. All relevant conflicts of interest that are identified are thoroughly vetted by EOCME for fair balance, scientific objectivity, and patient care recommendations. EOCME is committed to providing its learners with CME activities that promote improvements or quality in healthcare and not a specific proprietary business or a commercial interest.

The planning committee, staff, authors and editors listed below have identified no financial relationships or relationships to products or devices they or their spouse/life partner have with commercial interest related to the content of this CME activity:
Tamara Bleak, BSN, RN, MBA; Peter G. Davis, MD; Nicole R. Dobson, MD; Steven M. Donn, MD, FAAP; Michael Dunn, MD, FRCP(C); Kevin C. Dysart, MD; Elizabeth E. Foglia, MD, MSCE; Anjali Fortna; Samir Gupta, MD, DM, FRCPCH, FRCPI; Kerry Holland; Kevin Ives, MD; Lucky Jain, MD, MBA; Haresh Kirpalani, BM, MSc, FRCP(C); Brigitte Lemyre, MD, FRCPC; Brett J. Manley, MB BS (Hons), PhD; Lars Mense, MD; Amit Mukerji, MD, FRCP(C); Palani Murugesan; Charles C. Roehr, MD, PhD; Megan Suermann; Arjan B. te Pas, MD, PhD; Markus Waitz, MD; Stephen E. Welty, MD; Clyde J. Wright, MD.

The planning committee, staff, authors and editors listed below have identified financial relationships or relationships to products or devices they or their spouse/life partner have with commercial interest related to the content of this CME activity:
Jennifer Beck, PhD and her spouse/partner are both on the speakers' bureau for, are consultants/advisors for, and receive royalties/patents from, MAQUET Holding B.V. & Co KG.
Kevin Crezee, BS, RRT-NPS has stock ownership in, and an employment affiliation with, Mallinckrodt Pharmaceuticals.
Kimberly S. Firestone, MSc, RRT is on the speakers' bureau for MAQUET Holding B.V. & Co KG.
Angela Kribs, MD is a consultant/advisor for Chiesi Farmaceutici S.p.A.
Donald Null Jr, MD, FAAP is on the speakers' bureau for Mallinckrodt Pharmaceuticals.
Ravi Mangal Patel, MD, MSc on the speakers' bureau for MEDNAX Services, Inc.
Richard A. Polin, MD is a consultant/advisor for Fisher & Paykel Healthcare Limited; Discovery Labs, now Windtree Therapeutics, Inc; and Mallinckrodt Pharmaceuticals.
Howard Stein, MD is on the speakers' bureau for MAQUET Holding B.V. & Co KG.
Bradley A. Yoder, MD is on the speakers' bureau for Fisher & Paykel Healthcare Limited.

UNAPPROVED/OFF-LABEL USE DISCLOSURE

The EOCME requires CME faculty to disclose to the participants:

1. When products or procedures being discussed are off-label, unlabelled, experimental, and/or investigational (not US Food and Drug Administration [FDA] approved); and
2. Any limitations on the information presented, such as data that are preliminary or that represent ongoing research, interim analyses, and/or unsupported opinions. Faculty may discuss information about pharmaceutical agents that is outside of FDA-approved labelling. This information is intended solely for CME and is not intended to promote off-label use of these medications. If you have any questions, contact the medical affairs department of the manufacturer for the most recent prescribing information.

TO ENROLL

To enroll in the *Clinics in Perinatology* Continuing Medical Education program, call customer service at 1-800-654-2452 or sign up online at http://www.theclinics.com/home/cme. The CME program is available to subscribers for an additional annual fee of $235 USD.

METHOD OF PARTICIPATION

In order to claim credit, participants must complete the following:
1. Complete enrolment as indicated above.
2. Read the activity.
3. Complete the CME Test and Evaluation. Participants must achieve a score of 70% on the test. All CME Tests and Evaluations must be completed online.

CME INQUIRIES/SPECIAL NEEDS

For all CME inquiries or special needs, please contact elsevierCME@elsevier.com.

CLINICS IN PERINATOLOGY

ISSUE OF RELATED INTEREST

Clinics in Chest Medicine, December 2016 (Vol. 37, Issue 4)
Mechanical Ventilation
Neil R. MacIntyre, *Editor*
Available at: http://www.chestmed.theclinics.com

THE CLINICS ARE AVAILABLE ONLINE!
Access your subscription at:
www.theclinics.com

Foreword

Assisted Ventilation in Newborns: Less May Be More!

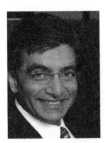

Lucky Jain, MD, MBA
Editor

For many of us who trained in the 1980s, it was an exciting time to be in neonatology, particularly for clinicians with a special interest in respiratory medicine. Surfactant was just around the corner[1]; newer ventilators were being introduced, and high-frequency ventilation and extracorporeal membrane oxygenation had gained traction as rescue therapies, while liquid ventilation[2] was ready to undergo human trials. These advances collectively contributed to a significant drop in mortality and growth of the subspecialty. Yet, unbeknownst to many, a culture was emerging in our neonatal intensive care units (NICUs) that would later prove to be harmful: we had begun to believe that early and more is better, and a preemptive aggressive approach to managing respiratory problems had taken off.

Since "prophylactic" surfactant therapy had been shown to be better than "rescue" treatment, we were trained to quickly intubate tiny babies in the delivery room and deliver the treatment. Once intubated, these babies often stayed on ventilators until multiple doses of surfactant had been given. Few centers were willing to give noninvasive support a decent trial, and efficacy of less-invasive approaches like bubble continuous positive airway pressure (CPAP) from centers like Columbia Presbyterian in New York were viewed with skepticism. No two centers agreed on the best approach, and significant differences in rates of bronchopulmonary dysplasia from various centers across the country were noticed and reported.[3] There was also a growing awareness of the harmful effects of hyperoxia, volutrauma, and ventilator-induced injury. Yet, attempts at standardizing therapies were unsuccessful because of the lack of randomized controlled trials and agreement on what constituted the right approach.

Since then, several large trials have confirmed the efficacy of a less-invasive approach to managing respiratory distress in newborns.[4,5] This has led to a proliferation of technologies and devices to deliver noninvasive respiratory support effectively. Many of these devices are relatively inexpensive and easy to use (**Fig. 1**)[6] and have led to considerable expansion of their application in developing countries. A kinder, gentler

Clin Perinatol 43 (2016) xv–xvii
http://dx.doi.org/10.1016/j.clp.2016.09.002
0095-5108/16/© 2016 Published by Elsevier Inc.

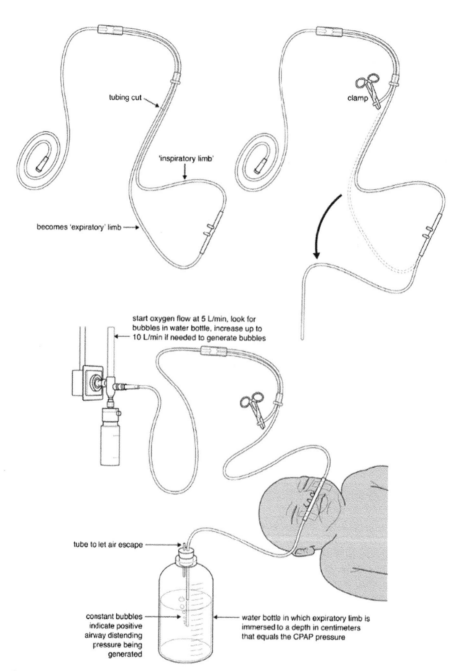

tubing cut

clamp

'inspiratory limb'

becomes 'expiratory' limb

start oxygen flow at 5 L/min, look for bubbles in water bottle, increase up to 10 L/min if needed to generate bubbles

tube to let air escape

constant bubbles indicate positive airway distending pressure being generated

water bottle in which expiratory limb is immersed to a depth in centimeters that equals the CPAP pressure

Fig. 1. An inexpensive bubble CPAP setup using modified nasal prongs. (*From* Duke T. CPAP: a guide for clinicians in developing countries. Pediatr Int Child Health 2014;34:7; with permission.)

approach to managing lung disease has finally found its rightful place in our NICUs. This issue of the *Clinics in Perinatology* underscores the growing need and awareness of noninvasive ventilation. Drs Yoder and Kirpalani are to be congratulated for bringing together a superb set of state-of-the-art articles on this topic. As always, I am grateful to the editors, authors, and the publishing team at Elsevier (Kerry Holland and Casey Jackson) for helping disseminate critical knowledge on this important topic through this issue of the *Clinics in Perinatology*.

Lucky Jain, MD, MBA
Emory University School of Medicine
Department of Pediatrics
Children's Healthcare of Atlanta
2015 Uppergate Drive
Atlanta, GA 30322, USA

E-mail address:
ljain@emory.edu

REFERENCES

1. Fujiwara T, Maeta H, Chida S, et al. Artificial surfactant therapy in hyaline membrane disease. Lancet 1980;1:55–9.
2. Wolfson MR, Shaffer TH. Liquid ventilation during early development: theory, physiologic processes and application. J Dev Physiol 1990;13:1–12.
3. Avery ME, Tooley WH, Keller JB, et al. Is chronic lung disease in the low birth weight infant preventable? A survey of eight centers. Pediatrics 1987;79:26–30.
4. Morley CJ, Davis PG, Doyle LW, et al. Nasal CPAP or intubation at birth for very preterm infants. N Engl J Med 2008;358:700–8.
5. Finer NN, Carlo WA, Walsh MC, et al. Early CPAP versus surfactant in extremely preterm infants. N Engl J Med 2010;362:1970–9.
6. Duke T. CPAP: a guide for clinicians in developing countries. Pediatr Int Child Health 2014;34:3–11.

Preface

Noninvasive Ventilation

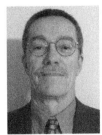 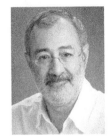

Bradley A. Yoder, MD   Haresh Kirpalani, BM, MSc, FRCPC
Editors

We are privileged to have participated in such a lineup of today's experts in noninvasive care. In this preface, we make only three brief, almost philosophical, comments.

First, we will simply excuse our backward glances at history as being of potential use. As Newton wrote to Hooke: "We see further by standing upon the shoulders of giants" (Isaac Newton in letter to Robert Hooke, 5 February 1676). As the story of the Prophet Elisha shows, interest in noninvasive support for infants has a long history extending back to the ancients. (In ancient times, the Prophet Elisha is said to have revived the Shunammite child by mouth-to-mouth breathing ["And he went and lay upon the child, putting his mouth upon his mouth... and the flesh of the child waxed warm." 2 Kings 4:32-34]).

Second, we are struck by a repetitive rediscovery of old therapies—but using new technology. Likely, this is because newborn lung disease is intimately tied to the limitations imposed by the physical properties of the thorax and respiratory mechanics. For example, jumping centuries ahead of Elisha, into the era of modern ventilation—even pioneers of intubated ventilation feared its consequences. But they were handicapped by fearsome devices. Llewellyn and colleagues,[1] in 1970, justified a randomized controlled trial (RCT) of nasal intermittent positive pressure ventilation (IPPV) saying: "Most centres use an oro-tracheal or naso-tracheal tube to apply intermittent positive pressure ventilation (IPPV). It has become evident that the advantages of such a technique must be weighed against its complications." However, **Fig. 1** indicates just how difficult that was, and, not surprisingly, there were complications, including cerebellar hemorrhages.[2]

Last, some collective humility is in order. Today, we consider ourselves to be very modern, because we embrace where possible, an RCT-supported evidence-based medicine. Yet our "forefathers and foremothers" had performed many important, if small and underpowered, RCTs of innovations in respiratory medicine.[1,3–5] This is a strange paradox, as one widely used therapy nowadays, continuous positive airway pressure (CPAP), remained untested for many years. A short reminder of this story is worthwhile.

Clin Perinatol 43 (2016) xix–xxii
http://dx.doi.org/10.1016/j.clp.2016.09.001
0095-5108/16/© 2016 Published by Elsevier Inc.

perinatology.theclinics.com

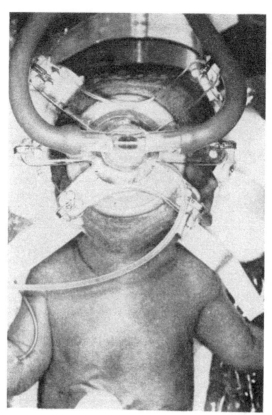

Fig. 1. Face mask in position with supporting harness. (*From* Llewellyn MA, Tilak KS, Swyer PR. A controlled trial of assisted ventilation using an oro-nasal mask. Arch Dis Child 1970;45(242):453–9; with permission.)

A key step was to recognize the newborn's glottic maneuvers, observed by Harrison and colleagues,[6] as a mechanism to retain lung volume. Others had used a positive end-expiratory pressure during endotracheal intubated ventilation.[7,8] But Gregory and colleagues[9] took the key step to enable spontaneously breathing infants to augment end-expiratory lung volume. They reported 20 infants treated with either intubated CPAP (n = 18) or chamber-delivered CPAP (n = 2) and a remarkable 80% survival rate.

As we look back, we can only lament the faltering steps our community took to move this revolution into a widespread, routine practice. It is true that the therapy was quite cumbersome (**Fig. 2**). Yet the delays in adoption of this approach seem inordinate. Avery and colleagues[10] raised a flag when observing a site-specific reduction in rates of bronchopulmonary dysplasia (BPD), but not death, could have been associated with CPAP therapy. Yet it was only in 2008 that the courageous and necessary RCT of Morley and colleagues[11] was reported. It had only (sic) taken 37 years after Gregory's initial signpost. Thankfully others soon followed him.

A sign of improvement has been that since then the power of RCTs has been more readily called upon. A great deal of time and effort have been put into the development and application of noninvasive ventilator (NIV) approaches to supporting respiratory function in neonates. Cumulatively, these trials show only a small reduction in rates

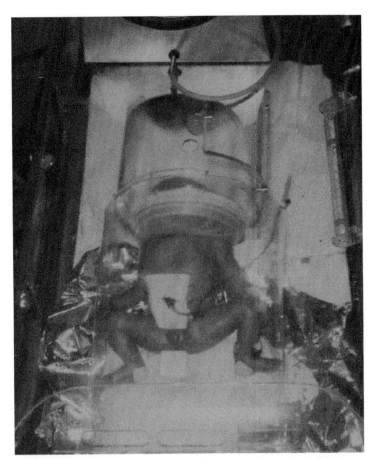

Fig. 2. The first infant treated in the Gregory Box in October 1971. (*From* Dunn PM. The early use of neonatal continuous positive airway pressure (CPAP) in Bristol. WEMJ 2016;115(1):1–3; with permission.)

of BPD, which remain relatively unchanged over the past decade. This has led to investigations of other NIV approaches, including nasal ventilation and high-flow nasal cannula therapy. Not only have available modes increased but also the interfaces through which these modes may be applied. In addition, supportive therapies that may assist a NIV approach, such as caffeine and minimally invasive surfactant, have a developing evidence base.

In the issue of *Clinics in Perinatology*, readers will find an up-to-date review of noninvasive approaches to supporting preterm respiratory function. This draws on the expertise of leading investigators in the field. This issue reviews the physiologic mechanisms by which the various approaches to NIV may support respiratory function; the evidence base supporting different NIV approaches; and adjunctive aspects of NIV therapy, including their use during neonatal transport and the application of other supportive therapies such as inhaled NO.

We greatly appreciate the expertise and efforts of the contributing authors, without whom this issue of *Clinics in Perinatology* would not be possible. They have at times slightly differing perspectives. Given our current level of technology, experience, and evidence, this is as it should be. We hope that the information conveyed in this issue will spark additional investigations into the application of NIV in an effort to improve the respiratory outcomes of our most fragile population of patients.

Bradley A. Yoder, MD
Department of Pediatrics
Division of Neonatology
University of Utah School of Medicine
PO Box 581289
Salt Lake City, UT 84158-1289, USA

Haresh Kirpalani, BM, MSc, FRCPC
Division of Neonatology
Children's Hospital of Philadelphia
3401 Civic Center Boulevard
Philadelphia, PA 19104, USA

E-mail addresses:
Bradley.Yoder@hsc.utah.edu (B.A. Yoder)
kirpalanih@email.chop.edu (H. Kirpalani)

REFERENCES

1. Llewellyn MA, Tilak KS, Swyer PR. A controlled trial of assisted ventilation using an oro-nasal mask. Arch Dis Child 1970;45(242):453–9.
2. Pape KE, Armstrong DL, Fitzhardinge PM. CNS pathology associated with mask ventilation. Pediatrics 1977;60(5):787–8.
3. Murdock AI, Linsao L, Reid MM, et al. Artificial mechanical ventilation in the respiratory distress syndrome: a controlled trial. Arch Dis Child 1970;45(243):624–33.
4. Reid DH, Tunstall ME, Mitchell RG. A controlled trial of artificial respiration in the respiratory-distress syndrome of the newborn. Lancet 1967;1(7489):532–3.
5. Silverman WA, Sinclair JC, Gaudy GM, et al. A controlled trial of management of respiratory distress syndrome in a body-enclosing respirator. I. Evaluation of safety. Pediatrics 1967;39(5):740–8.
6. Harrison VC, Heese Hde V, et al. The significance of grunting in hyaline membrane disease. Pediatrics 1968;41(3):549–59.
7. Ashbaugh DG, Petty TL, Bigelow DB, et al. Continuous positive-pressure breathing (CPPB) in adult respiratory distress syndrome. J Thorac Cardiovasc Surg 1969;57(1):31–41.
8. Llewellyn MA, Swyer PR. Positive expiratory pressure during mechanical ventilation in the newborn. Atlantic City (NJ): Program of the Society for Pediatric Research; 1970. p. 224.
9. Gregory GA, Kitterman JA, Phibbs RH, et al. Treatment of the idiopathic respiratory-distress syndrome with continuous positive airway pressure. N Engl J Med 1971;284(24):1333–40.
10. Avery ME, Tooley WH, Keller JB, et al. Is chronic lung disease in low birth weight infants preventable? A survey of eight centers. Pediatrics 1987;79(1):26–30.
11. Morley CJ, Davis PG, Doyle LW, et al, COIN Trial Investigators. Nasal CPAP or intubation at birth for very preterm infants. N Engl J Med 2008;358(7):700–8.

Physiologic Basis for Nasal Continuous Positive Airway Pressure, Heated and Humidified High-Flow Nasal Cannula, and Nasal Ventilation

CrossMark

Kevin C. Dysart, MD

KEYWORDS

- Nasal CPAP • High-flow nasal cannula • Nasal ventilation

KEY POINTS

- Non-invasive support modalities utilize different applications and mechanisms but share similar physiologic mechanisms of support.
- All modes assist care givers in avoiding mechanical ventilation and the associated injuries to the lungs and airways.
- None of the modalities can achieve the ideal goal of being the right therapy for all patients across the age and disease spectrum treated in the newborn intensive care unit setting.

PHYSIOLOGY OF NORMAL BREATHING AND PATHOPHYSIOLOGY ENCOUNTERED IN NEONATAL MEDICINE

Introduction

Many readers of this issue of *Clinics in Perinatology* will have extreme familiarity and knowledge concerning spontaneous breathing physiology in newborns and infants. Although this is undoubtedly the case, it does seem appropriate to review some basic principles regarding neonatal spontaneous ventilation to better understand the variety of pathophysiologies that are presented to neonatal care practitioners and the application of noninvasive respiratory therapies.

Although the disease process themselves represent a heterogeneous group of unique physiologic challenges, the therapeutic interventions that are noninvasive support are broken into 3 large categories, each of which supports spontaneous ventilation during both phases of the respiratory cycle leading to an improvement in patient

Disclosures: None.
Children's Hospital of Philadelphia, 34th and Civic Center Boulevard, Philadelphia, PA 19104, USA
E-mail address: DysartK@email.chop.edu

Clin Perinatol 43 (2016) 621–631
http://dx.doi.org/10.1016/j.clp.2016.07.001   perinatology.theclinics.com
0095-5108/16/© 2016 Elsevier Inc. All rights reserved.

comfort and ventilation efficiency. The goal of these therapeutic interventions is to avoid invasive mechanical support. Over the past 50 years in newborn medicine, our understanding of these different support modalities has allowed us to pursue these strategies at younger gestational ages and smaller birth weights, with significantly more success. The goal of all of these noninvasive therapies is to avoid ventilator-induced lung injury and improve patient outcomes.[1–6]

Control of Respiration

Control of ventilation is a complex feedback system between the central nervous system and the lungs through the result of alveolar ventilation that leads to normal gas tensions and pH in a healthy state. In a disease state, insufficient oxygen or elevated carbon dioxide concentrations in the blood result in abnormal responses of the feedback loop leading to either inability to correct the abnormalities or cessation of breathing. The lowered oxygen concentration in the blood stimulates chemoreceptors in both the carotid and aortic bodies, while elevated concentrations of carbon dioxide similarly elevate the concentrations of carbon dioxide in the cerebral spinal fluid. These changes stimulate central chemoreceptors in the medullary respiratory center via signaling through the glossopharyngeal and vagus nerves. In response, the phrenic and intercostal nerves, through descending corticospinal tracts, stimulate more frequent breathing. The same stimuli lead to an increase in the amplitude of respiration, leading ultimately to an increase in tidal volume. These changes ultimately lead to an increase in minute ventilation with the overall trend of normalizing the partial pressure of carbon dioxide and oxygen with the secondary impact of balancing the pH of the blood.[7]

It is well understood that neonates have an abnormal response through these pathways to rising partial pressures of carbon dioxide and falling concentrations of oxygen. Most neonatologists focus on the relationship between rising and falling partial pressures of carbon dioxide in newborn breathing patterns. The more preterm an infant is born, the more likely the infant will have significant apnea.[8] This apnea is in large part related to the preterm infant's inability to respond with a normal linear response to rising partial pressures of carbon dioxide. One of the most common medicinal therapies available to the neonatologist, caffeine, directly targets this abnormal response, normalizing the slope closer to that of healthy preterm infants without apnea, or full-term infants.

Neonates also demonstrate a significant abnormality in the way in which they respond to hypoxemia. Although the initial response of neonates is to increase respiratory drive, and thus minute ventilation, this response is only temporary. After approximately 1 to 2 minutes, neonates have hypoxemic depression of the respiratory drive. This results in a return to their initial state or even depression of the respiratory activity. This paradoxic response may play an important role in the apnea observed in preterm infants.[9]

Finally, it is important to note the impact of nasopharyngeal airway patency and pulmonary stretch receptors, and the interplay they have on respiratory timing and maintenance of minute ventilation. Neonates who suffer apnea often experience obstruction of the upper airway. This obstruction may be related to disrupted control in the neonate's ability to maintain a patent upper airway in the face of a more compliant tissue. The combination of this and abnormal timing of pharyngeal muscle activation, as compared with the diaphragmatic contraction, may predispose the upper airway to collapse, leading to the observed obstructions. Pulmonary stretch receptors also play an important role in maintaining appropriate lung inflation and preventing overdistention. These may be an important mechanism through which the therapeutic approaches discussed here influence respiratory timing and apnea.[9]

Although clearly the medicinal approach with caffeine is the most common in treating apnea of prematurity, clinicians often use all of the available noninvasive devices as well. Although synchronization with the infant's respiratory effort is unnecessary for therapies like high-flow nasal cannula and nasal continuous positive airway pressure (CPAP), treating apnea with nasal ventilation has been limited by the inability to match the infant's respiratory effort. As will be discussed elsewhere in this issue, specifically for nasal ventilation, the emerging use of neural-assist ventilation (NAVA) offers the hope of synchronization for future applications and clinical trials.

Mechanics of Respiration

Although it is challenging to discuss the entirety of respiratory physiology in health and disease, it is worth briefly reviewing the mechanics at work in both inspiration and expiration so that we may better understand the potential benefits of noninvasive ventilation support in newborns.

Respiratory Gas Conditioning

The crucial nature of the airway epithelium in conditioning atmospheric gases during spontaneous ventilation is well understood. The nasal, pharyngeal, and lower airways act in many important ways to continually maintain debris clearance, lubricate the airways through mucus production, and humidify the respiratory gas across a variety of ambient conditions.[10]

Upper Airway Function

During spontaneous breathing, the upper airway must continue to remain patent throughout both the inspiratory and expiratory phases of each breath. Pharyngeal muscle tone prevents collapse during inspiration, allowing gases to be entrained through the negative pressure created in the thorax. Without this active control and maintenance of patency, obstructive events become increasingly more likely. Preterm and term infants suffering respiratory distress, in which increasingly negative thoracic pressures and increased work of breathing demand more from the pharyngeal muscle tone, often experience airway obstructive events related to the inability of the pharynx and upper airway to maintain patency. All of the modalities discussed in this issue address this problem through similar mechanisms.

The upper airway also provides a small amount of dead space ventilation for preterm infants to deal with. This dead space represents wasted minute ventilation throughout the respiratory cycle. All of the therapies discussed potentially aid in diminishing the amount of wasted ventilation in infants suffering respiratory distress.

Spontaneous Breathing

Inspiration

If we start by considering the respiratory system when it is at rest, there is a negative pleural pressure while alveolar pressure is atmospheric and there is no flow in the system. The elastic recoils of both the lung and the chest wall are equal and opposite when the respiratory muscles are at rest. Even in this state, the newborn with respiratory distress is at a disadvantage as compared with older children and adults. An imbalance in these pressures often leads to a diminished residual volume and functional residual capacity, resulting in atelectasis. Starting from this disadvantaged point, the newborn infant then must generate the negative pleural pressure, via the contractile force of both the intercostal muscles and diaphragm, to create the subatmospheric alveolar pressure necessary to generate spontaneous minute ventilation. Combining this with a lung that achieves small volume changes as it relates to pressure changes, a chest wall that is too compliant due to its cartilaginous nature, and a diminished muscular force generating capacity, it becomes clear why inspiration is such a difficult task for a newborn infant with respiratory distress.[7]

Expiration

Once the inspiratory volume is achieved as a result of the previously discussed actions, expiration must begin. Expiration is mostly a passive process. Intercostal and diaphragmatic muscles relax and elastic recoil of the lung allows the generation of a positive alveolar pressure, compared with the airway opening, creating the egress of gas. Although many problems for newborns are generated during the inspiratory part of the breath, there are times in which the airways, needing to be rigid and withstand these fluctuating pressures, are cartilaginous and begin to collapse during expiration, trapping gas behind them. If this is untreated over multiple ventilation cycles, this gas trapping can become a significant problem for newborn infants. This problem often manifests itself at later ages in neonatal medicine, often when infants have established bronchopulmonary dysplasia. Early on in the newborn period, problems of airway resistance may make it more difficult for the passive expiration to occur.

Summary

It is in the support of both inspiration and expiration that noninvasive modalities provide the greatest amount of support in maintaining functional residual capacity and improving minute ventilation.

PHYSIOLOGY OF NONINVASIVE SUPPORT
Prevention of Mucosal Injury

A crucial function of noninvasive support modalities is their ability to condition the respiratory gases, by both warming to near body temperature, and humidifying the gas mixtures. Without this proper conditioning, patient discomfort and nasal mucosal injury, as well as pharyngeal and lower airway injury, are well described.

Early in the attempts to provide supplemental support to patients with respiratory distress, it became clear that appropriate conditioning was crucial for maintaining patient comfort and preventing injury related simply to inspiring a dry cold gas. Specifically in newborns, Greenspan and colleagues[11] published the negative impact on airway resistance of inspiring a cold dry gas. Subsequently, other investigators have described both alterations in airway resistance and injury to nasal and airway mucosa as a consequence of poorly conditioned respiratory gases during a variety of modes of ventilation support.[12,13]

Although all of the noninvasive therapies have systems in place to warm and humidify the respiratory gas, heated humidified-nasal cannula (HHFNC), achieves the higher flow rates applied to the nasopharynx through novel humidification systems. Although many clinicians simply refer to HHFNC as high-flow nasal cannula, the exclusion of the mentioning of the heating and humidification process that takes place ignores one of the most important aspects of the therapy as well as the mechanism through which we are able to deliver higher than traditional flow to newborns, without injuring the nasal mucosa or irritating both large and small airways. Traditionally, nasal cannula oxygen was limited to approximately 2 lpm of either 100% or blended oxygen. An additional limiting factor included the drying and irritating nature of the respiratory gas with the simple bubble humidifiers that were available at the time. The introduction of systems that could raise the relative humidity of the inspiratory gas to nearly 100% gave clinicians the ability to increase flow rates in their patients to better match the inspiratory work of breathing. These increased flow rates traditionally would have led to mucosal injury resulting in drying of the nasal and tracheal secretions as well as breakdown of mucosal integrity. Woodhead and colleagues[13] reported improvements in the appearance of the nasal mucosa when breathing with the assistance of HHFNC as compared with traditional nasal cannula after extubation.

There are 2 main systems, both proprietary, that have allowed for these advancements. Vapotherm Corporation (Exeter, NH) introduced a pass-through cartridge system that humidifies the inspiratory gas to nearly 100% relative humidity while warming the gas simultaneously. Fisher-Paykel (Fisher & Paykel Healthcare Limited, Auckland, New Zealand), a maker of heated and humidification circuits for nasal CPAP and nasal ventilation systems, have also adapted their technology to provide this through a nasal cannula. Both systems provide significant humidification and warming to allow all 3 modalities to be applied to patients in a wide physiologic range, without injuring the mucosa and preserving the important functions of the nasopharynx and airways.

Maintenance of Pharyngeal Tone

As mentioned previously, maintenance of the upper airway requires the active control of the pharyngeal muscles to prevent occlusion throughout both phases of the respiratory cycle. Although much of apnea treatment, especially in preterm infants, focuses on central apnea, the importance of obstructive apneic events cannot be overlooked. Infants suffering respiratory distress often have obstructive events, historically blamed on gastroesophageal reflux disease, that complicate the picture for infants trying to wean to room air and achieve a successful discharge.

The most common therapy for obstructive apnea to improve patency of the upper airway has been nasal CPAP. Nasal CPAP levels between 4 and 6 cm H2O have traditionally yielded success in treating obstructive apnea events.[14] This stabilization of pharyngeal tone becomes even more important when infants, suffering from respiratory distress syndrome need to develop more negative intrathoracic pressures to achieve spontaneous ventilation, putting greater demands on the nasopharynx.

Nasal intermittent ventilation augments nasal CPAP by providing phasic changes in pressures applied at the nasopharynx, thus augmenting the delivered pressure in attempts to stabilize the pharyngeal tone and prevent obstructive apneic events. Clinicians often use this modality as an escalation from nasal CPAP in attempt to stabilize infants after extubation, as well as to prevent reintubation after a successful extubation.[1,15,16]

Nasal cannula devices likely aid in the stabilization of pharyngeal tone through similar mechanisms by generating nasal pressures through the application of varying nasal flow rates. There is minimal evidence to support this hypothesis; however, because both animal and human models show clear evidence of elevations in pharyngeal and airway pressures as measured by esophageal balloons and direct pharyngeal and tracheal measurements, it is fair to assume that there is equal stabilization of the pharyngeal tone via the flow rates traditionally applied with HHFNC, 2 to 10 L per minute.[17–20]

Nasopharyngeal Deadspace Washout

The nasopharynx provides an important source of anatomic deadspace that can be diminished, likely through all 3 modalities of noninvasive support.

Similar to mechanisms that lead to improvements in gas exchange seen with tracheal gas insufflation, the provision of increased flow in the nasopharynx likely improves the washout of the nasopharyngeal dead space. This hypothesis is supported most strongly by literature surrounding high-flow nasal cannula therapy, but because the other 2 mechanisms, nasal CPAP as well as nasal intermittent mandatory ventilation, develop pressure within the circuit via flow generators, the flow in the nasopharynx washes clear carbon dioxide from the gas mixture at the end of expiration.

Entraining fresh gas thus eliminates the contribution of rebreathing from the nasopharynx.

Several studies have demonstrated the impact of increased flows in the nasopharynx on immediate improvement in the condition of patients receiving high-flow nasal cannula in both the adult and the neonatal time periods. Patients have been able to extubate successfully from higher levels of support or exercise with greater tolerance, while being able to maintain a static respiratory rate and title volume, implying that at the same minute ventilation, respiratory efficiency is considerably improved. These findings, in combination with bench research further supporting nasopharyngeal washout as a potential mechanism for flow support devices to improve respiratory distress, continues to support this as a potential mechanism for patient-level improvements when receiving noninvasive support modalities.[19,21–23]

Assisting the Inspiratory Work of Breathing

Generating the needed negative inventory pressure in the thorax to maintain spontaneous ventilation is an essential part of the support that any noninvasive modality brings to newborns and infants suffering respiratory distress. All 3 modalities assist ventilation, and maintain or improve ventilation, by alleviating the work of breathing necessary to improve overall ventilation efficiency. This improvement in ventilation efficiency improves patient comfort as well as allowing the infant to continue to spontaneously support ventilation without invasive methodologies. There are likely a handful of complementary ways in which all 3 modalities share common pathways to achieve this goal.

Warming and Humidifying the Respiratory Gas

As discussed previously, a major role of the nasopharynx, and the epithelium lining the upper airway, is to provide moisture and remove debris while warming the inspiratory gas such that it prevents a tracheal and bronchial response. All 3 modalities replace the warming and humidification process and spare the metabolic work necessary to continue spontaneous ventilation. It is possible that by presenting the airways with warmed and humidified gas that the necessary cellular work is reduced and overall metabolic balance is improved.[10,21]

Diminishing the Pressure Cost of Breathing

Diminishing the pressure cost of breathing, and thereby improving ventilation efficiency, may be the dominant mechanism through which newborn infants, both preterm and term, experience a direct benefit from the noninvasive therapies routinely applied in the clinical care of such infants. All 3 noninvasive modalities have been demonstrated to alter pharyngeal and thoracic pressure through the applications via mask or nasal cannula at the nasal opening. Of course the infant continues to spontaneously breath with the assistance of these therapies generating pressures that are both negative and positive to the end expiratory pressure created via the nasal application. This augmentation of pressure and flow in the nasopharynx has the ultimate effect of both stabilizing the lung and airways in expiration as well as augmenting nasopharyngeal flow, creating a situation in which the infant needs to create a less negative intrathoracic pressure to drive spontaneous ventilation while maintaining functional residual capacity.

Although providing supplemental oxygen via the use of a nasal cannula may have a long history in medicine, nasal CPAP may be the first therapy reported to assist ventilation for patients suffering respiratory distress. In the early part of the twentieth century, researchers described the positive impact of the application of positive airway pressure for patients. In the 1930s, physician Alvin Barach[24–28] conducted a series of trials with patients suffering respiratory distress as a consequence of reactive airway disease (RAD). He was specifically interested in modalities that could assist gas egress for patients with severe exacerbations of their underlying RAD. He was also interested in the use of helium is a carrier molecule for oxygen to facilitate ventilation in such patients taking advantage of helium's unique inert chemistry and physical characteristics. In one of his research publications, he described a blower system, with a warming unit, to facilitate the delivery of this Heliox mixture. During his description of the device, he admits that he was initially concerned that applying the pressure at the nasopharynx to deliver this gas mixture would make the egress of gas more difficult. To his surprise, patients who participated in his clinical trial reported the opposite, that indeed this application of pressure via his unique blower system facilitated the egress gas. Although the mechanism at play here was likely providing stability for the airways, both large and small, during expiration in patients who had significant RAD, it is likely that similar mechanisms assist infants suffering respiratory distress.[24–28]

It would take the better part of the next 40 years to come to a better understanding of the pathophysiology of respiratory distress in preterm infants. By the 1970s, Gregory and colleagues[4] had come to the understanding that infants suffering respiratory distress benefited from the application of CPAP, even noting that as compared with the ventilation technology of the time, infants treated with CPAP seem to be more comfortable clinically. In this era, CPAP was traditionally applied via an endotracheal tube, which of course had significant limitations, including infants having to spontaneously breathe through the fixed length resistor provided by the endotracheal tube.

Clinicians and researchers over the next 40 years invested significant amounts of time developing both simple and complicated systems to apply nasal CPAP. Systems such as "bubble CPAP" represent the simplest applications of the therapy, whereas proprietary systems, with patented technologies to improve the nasal interface and nasopharyngeal ventilation, represent more complicated systems to achieve the same end. Regardless of the system, both have similar impacts with improvements in ventilation efficiency. Currently there is little evidence that one system offers significant benefit over the other.[5,29–32]

Nasal intermittent mandatory ventilation offers many of the same benefits as nasal CPAP in the assistance of ventilation for infants suffering respiratory distress. Owen and Manley,[1] in a recent review, exhaustively cover all of the available comparisons in current research for the application of NIMV as compared with nasal CPAP. There is little current evidence that nasal intermittent mandatory ventilation systems offer significant benefit over nasal CPAP. In the largest randomized trial in which the 2 therapies were directly compared, there is no difference in the primary outcome survival to 36 weeks post menstrual age without bronchopulmonary dysplasia. The one area in which nasal intermittent mandatory ventilation may confer benefit is in preventing extubation failure in infants. Mechanistically, it is likely that nasal intermittent mandatory ventilation is providing cyclic nasal pressure support throughout the respiratory cycle. One intriguing future advantage of this modality of support may be the ability to improve synchronization. Being able to synchronize this phasic pressure support to the spontaneous respiratory cycle may prove to make this modality superior in improving ventilation efficiency by further diminishing the pressure cost of breathing.[1]

HHFNC likely offers similar benefits in improving ventilation efficiency, as mentioned previously. The application of flow rate between 2 and 10 lpm to the nasopharynx has been shown to develop nasopharyngeal pressures consistent with the application of nasal CPAP and nasal intermittent mandatory ventilation in both preterm and term infants as well as in animal models of respiratory disease. Frizzola and colleagues[20] previously reported the application of random nasal flows, delivered via a clinically available HHFNC system, and improvements in ventilation efficiency. This improvement manifested itself as a reduction in the needed negative intrathoracic pressure to create inspiration and physiologic levels of end expiratory pressure consistent with nasal CPAP applications between 5 and 8 cm H2O pressure. Other investigators have published similar findings in infants being treated with respiratory distress with end expiratory pressures that were comparable between nasal CPAP and HHFNC. There also seems to be equivalency in the clinical outcomes when directly comparing the 2 therapies in the treatment of newborn infants.[18,20,33–35]

Maintaining Functional Residual Capacity

One of the hallmarks of infants suffering respiratory distress is "grunting." This respiratory event is widely thought to represent an expiratory maneuver whose goal is to maintain end expiratory volume in a disease state characterized by low lung compliance and prevent closing of the lung.[36] Clinically, aside from the audible grunting, this is manifested as an increasing need for inspired oxygen, atelectasis of the lung, and carbon dioxide retention as the amount of anatomic and physiologic dead space rises. The application of an expiratory pressure helps to reverse many of these pathophysiologies. By stabilizing the large and small airways and the alveoli at end expiration, alveolar recruitment is maintained. This maintenance of alveolar recruitment often reverses the underlying end expiratory volume loss and improves supplemental oxygen requirements. As a consequence of the stabilization, the next breath occurs from a more favorable place in the pressure-volume relationship. Although the application of an expiratory pressure itself does not lead to a direct increase in alveolar minute ventilation, the improved lung volumes, as well as improved compliance, leads ultimately to improved inspiratory tidal volumes and a secondary improvement in alveolar minute ventilation results. This then results in lower ventilation rates and measured partial pressures of carbon dioxide.

Nasal intermittent mandatory ventilation works through similar mechanisms as nasal CPAP in reversing the pathophysiologies of respiratory distress. A helpful addition to this therapy would be improved methods of synchronization so as to support the entire respiratory cycle and provide improved outcomes.[1] In the current state, however, there is limited evidence to suggest that the phasic support provided at the nasopharynx is indeed leading to actual changes in tidal volumes. Due to the unsynchronized nature of the phasic pressure changes, there are likely times that the inspiratory cycle for both the infant and ventilator are delivered simultaneously. However, there are also times when there is direct competition because they are perfectly out of phase with one another. Regardless, maintaining functional residual capacity, improving oxygen need, and treating atelectasis are likely achieved with nasal intermittent mandatory ventilation.[1,37,38]

Similar to both of the previously discussed therapies, HHFNC provides not just inspiratory support but support at end expiration by raising end expiratory pressure. There are both animal and infant studies to support the generation of CPAP, and thus elevated end expiratory pressures. The generated pressures are similar to nasal CPAP across the HHFNC flow rates typically used to treat preterm and term infants with respiratory distress.[3,17,20]

SUMMARY

All 3 modalities that provide noninvasive support have demonstrated value for clinicians treating both preterm and term infants with a wide variety of pathophysiologies leading to respiratory distress and apnea. Whether the device is a pressure-regulated system using flow to generate pressures delivered at the nasopharynx or simple flow delivery systems to the nasopharynx, the mechanisms leading to improvement are similar across the modalities. The ability to support the inspiratory work of breathing needed to create a spontaneous breath, splint the nasopharynx to prevent collapse, improve both central and obstructive apneic events, while supporting end expiration with elevated pressures to maintain alveolar recruitment and prevent airway collapse, are crucial for all 3 modalities. The assistance provided by these modalities during spontaneous ventilation helps avoid the need for mechanical ventilation, allowing infants to avoid further lung injury associated with protracted mechanical ventilation courses.

REFERENCES

1. Owen LS, Manley BJ. Nasal intermittent positive pressure ventilation in preterm infants: equipment, evidence, and synchronization. Semin Fetal Neonatal Med 2016;21(3):146–53.
2. Wright CJ, Kirpalani H. Targeting inflammation to prevent bronchopulmonary dysplasia: can new insights be translated into therapies? Pediatrics 2011; 128(1):111–26.
3. Manley BJ, Dold SK, Davis PG, et al. High-flow nasal cannulae for respiratory support of preterm infants: a review of the evidence. Neonatology 2012;102(4):300–8.
4. Gregory GA, Kitterman JA, Phibbs RH, et al. Treatment of the idiopathic respiratory-distress syndrome with continuous positive airway pressure. N Engl J Med 1971;284(24):1333–40.
5. Davis PG, Henderson-Smart DJ. Nasal continuous positive airways pressure immediately after extubation for preventing morbidity in preterm infants. Cochrane Database Syst Rev 2003;(2):CD000143.
6. Davis PG, Lemyre B, De Paoli AG. Nasal intermittent positive pressure ventilation (NIPPV) versus nasal continuous positive airway pressure (NCPAP) for preterm neonates after extubation. Cochrane Database Syst Rev 2001;(3):CD003212.
7. Hansen JT, Koeppen BM. Netter's atlas of human physiology. 2002. Available at: http://158.69.150.236:1080/jspui/handle/961944/72970.
8. Gerhardt T, Bancalari E. Apnea of prematurity: I. Lung function and regulation of breathing. Pediatrics 1984;74(1):58–62. Available at: http://eutils.ncbi.nlm.nih.gov/entrez/eutils/elink.fcgi?dbfrom=pubmed&id=6429625&retmode=ref&cmd=prlinks.
9. Miller M, Martin RJ. Pathophysiology of apnea of prematurity. Fetal Neonatal Physiol 2004;1(91):998–1011.
10. Negus VE. Humidification of the air passages. Acta Otolaryngol 2009;41:74–83.
11. Greenspan JS, Wolfson MR, Shaffer TH. Airway responsiveness to low inspired gas temperature in preterm neonates. J Pediatr 1991;118(3):443–5.
12. Fontanari P, Burnet H, Zattara-Hartmann MC, et al. Changes in airway resistance induced by nasal inhalation of cold dry, dry, or moist air in normal individuals. J Appl Physiol (1985) 1996;81(4):1739–43. Available at: http://eutils.ncbi.nlm.nih.gov/entrez/eutils/elink.fcgi?dbfrom=pubmed&id=8904594&retmode=ref&cmd=prlinks.
13. Woodhead DD, Lambert DK, Clark JM, et al. Comparing two methods of delivering high-flow gas therapy by nasal cannula following endotracheal extubation: a prospective, randomized, masked, crossover trial. J Perinatol 2006;26(8):481–5.

14. Miller MJ, Carlo WA, Martin RJ. Continuous positive airway pressure selectively reduces obstructive apnea in preterm infants. J Pediatr 1985;106(1):91–4. Available at: http://eutils.ncbi.nlm.nih.gov/entrez/eutils/elink.fcgi?dbfrom=pubmed&id=3917503&retmode=ref&cmd=prlinks.

15. Gizzi C, Papoff P, Giordano I, et al. Flow-synchronized nasal intermittent positive pressure ventilation for infants <32 weeks' gestation with respiratory distress syndrome. Crit Care Res Pract 2012;2012(2):301818.

16. Moretti C, Giannini L, Fassi C, et al. Nasal flow-synchronized intermittent positive pressure ventilation to facilitate weaning in very low-birthweight infants: unmasked randomized controlled trial. Pediatr Int 2008;50(1):85–91.

17. Jassar RK, Vellanki H, Zhu Y, et al. High flow nasal cannula (HFNC) with Heliox decreases diaphragmatic injury in a newborn porcine lung injury model. Pediatr Pulmonol 2014;49(12):1214–22.

18. Saslow JG, Aghai ZH, Nakhla TA, et al. Work of breathing using high-flow nasal cannula in preterm infants. J Perinatol 2006;26(8):476–80.

19. Dysart KC, Miller TL, Wolfson MR, et al. Research in high flow therapy: mechanisms of action. Respir Med 2009;103(10):1400–5.

20. Frizzola M, Miller TL, Rodriguez ME, et al. High-flow nasal cannula: impact on oxygenation and ventilation in an acute lung injury model. Pediatr Pulmonol 2011;46(1):67–74.

21. Holleman-Duray D, Kaupie D, Weiss MG. Heated humidified high-flow nasal cannula: use and a neonatal early extubation protocol. J Perinatol 2007;27(12):776–81.

22. Byerly FL, Haithcock JA, Buchanan IB, et al. Use of high flow nasal cannula on a pediatric burn patient with inhalation injury and post-extubation stridor. Burns 2006;32(1):121–5.

23. Dewan NA, Bell CW. Effect of low flow and high flow oxygen delivery on exercise tolerance and sensation of dyspnea. A study comparing the transtracheal catheter and nasal prongs. Chest 1994;105(4):1061–5. Available at: http://eutils.ncbi.nlm.nih.gov/entrez/eutils/elink.fcgi?dbfrom=pubmed&id=8162725&retmode=ref&cmd=prlinks.

24. Barach AL, Eckman M. The use of helium as a new therapeutic gas*. Anesth Analg 1935;14:210–5.

25. Diblasi RM. Nasal continuous positive airway pressure (CPAP) for the respiratory care of the newborn infant. Respir Care 2009;54(9):1209–35. Available at: http://eutils.ncbi.nlm.nih.gov/entrez/eutils/elink.fcgi?dbfrom=pubmed&id=19712498&retmode=ref&cmd=prlinks.

26. Barach AL. The use of helium in the treatment of asthma and obstructive lesions in the larynx and trachea. Ann Intern Med 1935;9(6):739–65.

27. Dunn PM. Dr von Reuss on continuous positive airway pressure in 1914. Arch Dis Child 1990;65(1 Spec No):68. Available at: http://www.ncbi.nlm.nih.gov/pmc/articles/PMC1590176/.

28. Barach AL. Rare gases not essential to life. Proc Soc Exp Biol Med 1934;32:462–4.

29. Tagare A, Kadam S, Vaidya U, et al. Bubble CPAP versus ventilator CPAP in preterm neonates with early onset respiratory distress–a randomized controlled trial. J Trop Pediatr 2013;59(2):113–9.

30. Yagui ACZ, Vale LAPA, Haddad LB, et al. Bubble CPAP versus CPAP with variable flow in newborns with respiratory distress: a randomized controlled trial. J Pediatr (Rio J) 2011;87(6):499–504.

31. Yadav S, Thukral A, Sankar MJ, et al. Bubble vs conventional continuous positive airway pressure for prevention of extubation failure in preterm very low birth weight infants: a pilot study. Indian J Pediatr 2012;79(9):1163–8.

32. Stefanescu BM, Murphy WP, Hansell BJ, et al. A randomized, controlled trial comparing two different continuous positive airway pressure systems for the successful extubation of extremely low birth weight infants. Pediatrics 2003;112(5): 1031–8.

33. Manley BJ, Owen LS, Doyle LW, et al. High-flow nasal cannulae in very preterm infants after extubation. N Engl J Med 2013;369(15):1425–33.

34. Wilkinson D, Andersen C, O'Donnell CP, et al. High flow nasal cannula for respiratory support in preterm infants. Cochrane Database Syst Rev 2011;(5):CD006405.

35. Manley BJ, Owen L, Doyle LW, et al. High-flow nasal cannulae and nasal continuous positive airway pressure use in non-tertiary special care nurseries in Australia and New Zealand. J Paediatr Child Health 2012;48(1):16–21.

36. Harrison VC, Heese Hde V, Klein M. The significance of grunting in hyaline membrane disease. Pediatrics 1968;41(3):549–59.

37. Lemyre B, Davis PG, De Paoli AG, et al. Nasal intermittent positive pressure ventilation (NIPPV) versus nasal continuous positive airway pressure (NCPAP) for preterm neonates after extubation. Cochrane Database Syst Rev 2014;9:CD003212.

38. Demauro SB, Millar D, Kirpalani H. Noninvasive respiratory support for neonates. Curr Opin Pediatr 2014;26(2):157–62.

Sustained Lung Inflation
Physiology and Practice

Elizabeth E. Foglia, MD, MSCE[a],*, Arjan B. te Pas, MD, PhD[b]

KEYWORDS

- Sustained inflation • Lung aeration • Bronchopulmonary dysplasia • Preterm

KEY POINTS

- Lung aeration is essential for successful transition after birth.
- The optimal method to safely and effectively aerate the preterm lung is unknown.
- Sustained inflation is a promising alternative strategy to intermittent positive pressure ventilation with positive end-expiratory pressure.
- There are insufficient data to recommend sustained inflation for routine clinical use at this point.

INTRODUCTION

Aerating the lung is critical for successful neonatal transition after birth. The fetus has liquid-filled lungs, and the newly born infant must rapidly clear this lung liquid to aerate the lungs, establish a functional residual capacity (FRC), and provide a surface for gas exchange. Lung aeration then triggers a cascade of physiologic changes, including decreased pulmonary vascular resistance, increased pulmonary blood flow, and ultimately the transition from fetal to neonatal circulation.

Most term infants begin to establish the FRC with the first spontaneous breaths after birth. Vyas and colleagues[1] demonstrated that the tidal volume of these first inspirations is closely associated with gains in FRC. Conversely, preterm infants must overcome multiple physiologic challenges to aerate the lung. These include a compliant chest wall and weak musculature,[2–4] immature epithelial sodium channels,[5,6] and immature surfactant composition and production.[7] Accordingly, almost all extremely preterm infants require respiratory support during neonatal transition.[8] At present,

Disclosures: The authors have no financial conflicts of interest to disclose. The authors are both investigators on the ongoing SAIL (Sustained Aeration of Infant Lungs) trial, Clinicaltrials.gov Identifier NCT02139800.

a Division of Neonatology, The Children's Hospital of Philadelphia, The Hospital of the University of Pennsylvania, The University of Pennsylvania Perelman School of Medicine, 8th Floor Ravdin Building, 3400 Spruce Street, Philadelphia, PA 19104, USA; b Division of Neonatology, Department of Pediatrics, Leiden University Medical Center, Albinusdreef 2, 2300 RC, Leiden, Netherlands
* Corresponding author.
E-mail address: foglia@email.chop.edu

the best method of promoting lung aeration while avoiding trauma to the fragile preterm lung is unknown.

The current standard practice to facilitate lung aeration is intermittent positive pressure ventilation (IPPV) with positive end-expiratory pressure (PEEP) in apneic infants and continuous positive airway pressure (CPAP) alone in spontaneously breathing infants.[9] Both CPAP and PEEP promote lung liquid clearance from the alveoli, defend gains in the FRC, and reduce atelectrauma. Ultimately, these all facilitate lung recruitment.

An alternative approach to clear lung liquid and aerate the lung is "sustained inflation" (SI), in which an initial inflating pressure is held for a prolonged duration. Here, we review the physiology supporting SI as a strategy to promote lung aeration and the available clinical evidence for the efficacy and safety of SI in preterm infants.

PHYSIOLOGY
Physiologic Rationale for Sustained Inflation

The recent progress in understanding the mechanisms regulating lung aeration at birth[10,11] has led to recognition that the respiratory transition consists of different phases: (1) lung liquid clearance and aeration of distal airways, (2) prevention of lung liquid reentry, and (3) gas exchange and homeostasis.[12] Thus, the initial respiratory support should promote lung liquid clearance and lung aeration. This is not only critical for establishing pulmonary gas exchange, but also for initiating the cardiovascular changes necessary for transition to the postnatal circulation.[13]

Although the interacting mechanism is currently unknown, it has become clear that the lung aeration, and not oxygenation per se, is responsible for the increase in pulmonary blood flow and heart rate after birth.[13] Further, uniform lung aeration is needed to avoid large ventilation-perfusion mismatch, which can occur in a partially aerated lung.[14]

Lung Liquid Clearance

The volume of airway liquid at birth depends on how much is cleared before birth, which depends on the mode and timing of delivery. However, at birth the airways are always partly filled with a significant amount of liquid, and this must be cleared. After birth, airway liquid clearance is driven by an increased transepithelial pressure gradient, which is generated by creating a subatmospheric pressure around the distal airway. When infants fail to create this, the pressure gradient can be achieved by applying positive pressure to the airways.[10] The airway resistance is approximately 100 times higher when airways are filled with liquid than with air; this resistance can be overcome by using either higher pressures or longer inflations.

Using high pressures with short inflation times will contribute to heterogeneous lung aeration, as air will flow initially to the low-resistance, aerated lung rather than the high-resistance, liquid-filled lung. This results in overdistention and injury to already aerated regions.[15,16] A theoretically better alternative is to prolong the time over which the inflation pressure is applied (SI). Although lung aeration initially occurs in a nonuniform pattern during an SI, if the inflation is long enough, most of the lung will aerate before the inflation has ceased.

PRECLINICAL DATA
Preterm Animal Models

Using phase-contrast radiographic imaging in a preterm rabbit model, te Pas and colleagues[16] demonstrated that an initial SI can uniformly aerate the lung and fully recruit an FRC and the tidal volumes given by tidal ventilation after SI. (**Fig. 1**) In a preterm lamb model, Sobotka and colleagues[17] compared an initial SI of 40 cm H_2O (for either 1 minute or until a volume of 20 mL/kg was administered) with standard ventilation. Lambs treated with SI demonstrated better lung function and more stable cerebral oxygen delivery without impeding pulmonary blood flow.

There are limited experimental data on the effect of SI on initial lung injury. In preterm rabbits, early injury markers were reduced following a 10-second SI of 30 cm H_2O, compared with repetitive inflations.[18] However, in a preterm lamb model, an SI was just as injurious as conventional IPPV.[19] Peak inflating pressures used in that study were high (50 cm H_2O), which could have contributed to injury by causing overdistention.[19] Another recent preterm lamb study indicated that a prolonged (over minutes) lung recruitment strategy that used stepwise increases (to 20 cm H_2O) and decreases in PEEP was a more effective strategy than an SI for improving respiratory function at birth.[20] However, considering that this strategy will be applied for minutes and that high PEEP levels can have severe effects on the pulmonary blood flow,[21] this approach is likely to have a major detrimental impact on cardiovascular function.

Many factors could influence both the required pressure and duration for SI to achieve uniform lung aeration without overinflating and injuring lung regions. So far in the imaging studies, where lung distension was accurately monitored, overdistention did not occur.[15,16] When using an inflation pressure of 30 cm H_2O in a preterm rabbit, 90% of the lung was aerated by 14 seconds, but there was much variation between animals.

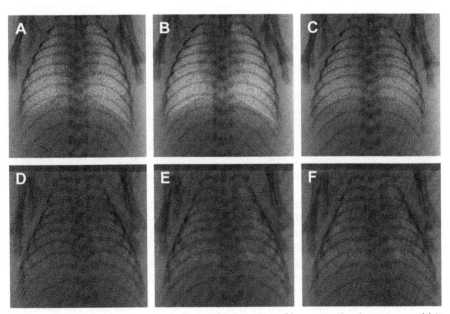

Fig. 1. Example of phase-contrast radiographic imaging of lung aeration in preterm rabbits using initial SI of 15 seconds (*A–C*) versus positive pressure ventilation with inflation time of 1 second (*D–F*). First image is taken after 7 seconds (*A, D*), the second at end of inspiration at 15 seconds (*B, E*), and the last image is taken at end of expiration after 15 seconds (*C, F*). Lung aeration is larger and more uniform during (*A, D*) and at the end of SI (*B, E*), and FRC is higher after SI (*C, F*). (*From* te Pas AB, Siew M, Wallace MJ, et al. Effect of sustained inflation length on establishing functional residual capacity at birth in ventilated premature rabbits. Pediatr Res 2009;66(3):295–300; with permission.)

The effect of gestational age and lung liquid volumes present on inflation pressure and duration needed to achieve lung aeration was recently investigated in a preterm rabbit model.[22] More immature kittens required higher starting pressures and longer duration to achieve the set inflation volume. An increased lung liquid volume did not increase the pressure needed, but required a longer duration. However, the lung liquid volume had no influence on the pressure and duration in the most immature kitten (27 days, comparable to 24 weeks' gestational age of a human infant). Possibly these kittens had smaller distal gas exchange surface area, which is then the dominant factor determining the rate of liquid movement across the epithelium.[22]

Asphyxiated Animal Models

Klingenberg and colleagues[23] demonstrated that an initial 30-second SI led to faster recovery of heart rate, blood pressure, and oxygenation in asphyxiated lambs when compared with standard repetitive inflations. The increase in heart rate was already noticed within 5 seconds of initiating the SI. This experiment was repeated using different oxygen contents.[24] Although in the immediate postasphyxiated period some oxygen was needed for increase in pulmonary blood flow and the heart rate recovery, the concentration needed was minimal: an equivalent improvement was detected when 5% or 21% of oxygen was used. Increasing the oxygen to 100% did not lead to further improvement. It is likely that the effect of lung aeration on pulmonary blood flow is supplemented by a direct effect of oxygen on myocardium and the pulmonary vasculature, for which only a small amount of oxygen is needed. Asphyxiated infants are unable to autoregulate the cerebral vessels. Increased cerebral blood flow resulting from rebound tachycardia and hypertension following SI may increase the risk for intracranial hemorrhages.[23,24] Administering 100% oxygen would then also increase the cerebral oxygen delivery, increasing the risk for hyperoxia-induced brain injury.[24]

HUMAN STUDIES: PHYSIOLOGIC RESPONSE TO SUSTAINED INFLATION
Respiratory Function Measurements

When Vyas and colleagues[25] applied SIs of 5 seconds to asphyxiated infants at birth, the inflation volumes were nearly twofold larger than when 1-second inflations were applied, and an SI always led to formation of FRC. However, in this study and in all animal studies, the SI was applied after intubation, whereas current studies apply SI via facemask in the delivery room (DR).

van Vonderen and colleagues[26] analyzed airflow and volume changes in preterm infants treated with SI after birth. They observed that often large mask leak and airway obstruction occurred, and the SI was not effective unless the infants were spontaneously breathing. As most of the FRC gain occurred when breaths were taken, the role of spontaneous breathing appears to be important for the SI to be clinically effective. The investigators hypothesized that active glottis adduction at birth might prevent air from entering the lung during an SI. Before birth, active glottis adduction during apnea is needed for lung expansion and lung growth.[27] It is possible that this pattern of activity temporarily persists at birth.

Near Infrared Spectroscopy

Fuchs and colleagues[28] measured hemodynamic changes in preterm infants treated with SI after birth. Of 24 infants, 16 (75%) required a second SI for persistent bradycardia or hypoxemia after the first SI; only 2 infants required a third SI. Rise in heart rate, signaling an effective SI, led to a rapid rise in cerebral tissue oxygen saturation.

Schwaberger and colleagues[29] randomized 40 preterm infants in a pilot trial comparing SI with "standard" respiratory care on cerebral blood volume measurements measured with near infrared spectroscopy. Although cerebral blood volume decreased in the first 15 minutes after birth in control infants, cerebral blood volume remained essentially unchanged in the SI-treated infants. These preliminary data accentuate the need for future studies that include both physiologic and clinical outcomes following SI in preterm infants.

OBSERVATIONAL HUMAN STUDIES

Vyas and colleagues[25] reported the effect of SI more than 30 years ago, but SI remained understudied for decades. There is now a renewed clinical interest in this intervention, with a special focus in preterm infants.

Three observational studies have compared outcomes of preterm infants treated with SI with controls. These studies differ regarding population, the definition of SI, respiratory interventions in the control group, and outcomes (**Table 1**).

In 1999, Lindner and colleagues[30] compared outcomes of 123 extremely low birth weight infants born before and after a new DR protocol was implemented. The "old" protocol used IPPV via bag and facemask, followed by intubation and mechanical ventilation for ongoing respiratory distress. In the "new" protocol, 1 to 2 SIs were applied via nasopharyngeal tube, before transitioning to nasal CPAP or ongoing IPPV (if necessary). Following introduction of the new protocol, infants were less often intubated in the DR (40% vs 84%, $P<.001$) or during their hospital stay (75% vs 93%, $P<.01$). In addition, fewer infants treated with the new protocol developed bronchopulmonary dysplasia (BPD) (12% vs 32%, $P<.05$). However, the new protocol introduced many interventions to DR care of the preterm, including an individualized approach to intubation in the DR, more nasal CPAP use, and novel thermoregulation interventions. Thus, the individual effect of SI on the observed outcome improvements is uncertain.

Lista and colleagues[31] published their experience implementing SI in the DR management of preterm infants less than 32 weeks' gestation. They compared outcomes of 119 historical controls with 89 infants treated with SI. Other respiratory interventions were similar between groups. Infants treated with SI experienced less need for mechanical ventilation during hospitalization (51% vs 76%, $P<.0001$), shorter duration of mechanical ventilation (5 ± 11 vs 11 ± 19 days, $P = .008$), and less treatment with postnatal steroids (10% vs 25%, $P = .01$). In addition, fewer infants treated with SI developed BPD (7% vs 25%, $P = .004$). Neonatal morbidities, such as pneumothorax, patent ductus arteriosus, and severe intraventricular hemorrhage, did not significantly differ between groups.

Grasso and colleagues[32] compared 78 infants ≤34 weeks' gestation treated with a single SI followed by IPPV (as needed) with 78 historical controls treated with IPPV. Both cohorts received CPAP in the DR. Infants treated with SI were less likely to be intubated in the DR (6% vs 21%; $P<.01$) or to require mechanical ventilation during hospitalization (14% vs 55%; $P \leq .001$). There were no significant differences between groups regarding mortality, pneumothorax, intraventricular hemorrhage, and BPD.

These studies are all limited by their use of historical controls. In addition, some of these protocols were a package of interventions, making it challenging to isolate the individual effect of SI on clinical outcomes. Nonetheless, these studies demonstrate that treating preterm infants with SI is feasible and safe, and they provide essential preliminary data for randomized controlled trials (RCTs) of SI in this population.

Table 1
Observational studies of preterm infants treated with sustained inflation compared with historical controls

Study	Lindner et al,[30] 1999	Lista et al,[31] 2011	Grasso et al,[32] 2015
Sustained inflation group			
Population	67 infants: BW <1000 g and ≥24 wk gestation	89 infants: <32 wk gestation	78 infants: BW ≤2000 g and ≤34 wk gestation
Intervention	First SI: 20 cm H_2O × 15 s Up to 1 more SI: 25 cm H_2O × 15 s PEEP 4–6 cm H_2O	First SI: 25 cm H_2O × 15 s Up to 1 more SI: 25 cm H_2O × 15 s PEEP 5 cm H_2O	One SI: 25 cm H_2O × 15 s PEEP 4 cm H_2O
Control group			
Population	56 infants: BW <1000 g and ≥24 wk gestation	119 infants: <32 wk gestation	78 infants: BW ≤2000 g and ≤34 wk gestation
Intervention	IPPV via facemask, followed by intubation and mechanical ventilation for respiratory distress	CPAP 5 cm H_2O or IPPV (PIP <25 cm H_2O) with PEEP 5 cm H_2O	IPPV with initial PIP 30–40 cm H_2O, then 20 cm H_2O with PEEP 5 cm H_2O
Outcomes	SI group with less • Intubation in DR: 40% vs 84%, P<.001 • BPD: 12% vs 32%, P<.05	SI group with less • Mechanical ventilation: 51% vs 76%, P<.0001 • BPD: 7% vs 25%, P = .004	SI group with less • Intubation in DR: 6% vs 21%, P<.01 • Mechanical ventilation: 14% vs 55%, P≤.001
Comments	Other treatment differences: Individualized intubation criteria in DR, thermoregulation protocol	Infants in control group retrospectively enrolled, infants in SI group prospectively enrolled	High initial PIP for IPPV

Abbreviations: BPD, bronchopulmonary dysplasia; BW, birth weight; CPAP, continuous positive airway pressure; DR, delivery room; IPPV, intermittent positive pressure ventilation; PEEP, positive end-expiratory pressure; PIP, peak inspiratory pressure; SI, sustained inflation.
Data from Refs.[30–32]

RANDOMIZED CONTROLLED TRIALS
Overview

There are 5 published RCTs of SI in preterm infants. These trials vary in design, population, control interventions, and outcomes (**Table 2**). Perhaps most importantly, the definition of SI itself differs across these trials: peak inflation pressures range from 20 to 30 cm H_2O, the duration of SI ranges from 5 to 15 seconds, and the number of inflations range from 1 to 3 (**Fig. 2**).

Efficacy

Lindner and colleagues[33] enrolled 61 preterm infants in a single-site RCT comparing SI with IPPV. This study was closed early due to slow recruitment and did not reach the targeted sampled size of 110. Thus, the study was underpowered to detect a difference in the primary outcome, intubation and mechanical ventilation in the first 48 hours after birth (61% SI vs 70% IPPV, $P = .59$). There were no significant differences between groups in mortality, air leaks, or chronic lung disease.

Harling and colleagues[34] randomized 52 preterm infants requiring resuscitation to receive either a 5-second SI or 2-second "conventional" lung inflation as the first assisted breath after birth. There were no significant differences between treatment groups in the primary outcome, cytokine markers of lung inflammation. The incidence of BPD and death were similar between treatment groups, although the study was not powered to detect differences in these outcomes. It is likely that the experimental inflations compared in this trial (5 seconds) were too similar to the control inflations (2 seconds) to result in significant differences in outcomes between treatment groups.

te Pas and Walther[35] enrolled 207 preterm infants in a trial comparing 2 DR respiratory protocols. In the SI treatment arm, respiratory support was delivered with a T-piece via nasopharyngeal tube, and nasal CPAP was initiated after 1 to 2 SIs. In the control group, infants were treated with IPPV via self-inflating bag and facemask, and CPAP was not used in the DR. The primary outcome, mechanical ventilation in the first 72 hours after birth, was significantly lower in the SI group compared with control infants (37% vs 51%, odds ratio [OR] 0.57, 95% confidence interval [CI] 0.32–0.98). In addition, the incidence of moderate-severe BPD among survivors was lower in the SI group (9% vs 19%, OR 0.41, 95% CI 0.18–0.96). Because many aspects of respiratory care differed between treatment arms, it is difficult to isolate the causal effect of SI on these clinical outcomes.

The multisite SLI (Sustained Lung Inflation) trial randomized 291 preterm infants to receive either SI or nasal CPAP, with subsequent care according to Neonatal Resuscitation Program guidelines. This trial differed from the other published trials in that all eligible infants were enrolled regardless of cardiorespiratory status. Infants in the SI treatment arm experienced a significant reduction in the primary outcome, mechanical ventilation in the first 72 hours after birth (53% vs 65%, unadjusted OR 0.62, 95% CI 0.38–0.99). There were no significant differences between groups in the secondary outcomes of BPD or death.[36]

Mercadante and colleagues[37] performed a single-site RCT of SI in late preterm infants 34-36^{6/7} weeks' gestation. In the SI treatment arm, infants received a single prophylactic SI and then were transitioned to CPAP, regardless of respiratory status after birth. Subsequent care was guided by the infant's clinical status. In the control arm, treatment was based on Neonatal Resuscitation Program (NRP) guidelines, with respiratory interventions guiding the infant's clinical status. There was no significant difference in the primary outcome: need for respiratory support during hospitalization (11% vs 9%, relative risk [RR] 1.24, 95% CI 0.51–2.99). Secondary outcomes,

Table 2
Randomized trials of sustained inflation in preterm infants

Study	Lindner et al,[33] 2005	Harling et al,[34] 2005	te Pas et al,[35] 2007	Lista et al,[36] 2015	Mercadante et al,[37] 2016
Sample size	n = 61 infants	n = 52 infants	n = 207 infants	n = 291 infants	n = 185
Population	GA: 25–28 6/7 wk plus clinical eligibility criteria	GA: <31 wk plus clinical eligibility criteria	GA: 25–32 6/7 wk plus clinical eligibility criteria	GA: 25–28 6/7 wk No clinical eligibility criteria	GA: 34–36 6/7 wk No clinical eligibility criteria
Consent	Antenatal	Antenatal	Antenatal	Antenatal	Antenatal
Randomization	After birth, based on clinical criteria	Before birth; enrollment based on clinical criteria	Before birth; enrollment based on clinical criteria	After birth	Before birth
Sustained inflation					
Definition	20 cm H_2O × 15 s Up to 2 more SI: 25 cm H_2O × 15 s, 30 cm H_2O × 15 s	25–30 cm H_2O × 5 s	20 cm H_2O × 10 s Up to 1 more SI: 25 cm H_2O × 10 s	25 cm H_2O × 15 s Up to 1 more SI: 25 cm H_2O × 15 s	25 cm H_2O × 15 s Up to 1 more SI: 25 cm H_2O × 15 s
PEEP/CPAP	4–6 cm H_2O	3–4 cm H_2O	5–6 cm H_2O	5 cm H_2O	5 cm H_2O
Interface, device	NP tube, ventilator	Facemask or ETT, T-piece	NP tube, T-piece	Facemask, T-piece	Facemask, T-piece

Control intervention

Intervention	IPPV: PIP 20 cm H_2O, escalating to 25, 30 cm H_2O	IPPV: PIP 25–30 cm H_2O × 2 s	IPPV: initial PIP 30–40 cm H_2O, then ≤20 cm H_2O	Nasal CPAP 5 cm H_2O, further resuscitation according to NRP	Resuscitation according to NRP
PEEP/CPAP	4–6 cm H_2O	3–4 cm H_2O	No PEEP or CPAP in DR	5 cm H_2O	As needed, per NRP
Interface, device	NP tube, ventilator	Facemask or ETT, T-piece	Facemask, self-inflating bag	Facemask, T-piece	Facemask, T-piece
Primary outcome	Intubation within first 48 h of life: SI (61%) vs IPPV (70%), OR 0.68 (0.23–1.97)	Cytokines in BAL at 12 HOL: no significant differences	Intubation within 72 h after birth: SI (37%) vs IPPV (51%), OR 0.57 (0.32–0.98)	Intubation within 72 h after birth: SI (53%) vs CPAP (65%), OR 0.62 (0.38–0.99)	Any respiratory support in the NICU: SI (11%) vs control (9%), RR 1.24 (0.51–2.99)
Comments	Closed early, underpowered	Minimal treatment differences	Different devices and interfaces	Prophylactic approach to SI	Prophylactic approach to SI

Abbreviations: BAL, bronchoalveolar lavage; BPD, bronchopulmonary dysplasia; CPAP, continuous positive airway pressure; DR, delivery room; ETT, endotracheal tube; GA, gestational age; HOL, hours of life; IPPV, intermittent positive pressure ventilation; NICU, Neonatal Intensive Care Unit; NP, nasopharyngeal; NRP, Neonatal Resuscitation Program; OR, odds ratio; PEEP, positive end-expiratory pressure; PIP, peak inspiratory pressure; RR, relative risk; SI, sustained inflation.
Data from Refs.[33–37]

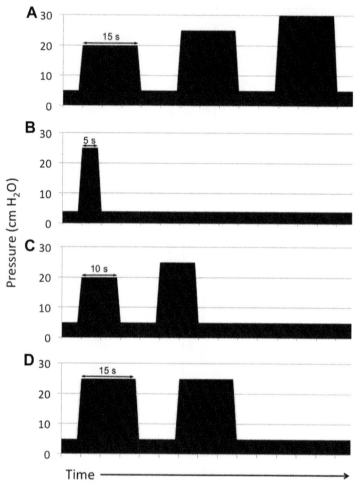

Fig. 2. Peak pressures, duration, and number of SI protocols used in published RCTs. (*A*) Lindner et al,[33] 2005; (*B*) Harling et al,[34] 2005; (*C*) te Pas and Walther,[35] 2007; (*D*) Lista et al,[36] 2015 and Mercadante et al,[37] 2016. For all trials, all enrolled infants received the first SI, subsequent SIs applied according to clinical response.

such as neonatal intensive care unit admission and length of hospital stay, did not significantly differ between groups.

Safety

The major safety concern for SI is the potential for air leaks. None of the individual trials found a significant increase in the incidence of air leaks following SI. In the Italian SLI trial, there was a higher, but nonsignificant, increase in pneumothorax in the SI arm compared with controls (6% vs 1%, OR 4.57, 95% CI 0.97–21.5).[36] In the RCT of late preterm infants,[37] air leaks occurred in 3 (3%) of 93 infants treated with SI, compared with 0 of 92 infants in the control group (*P* = .08). Of note, in both of these trials, infants were randomized irrespective of respiratory status, and all infants in the SI group received SI. Speculatively, this prophylactic approach to SI may increase the risk of air leaks. In the SLI trial, the median age at pneumothorax in the SI group was 70 hours. This late timing of pneumothorax raises the question of whether the SI itself caused the air leaks. It is possible that other factors, such as less surfactant use in the SI arm, contributed to the increase in air leaks.

META-ANALYSIS

Two meta-analyses of SI trials have been published.[38,39] O'Donnell and colleagues[38] included trials comparing SI (defined as inflations >1 second) with IPPV (defined as inflations ≤1 second) in term or preterm infants. Only 2 trials, with a total of 352 enrolled infants, were eligible for inclusion.[33,36] There was no significant difference in the primary outcome of death during hospitalization (RR 1.59, 95% CI 0.81–3.10), or the secondary pulmonary outcomes of intubation in the first 3 days of life or chronic lung disease.

Schmölzer and colleagues[39] included 4 trials comprising 611 preterm infants in their meta-analysis.[33–36] For the outcome of mechanical ventilation within 72 hours after birth, this analysis favored SI (RR 0.87, 95% CI 0.77–0.97). The absolute risk reduction was −0.10 (95% CI −0.17 to −0.03), giving a number needed to treat of 10. There were no significant differences in the outcomes of BPD, death, or the composite outcomes of BPD/death.

In the analysis by O'Donnell and colleagues,[38] the rate of pharmacologic therapy for a patent ductus arteriosus was significantly higher in the SI group (RR 1.27, 95% CI 1.03–1.56). Schmölzer and colleagues[39] found a similar result for the outcome of medical or surgical therapy for patent ductus arteriosus (RR 1.27, 95% CI 1.05–1.54). Neither meta-analysis demonstrated a significant difference in air leaks, severe intraventricular hemorrhage, or other measured neonatal outcomes.

SUMMARY

There is a strong rationale for using SI to support the initial phase of respiratory transition in preterm infants, and the pulmonary and hemodynamic effects of SI in experimental studies are promising. However, there is residual uncertainty regarding the optimal method of delivering SI, the target patient population for this intervention, and the physiologic response to SI (**Box 1**). Finally, it remains to be seen whether SI

Box 1
Ongoing questions about sustained inflation

- Definition of sustained inflation
  - Peak pressure
  - Duration
  - Number
- Prophylactic versus rescue approach
- Role of spontaneous breathing on the efficacy of sustained inflation
- Impact on physiologic outcomes
  - Respiratory function measurements
  - Oxygen and tissue saturation
- Impact on relevant clinical outcomes
  - Air leaks
  - Bronchopulmonary dysplasia
  - Death

improves clinically significant outcomes in preterm infants. Further studies, including both physiologic and clinical outcomes, may fill these knowledge gaps.

Two RCTs of SI with the primary outcome of BPD or death in preterm infants are ongoing. Schmölzer and colleagues[39] recently completed a single-site RCT of SI versus IPPV on the outcome of BPD in infants less than 33 weeks' gestation; results are not yet published.[40] The ongoing SAIL (Sustained Aeration of Infant Lungs) trial is an international multisite RCT comparing SI with IPPV on the primary outcome of BPD or death in 600 infants from 23-26[6/7] weeks' gestation.[41] These trials will inform our understanding of the long-term pulmonary outcomes following SI in preterm infants.

Current Recommendations

At present, SI is a promising experimental therapy, but there are insufficient data to support the use of SI in clinical practice. Accordingly, the 2015 International Liaison Committee on Resuscitation neonatal treatment recommendations do not include the use of SI in preterm infants after birth.[42] Further experimental data and results from well-designed RCTs are needed to determine whether and how SI should be used to optimize neonatal transition in preterm infants after birth.

REFERENCES

1. Vyas H, Field D, Milner AD, et al. Determinants of the first inspiratory volume and functional residual capacity at birth. Pediatr Pulmonol 1986;2(4):189–93.
2. Heldt GP, McIlroy MB. Distortion of chest wall and work of diaphragm in preterm infants. J Appl Physiol (1985) 1987;62(1):164–9.
3. Heldt GP, McIlroy MB. Dynamics of chest wall in preterm infants. J Appl Physiol (1985) 1987;62(1):170–4.
4. Deoras KS, Greenspan JS, Wolfson MR, et al. Effects of inspiratory resistive loading on chest wall motion and ventilation: differences between preterm and full-term infants. Pediatr Res 1992;32(5):589–94.
5. Janér C, Helve O, Pitkänen OM, et al. Expression of airway epithelial sodium channel in the preterm infant is related to respiratory distress syndrome but unaffected by repeat antenatal beta-methasone. Neonatology 2010;97(2):132–8.
6. Barker PM, Gowen CW, Lawson EE, et al. Decreased sodium ion absorption across nasal epithelium of very premature infants with respiratory distress syndrome. J Pediatr 1997;130(3):373–7.
7. Obladen M. Factors influencing surfactant composition in the newborn infant. Eur J Pediatr 1978;128(3):129–43.
8. Aziz K, Chadwick M, Baker M, et al. Ante- and intra-partum factors that predict increased need for neonatal resuscitation. Resuscitation 2008;79(3):444–52.
9. Committee on Fetus and Newborn. Respiratory support in preterm infants at birth. Pediatrics 2014;133(1):171–4.
10. Siew ML, te Pas AB, Wallace MJ, et al. Positive end-expiratory pressure enhances development of a functional residual capacity in preterm rabbits ventilated from birth. J Appl Physiol (1985) 2009;106(5):1487–93.
11. Siew ML, Wallace MJ, Allison BJ, et al. The role of lung inflation and sodium transport in airway liquid clearance during lung aeration in newborn rabbits. Pediatr Res 2013;73(4 Pt 1):443–9.
12. Hooper SB, te Pas AB, Kitchen MJ. Respiratory transition in the newborn: a three-phase process. Arch Dis Child Fetal Neonatal Ed 2016;101(3):F266–71.

13. Lang JAR, Pearson JT, Binder-Heschl C, et al. Increase in pulmonary blood flow at birth; role of oxygen and lung aeration. J Physiol 2015;594(5):1389–98.

14. Lang JAR, Pearson JT, te Pas AB, et al. Ventilation/perfusion mismatch during lung aeration at birth. J Appl Physiol (1985) 2014;117(5):535–43.

15. te Pas AB, Siew M, Wallace MJ, et al. Establishing functional residual capacity at birth: the effect of sustained inflation and positive end-expiratory pressure in a preterm rabbit model. Pediatr Res 2009;65(5):537–41.

16. te Pas AB, Siew M, Wallace MJ, et al. Effect of sustained inflation length on establishing functional residual capacity at birth in ventilated premature rabbits. Pediatr Res 2009;66(3):295–300.

17. Sobotka KS, Hooper SB, Allison BJ, et al. An initial sustained inflation improves the respiratory and cardiovascular transition at birth in preterm lambs. Pediatr Res 2011;70(1):56–60.

18. Wallace MJ, Zahra VA, te Pas AB, et al. A sustained inflation at birth reduces markers of lung injury. J Paediatr and Child Health 2012;48(Suppl 1):67.

19. Hillman NH, Kemp MW, Noble PB, et al. Sustained inflation at birth did not protect preterm fetal sheep from lung injury. Am J Physiol Lung Cell Mol Physiol 2013; 305(6):L446–53.

20. Tingay DG, Bhatia R, Schmölzer GM, et al. Effect of sustained inflation vs. step-wise PEEP strategy at birth on gas exchange and lung mechanics in preterm lambs. Pediatr Res 2014;75(2):288–94.

21. Crossley KJ, Morley CJ, Allison BJ, et al. Blood gases and pulmonary blood flow during resuscitation of very preterm lambs treated with antenatal betamethasone and/or Curosurf: effect of positive end-expiratory pressure. Pediatr Res 2007; 62(1):37–42.

22. te Pas AB, Kitchen MJ, Lee K, et al. Optimizing lung aeration at birth using a sustained inflation and positive pressure ventilation in preterm rabbits. Pediatr Res 2016;80(1):85–91.

23. Klingenberg C, Sobotka KS, Ong T, et al. Effect of sustained inflation duration; resuscitation of near-term asphyxiated lambs. Arch Dis Child Fetal Neonatal Ed 2013;98(3):F222–7.

24. Sobotka KS, Ong T, Polglase GR, et al. The effect of oxygen content during an initial sustained inflation on heart rate in asphyxiated near-term lambs. Arch Dis Child Fetal Neonatal Ed 2015;100(4):F337–43.

25. Vyas H, Milner AD, Hopkin IE, et al. Physiologic responses to prolonged and slow-rise inflation in the resuscitation of the asphyxiated newborn infant. J Pediatr 1981;99(4):635–9.

26. van Vonderen JJ, Hooper SB, Hummler HD, et al. Effects of a sustained inflation in preterm infants at birth. J Pediatr 2014;165(5):903–8.

27. Harding R, Bocking AD, Sigger JN. Influence of upper respiratory tract on liquid flow to and from fetal lungs. J Appl Physiol (1985) 1986;61(1):68–74.

28. Fuchs H, Lindner W, Buschko A, et al. Cerebral oxygenation in very low birth weight infants supported with sustained lung inflations after birth. Pediatr Res 2011;70(2):176–80.

29. Schwaberger B, Pichler G, Avian A, et al. Do sustained lung inflations during neonatal resuscitation affect cerebral blood volume in preterm infants? A random-ized controlled pilot study. PLoS One 2015;10(9):e0138964.

30. Lindner W, Vossbeck S, Hummler H, et al. Delivery room management of extremely low birth weight infants: spontaneous breathing or intubation? Pediat-rics 1999;103(5 Pt 1):961–7.

31. Lista G, Fontana P, Castoldi F, et al. Does sustained lung inflation at birth improve outcome of preterm infants at risk for respiratory distress syndrome? Neonatology 2011;99(1):45–50.
32. Grasso C, Sciacca P, Giacchi V, et al. Effects of Sustained Lung Inflation, a lung recruitment maneuver in primary acute respiratory distress syndrome, in respiratory and cerebral outcomes in preterm infants. Early Hum Dev 2015;91(1):71–5.
33. Lindner W, Högel J, Pohlandt F. Sustained pressure—controlled inflation or intermittent mandatory ventilation in preterm infants in the delivery room? A randomized, controlled trial on initial respiratory support via nasopharyngeal tube. Acta Paediatr 2005;94(3):303–9.
34. Harling AE, Beresford MW, Vince GS, et al. Does sustained lung inflation at resuscitation reduce lung injury in the preterm infant? Arch Dis Child Fetal Neonatal Ed 2005;90(5):F406–10.
35. te Pas AB, Walther FJ. A randomized, controlled trial of delivery-room respiratory management in very preterm infants. Pediatrics 2007;120(2):322–9.
36. Lista G, Boni L, Scopesi F, et al. Sustained lung inflation at birth for preterm infants: a randomized clinical trial. Pediatrics 2015;135(2):e457–64.
37. Mercadante D, Colnaghi M, Polimeni V, et al. Sustained lung inflation in late preterm infants: a randomized controlled trial. J Perinatol 2016;36(6):443–7.
38. O'Donnell CP, Bruschettini M, Davis PG, et al. Sustained versus standard inflations during neonatal resuscitation to prevent mortality and improve respiratory outcomes. Cochrane Database Syst Rev 2015;(7):CD004953.
39. Schmölzer GM, Kumar M, Aziz K, et al. Sustained inflation versus positive pressure ventilation at birth: a systematic review and meta-analysis. Arch Dis Child Fetal Neonatal Ed 2015;100(4):F361–8.
40. Assessment of lung aeration at birth. Clinicaltrials.gov Identifier NCT01739114. Available at: https://clinicaltrials.gov/ct2/show/NCT01739114?term=sustained+inflation&rank=3. Accessed March 1, 2016.
41. Foglia EE, Owen LS, Thio M, et al. Sustained Aeration of Infant Lungs (SAIL) trial: study protocol for a randomized controlled trial. Trials 2015;16:95.
42. Perlman JM, Wyllie J, Kattwinkel J, et al. Part 7: neonatal resuscitation: 2015 International Consensus on Cardiopulmonary Resuscitation and Emergency Cardiovascular Care Science With Treatment Recommendations. Circulation 2015;132(16 Suppl 1):S204–41.

Continuous Positive Airway Pressure

To Bubble or Not to Bubble?

Samir Gupta, MD, DM, FRCPCH, FRCPI[a],*, Steven M. Donn, MD[b]

KEYWORDS

- Continuous positive airway pressure, CPAP • Bubble CPAP • Ventilation
- Respiratory support

KEY POINTS

- Bubble continuous positive airway pressure (CPAP) has physiologic properties that could facilitate gas exchange.
- Bubble CPAP (bCPAP) has been successfully used in resource-poor settings.
- bCPAP is reported to improve success after extubation in preterm babies ventilated for less than 2 weeks.
- The success on CPAP is dependent on good nursing care and clear management protocols for weaning and escalation of care.
- Minimizing nasal injuries and improvising systems for optimizing CPAP delivery should be the focus of further investigations.

INTRODUCTION

Adaptation from intrauterine to extrauterine life involves changes in the physiology of every organ and system. It is a complex process, but most babies born at term gestation have a smooth transition. However, babies born prematurely are at a disadvantage, not only because of immaturity of their organ systems but also because the adaptive changes required for extrauterine survival create additional demands. Cardiorespiratory adaptation and establishment of adequate gas exchange are mandatory for intact survival.

A major development in neonatal respiratory support occurred with the introduction of continuous positive airway pressure (CPAP) by Gregory and colleagues[1] in 1971 to

Disclosures: None.
Conflict of Interest: None.
[a] Department of Paediatrics, University Hospital of North Tees, Durham University, Hardwick road, Stockton-on-Tees, TS19 8PE, United Kingdom; [b] Division of Neonatal-Perinatal Medicine, C.S. Mott Children's Hospital, University of Michigan Health System, 1540 East Hospital Drive, Ann Arbor, MI 48109, USA
* Corresponding author.
E-mail address: Samir.gupta@nth.nhs.uk

Clin Perinatol 43 (2016) 647–659
http://dx.doi.org/10.1016/j.clp.2016.07.003
perinatology.theclinics.com
0095-5108/16/© 2016 Elsevier Inc. All rights reserved.

support spontaneously breathing infants using bubble CPAP (bCPAP, F&P Health-care, Auckland, New Zealand). Since then, CPAP has been used either after extubation, or as a primary mode of respiratory support, in babies with respiratory distress syndrome (RDS) who exhibit sufficient respiratory drive.[2]

CPAP can be delivered using various devices. These devices can be broadly grouped into continuous flow and variable flow systems. bCPAP and ventilator-derived CPAP are continuous flow systems. Variable flow devices include the infant flow driver (IFD, Infant flow nCPAP system, Care Fusion, Yorba Linda, CA), Benveniste gas jet valve CPAP, Aladdin, and Arabella systems. The use of CPAP augments breathing and gas exchange and decreases the risk of ventilator-induced lung injury (VILI). However, its success is dependent on intact respiratory drive and lung disease that is not severe enough to warrant mechanical ventilation.[2]

PHYSIOLOGIC BASIS OF BUBBLE CONTINUOUS POSITIVE AIRWAY PRESSURE

CPAP is a form of continuous distending pressure, which facilitates the maintenance of increased transpulmonary pressure during the entire respiratory cycle. When positive pressure is applied to the airways of spontaneously breathing infants, it helps to maintain functional residual capacity (FRC) and assist gas exchange.[2]

FRC is the volume of air present in the lungs at the end of passive expiration. At FRC, the elastic recoil forces of the lungs and chest wall are equal but opposite, and there is no exertion by the diaphragm or other respiratory muscles. The loss of FRC can be partially compensated by the application of CPAP to maintain lung volume and prevent ventilation/perfusion mismatch and hypercarbia.[3]

The following physiologic principles underlying the effectiveness of CPAP in newborns have been described[2]:

- Abolition of upper airway occlusion and decrease in resistance
- Improvement in diaphragmatic activity
- Improvement in lung compliance and decreased airway resistance
- Increased tidal volume in stiff lungs with low FRC
- Conservation of surfactant on the alveolar surface

bCPAP uses air or blended gas that is heated and humidified and then delivered to the infant through a low-resistance nasal prong, mask, or cannula. The distal end of the expiratory tubing is submersed underwater, and the CPAP pressure generated is equal to the depth of submersion. Varying the depth of the underwater expiratory tube thus varies the CPAP pressure (**Fig. 1**). The generation of bubbling in the water chamber by exhaled gas has been hypothesized to produce chest vibrations that may enhance gas exchange.[4] With this principle, bCPAP may be an effective and inexpensive option for providing respiratory support to premature infants.

One of the mechanisms of bCPAP is the generation of "bubbles" by the gas escaping the submersed expiratory tube. The applied gas flow rate has been observed to affect the degree of bubbling, and it has been suggested that oscillations from bubbling affect the pressure amplitude and contribute to gas exchange by delivering low-amplitude, high-frequency oscillations to the lungs.[5]

Lee and colleagues[6] tested the hypothesis that bCPAP contributes to gas exchange. In a randomized crossover trial, they enrolled 10 preterm babies ready for extubation to bCPAP or ventilator-derived CPAP. They reported a 39% reduction in minute volume ($P<.001$) and a 7% reduction in respiratory rate ($P = .004$) with no change in transcutaneous CO_2 or pulse oximetry during bCPAP. The calculation of minute ventilation in this

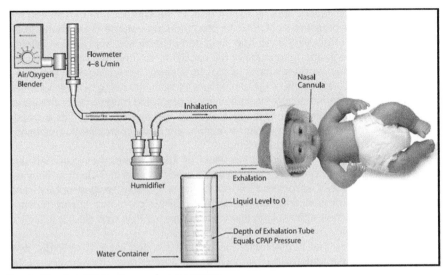

Fig. 1. Simple bCPAP setup and components.

study has been questioned, but the study concluded that chest vibrations produced by bCPAP might have contributed to improved gas exchange.

Morley and colleagues[7] challenged the findings of Lee in a crossover trial of 27 pre-term babies (median gestational age 27 weeks) at a bCPAP pressure of 6 cm H_2O. They observed a median (interquartile range) pressure amplitude of 2.7 cm H_2O (2.5–4.0) for slow bubbling (flow of 3 L/min) and 6 cm H_2O (4.6–7.1) for vigorous, high-amplitude bubbling (flow of 6 L/min). They also reported slightly lower pressure with slow bubbling compared with vigorous bubbling (5.28 vs 5.98 cm H_2O; $P<.001$) (**Fig. 2**). In this study, they did not find any effect of bubbling on respiratory rate or minute ventilation.

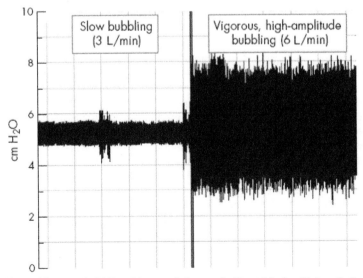

Fig. 2. Effect of flow on bubbling (slow and vigorous). (*From* Morley CJ, Lau R, De Paoli A, et al. Nasal continuous positive airway pressure: does bubbling improve gas exchange? Arch Dis Child Fetal Neonatal Ed 2005;90:F343–4; with permission.)

Pillow and Travadi[8] tested another hypothesis, of superimposition of noise on the underlying constant pressure in bCPAP to promote lung volume recruitment, in an in vitro lung model. They examined how lung compliance and applied flow altered the frequency, content, and magnitude of the oscillatory component of bCPAP pressure waveforms. They reported that in a closed system, increasing flow increased both the mean pressure and the range of pressure oscillations during bCPAP, whereas decreased compliance increased the frequency content and magnitude of the transmitted oscillatory pressures. They suggested that the use of bCPAP in a poorly compliant lung may promote lung volume recruitment through stochastic resonance and thus augment efficiency of gas mixing.

Pillow and colleagues[9] also tested the effect of the flow rate during bCPAP and compared it to constant pressure CPAP using 3 study groups in 34 lambs. They reported that bCPAP was associated with a higher pH, Pao_2, oxygen uptake, and decreased alveolar protein and concluded that bCPAP promotes airway patency and may offer protection against lung injury. However, the flow rate did not influence the 3-hour outcomes.

Another hypothesis that bCPAP use after extubation decreases lung injury, and that alterations to lung nitric oxide synthase (NOS) 3 expression may be one of the underlying mechanisms. Wu and colleagues[10] compared gas exchange, lung injury severity, and lung NOS expression between rats with VILI treated with either bCPAP or spontaneous breathing. They reported that bCPAP decreases lung injury possibly secondary to attenuation of lung NOS3 expression.

The gas flow rate is an important variable in bCPAP. At low CPAP (4–6 cm H_2O), the delivered pressures are reduced at higher flow rates, but at higher CPAP pressures (7–9 cm H_2O), the delivered pressures are higher as flow is increased. Reduction in delivered CPAP pressure could be secondary to increased resistance during spontaneous breathing or insufficient flow to meet inspiratory demand.[11] Also, fixed flows are reported to be more effective than titrated flow (flow just sufficient to create bubbling) for CPAP pressures in the 4- to 6 cm H_2O range.[12] The oropharyngeal temperature and absolute humidity were also delivered per specifications using bCPAP testing on a neonatal mannequin, whereas the variable flow device could not achieve this.[13]

One of the concerns of CPAP is intragastric gas delivery leading to "CPAP belly." Tyagi and colleagues[14] measured intragastric pressures and parameters of respiratory distress in 27 babies receiving bCPAP at 6 cm H_2O. They reported improvement in Downe score, oxygen saturation, and venous blood gases but did not find any increase in intragastric pressure. This finding suggests that bCPAP does not produce "CPAP belly," and there should be co-morbidities to account for this clinical phenomenon.

The nasal interface is another key to the success of CPAP. With bCPAP, the choice of nasal interface is limited. Bi-nasal prongs have been reported to be better than single-nasal prongs.[15] To deliver bCPAP using bi-nasal prongs, the choices are limited to the Fisher and Paykel or Hudson prongs. Bushell and colleagues[16] compared these 2 interfaces in a crossover trial and reported that both were equally effective in achieving the desired bCPAP pressures and targeted oxygen saturation. Nasal masks have also been reported to reduce extubation failures, and the practice of alternating nasal mask and nasal prongs is widely used to minimize nasal injuries.[17]

One of the limitations of bCPAP systems is the lack of pressure alarms and pressure-release valves. Large volumes of condensate in the exhalation limb of the patient circuit are also frequently observed. Youngquist and colleagues[18] reported that condensate in the exhalation limb of the patient circuit during bCPAP could significantly increase pressure delivered to the patient. Hence, emptying fluid from the exhalation limb every 2 to 3 hours is a good practice.

Components of the bCPAP circuit can also affect amplitude and frequency of noise, which in turn can impact lung recruitment. Wu and colleagues[19] reported that increasing the size and submersion depth of the expiratory limb of a CPAP circuit and decreasing the diameter of the bubble generator bottle intensified the magnitude but diminished the frequency of noise transmitted to a lung model.

bCPAP applies small-amplitude, high-frequency oscillations in airway pressure (Delta Paw). The increase in Delta Paw could affect the degree of respiratory support. Diblasi and colleagues[20,21] modified the bubbler exit angle and compared it at 135° (high-amplitude bCPAP) versus 0° (low-amplitude bCPAP). In this animal study, they observed that Pao_2 levels were higher ($P<.007$) with higher amplitudes, and that $Paco_2$ levels did not differ ($P = .073$).

FACTORS AFFECTING THE SUCCESS OF BUBBLE CONTINUOUS POSITIVE AIRWAY PRESSURE

The physiologic variables help in the understanding and optimization of a CPAP system, and diligent monitoring is necessary to achieve the intended results. However, there are several factors that can enhance the chances for success. These factors include optimizing delivery of CPAP and using adjuncts to improve outcomes.

Selection of Nasal Interface

The success of bCPAP is to a large extent dependent on the appropriate selection of a nasal interface. The small size prongs have the potential to move and result in nasal septal injury. They increase airway resistance and the chance of air leak around them, which hampers the delivery of the desired pressure. To the contrary, if the prongs are too large, they can impede blood flow to the nasal mucosa and cause damage. The correct size prongs should fit snugly in the nares without pinching the septum or causing blanching and should avoid contact with the nasal septum.

Monitoring and Preventing Nasal Injury

Good nursing care is the mainstay of success, particularly in infants requiring prolonged support with bCPAP. A nasal injury scoring system (**Table 1**) to document integrity of skin, septum, and other anatomic structures is helpful. Monitoring every 4 to 6 hours and early intervention are the most important variables. Strategies to minimize injury include use of protective barriers such as "cannulaide" or lyofoam, and alternating the use of prongs and masks may also attenuate injury.

Fixation of the Nasal Interface

It is important to have the nasal prongs, mask, or tubing properly positioned to reduce pressure on the nose and face and to avoid leaks. When properly positioned, the corrugated tubing should not touch the infant's skin, and there should be no lateral pressure on the nasal septum. Depending on the type of interface, the corrugated tubing should be affixed to the forehead or above the ears using an appropriate size snug pre-made cap or stockinet to securely hold the tubing in place.

Table 1
Nasal injury scoring chart

	Date/Time of Observation
Tip of nose	0: Normal 1: Red 2: Red + indent 3: Red/indent/skin breakdown 4: As above + tissue loss
Nasal septum	0: Normal 1: Red 2: Red + indent 3: Red/indent/skin breakdown 4: As above + tissue loss
Nostrils	0: Normal 1: Enlarged 2: Enlarged and prong shape 3: Red, bleeding 4: As above + skin breakdown
Nose shape	0: Normal 1: Pushed up/back but normal 2: Pushed up and shortened. No normal orientation when prongs removed

Data from Alsop E, Cook J, Gupta S. Nasal Injuries in Preterm Infants: Comparison of the Infant Flow Driver to Bubble CPAP. E-PAS 2008: 4456.4

Bubbling and System Check

bCPAP systems work on the continuous flow principle. If the baby stops breathing or the nasal interface is blocked or displaced, bubbling will cease. There is no provision on currently available systems for alarms. Intermittent checks and documentation of system performance are mandatory. Some commercially available systems have a built-in mechanism to allow water to decant into the attached container if the level rises above the set reference mark. If indigenous systems are used, regular decanting and changing of water are essential to prevent inadvertent high CPAP and the risk of infection. There is also the provision of measuring pressure close to mouth in the commercial systems for more precise monitoring. Regular suctioning of the nasal passages and cleaning of the prongs also contribute to good practice.

Optimizing Continuous Positive Airway Pressure Delivery

Unlike variable flow CPAP, where the pressures are delivered primarily at the nasal interface, bCPAP delivery depends on the baby breathing through the submersed expiratory tubing. If the baby's mouth is open, the flow can leak, causing a drop in pressure. To limit this, a pacifier or a chin strap can be used. Closure of mouth has been demonstrated to increase the pressure in the pharynx by 2 to 3 cm H_2O[22] **(Fig. 3)**. Regular aspiration of air from the stomach through an indwelling nasogastric tube and leaving the nasogastric tube to vent are routine practices to avoid inadvertent gastric distension.

Weaning from Bubble Continuous Positive Airway Pressure

The commonly used methods are pressure weaning and "seesaw" weaning. To use either method, the baby should be stable on CPAP support with no significant apnea

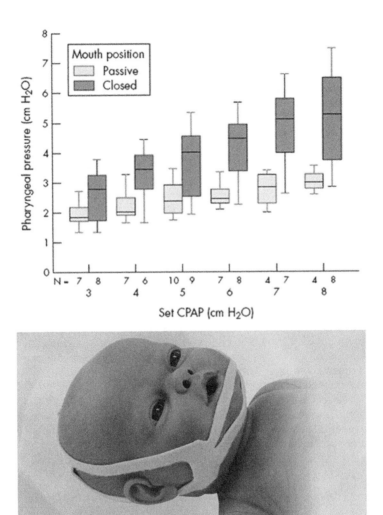

Fig. 3. Set pressure versus pharyngeal pressure in passive and closed mouth positions. ((*Top*) *From* De Paoli AG, Lau R, Davis PG, et al. Pharyngeal pressure in preterm infants receiving nasal continuous positive airway pressure. Arch Dis Child Fetal Neonatal Ed 2005;90:F79–81; with permission. (*Bottom*) *Courtesy of* Neotech Products, Valencia, CA; with permission.)

or bradycardia. Using pressure weaning, attempts are made to reduce CPAP by 1 cm H_2O at least every 12 hours until the baby is reaches 4 cm H_2O, and if stable, CPAP can be discontinued. Using seesaw weaning, CPAP is removed for increasing intervals of time without reducing pressure and finally discontinued. Pressure weaning has been reported to be superior to seesaw weaning.[23]

Escalating Treatment and Continuous Positive Airway Pressure Failure

The clinical and hemodynamic criteria are commonly used to declare failure of CPAP or to escalate the level of CPAP support. If a baby develops frequent minor apnea (>1 per hour, of self-recovering desaturation or bradycardia) or an episode of major apnea requiring intervention, support should be escalated.[24] Increasing oxygen requirement (>40% at bCPAP of 6–8 cm H_2O) is usually an indication for intubation and mechanical ventilation.[25] If the oxygen requirement increases by more than 10% during weaning, it warrants increasing CPAP to the previous level until the baby is stable. Poor gas exchange (pH < 7.2; Pco_2 > 60 mm Hg) is also an indication for escalating CPAP support.

CLINICAL TRIALS OF BUBBLE CONTINUOUS POSITIVE AIRWAY PRESSURE
Cohort and Observational Studies of Continuous Positive Airway Pressure Device Comparisons

The cohort study by Narendran and colleagues[26] incorporated the introduction of bCPAP in one hospital and conventional nasal continuous positive airway pressure (nCPAP) at another for the management of preterm babies with RDS (birth weights 401–1000 g). The data were collected on all extremely low-birth-weight babies and compared to historical controls and also between the hospitals. They reported a reduction in delivery room intubations with the use of both bCPAP and conventional nCPAP compared to historical controls (P<.001). They also reported a significant reduction in the use of postnatal steroids with bCPAP and a trend toward a reduction in chronic lung disease with bCPAP.

In an observational study from Canada, Pelligra and colleagues[27] reported a comparison during 2 time periods. The first used ventilator-derived CPAP with a nasopharyngeal tube, and the second used bCPAP. Data from 821 babies less than 32 weeks (397 babies in period 1, and 424 babies in period 2) were analyzed. There was a significant reduction in the use of exogenous surfactant, postnatal steroids, and the duration of mechanical ventilation with the use of bCPAP.

In another observational study, Massaro and colleagues[28] collected data on 36 preterm babies less than 2000 g who were solely managed with nCPAP over a period of 16 months. They grouped the babies into those who received bCPAP support and those who received ventilator-derived CPAP at the same pressures. The groups were demographically equivalent. The investigators reported no differences in the duration of CPAP support and other clinical outcomes, except that babies managed on bCPAP required oxygen for a shorter duration.

Randomized Trials Comparing Continuous Positive Airway Pressure Devices

Randomized controlled trials performed at birth
Mazzella and colleagues[29] compared IFD CPAP with bi-nasal prongs and bCPAP through a single nasopharyngeal tube. They randomized 36 preterm infants less than 36 weeks' gestation at less than 12 hours of age to receive one of the CPAP methods. They reported a significant beneficial effect on both oxygen requirement and respiratory rate (P<.0001) with IFD CPAP, compared to bCPAP, and a trend toward a decreased need for mechanical ventilation. This study, however, was limited by a small sample size and the use of different nasal interfaces.

McEvoy and colleagues[30] randomized 53 spontaneously breathing preterm babies between 25 and 32 weeks' gestation to receive either bCPAP or ventilator-derived CPAP using Hudson prongs after initial stabilization. The respiratory measurements (FRC and compliance) and CPAP failure through 7 days were compared. They observed no differences between groups.

Tagare and colleagues[31] compared the efficacy and safety of bCPAP with ventilator-derived CPAP in preterm neonates with RDS. Babies with a Silverman-Anderson score greater than or equal to 4 and oxygen requirement greater than 30% within first 6 hours of life were randomly allocated to bCPAP or ventilator-derived CPAP, and the proportion of neonates succeeding was compared. A higher percentage of infants was successfully treated with bCPAP (83% vs 63%, $P = .03$), suggesting superiority of bCPAP for this indication.

In a prospective randomized clinical trial performed by Hosseini and colleagues,[32] 161 preterm infants (28–37 weeks of gestational age) with RDS were randomized in the first hour of life to bCPAP or MediJet system CPAP (Med-CPAP). Short bi-nasal prongs were used in both groups and CPAP was set at 5 to 6 cm H_2O. The primary outcome was duration of CPAP support. There was no difference between the 2 systems.

Yagui and colleagues[33] compared bCPAP and IFD CPAP in 40 babies with birth weight greater than 1500 g. They reported no differences between the groups with regard to demographic data and CPAP failure (21.1% and 20.0% for IFD CPAP and bCPAP, respectively; $P = 1.000$).

Mazmanyan and colleagues[34] randomized 125 infants less than 37 weeks' gestation to bCPAP or IFD CPAP after stabilization at birth in a resource-poor setting. They reported bCPAP equivalent to IFD CPAP in the total number of days CPAP was required, within a margin of 2 days. The results of this trial should be interpreted with caution in extremely to moderately premature babies, because the study group was more mature, but it is a reassuring finding for a population of larger babies in a developing country. The median days (range) for days on CPAP were 0.8 days (0.04–17.5) on bCPAP, and 0.5 days (0.04–5.3) on IFD CPAP.

The trial by Bhatti and colleagues[35] compared Jet-CPAP (variable flow) and bCPAP in 170 preterm newborns less than 34 weeks' gestation with the onset of respiratory distress within 6 hours of birth. CPAP failure rates within 72 hours were similar (29% vs 21%; relative risk 1.4 [0.8–2.3], $P = .25$). Mean (95% confidence intervals [CI]) time to CPAP failure was 59 hours (54–64) in the Jet-CPAP group compared with 65 hours (62–68) in the bCPAP group. In this well designed trial, no difference was reported between the 2 study devices; however, the investigators did not stratify babies by severity of respiratory illness or gestational age.

bCPAP was compared with nasal BiPAP (Bilevel positive airway pressure) by Sadeghnia and colleagues[36] in a randomized controlled trial in 70 very-low-birth-weight babies. They reported no difference in the average duration of noninvasive respiratory support, complications of prematurity (such as chronic lung disease, intraventricular hemorrhage, death, and the number of doses of surfactant), as well as the duration of supplementary oxygen.

Randomized trials of continuous positive airway pressure after extubation

In a study by Sun and colleagues[37] among babies greater than 30 weeks' gestation and birth weight greater than 1250 g, the results favored IFD CPAP over ventilator-derived CPAP. In another study, Stefanescu and colleagues examined 162 extremely low birth weight infants and compared IFD CPAP with ventilator-derived CPAP using INCA prongs. They did not find any difference in the extubation success rate between the 2 study groups.[38]

These trials did not stratify babies by duration of ventilation. It has been reported that nCPAP support has advantages over just supplemental oxygen if the duration of ventilation is less than or equal to 14 days. The demographic differences in the aforementioned trials make it difficult to draw conclusions, but the results suggest that IFD CPAP is either superior to or has similar efficacy to ventilator-derived CPAP when used after extubation. De Paoli and colleagues[39] have stressed in their meta-analysis that a comparable nasal interface is required to allow comparison of CPAP generation systems in randomized trials.

In a subsequent trial, Gupta and colleagues[40] randomized 140 preterm infants 24 to 29 weeks' gestation or 600 to 1500 g at birth to receive bCPAP or IFD CPAP following the first attempt at extubation. Infants were stratified according to duration of initial ventilation ($\leq$14 days or >14 days). Babies were extubated when they passed the minute ventilation test used to objectively assess readiness for extubation.[41] The primary outcome of the study was the need for reintubation within72 hours. If an infant required reintubation, the originally assigned CPAP device was used until the infant was no longer requiring respiratory support. Although there was no statistically significant difference in the extubation failure rate (16.9% on bCPAP, 27.5% on IFD CPAP) for the entire study group, the median duration of CPAP support was 50% shorter in the infants on bCPAP, median 2 days (95% CI, 1–3 days) on bCPAP versus 4 days (95% CI, 2–6 days) on IFD CPAP (P = .031). In infants ventilated for less than or equal to 14 days (n = 127), the extubation failure rate was significantly lower with bCPAP (14.1%; 9/64) compared to IFD CPAP (28.6%; 18/63) (P = .046).

This well designed clinical trial suggests the superiority of post-extubation bCPAP over IFD CPAP in preterm babies less than 30 weeks, who are initially ventilated for less than 14 days. In this trial, similar nasal interfaces were used, stratification by duration of ventilation was performed, a similar weaning approach was utilized, and enrollment occurred after an objective assessment for readiness for extubation.

SUMMARY

nCPAP is increasingly used for respiratory support in preterm babies at birth and after extubation from mechanical ventilation. Various CPAP devices are available that can be broadly split into continuous flow and variable flow. There are potential physiologic differences between systems, and the choice of a CPAP device is too often guided by individual experience and preference rather than by evidence. When interpreting the evidence, clinicians should take into account the pressure generation sources, nasal interface, and the factors affecting the delivery of pressure, such as mouth position and respiratory drive. With increasing use of these devices, better monitoring techniques are required to assess the efficacy and early recognition of babies who are failing and in need of escalated support.

bCPAP seems to have physiologic properties that could facilitate gas exchange. The evidence from studies suggests it is comparable to continuous or variable flow CPAP for management of RDS at birth, even in resource-poor settings. bCPAP seems to have better success when used post-extubation among infants who received ventilation for up to 14 days. Care and familiarity with CPAP further increases the likelihood of success. Further work on minimizing nasal injuries and optimizing support will be foci of further investigation.

REFERENCES

1. Gregory GA, Kitterman JA, Phibbs RH, et al. Treatment of the idiopathic respiratory-distress syndrome with continuous positive airway pressure. N Engl J Med 1971;284:1333–40.
2. Gupta S, Donn SM. Continuous positive airway pressure: physiology and comparison of devices. Semin Fetal Neonatal Med 2016;21(3):204–11.
3. De Paoli AG, Morley C, Davis PG. Nasal CPAP for neonates: what do we know in 2003? Arch Dis Child Fetal Neonatal Ed 2003;88:F168–72.
4. Martin S, Duke T, Davis P. Efficacy and safety of bubble CPAP in neonatal care in low and middle income countries: a systematic review. Arch Dis Child Fetal Neonatal Ed 2014;99:F495–504.
5. Poli JA, Richardson CP, DiBlasi RM. Volume oscillations delivered to a lung model using 4 different bubble CPAP systems. Respir Care 2015;60:371–81.

6. Lee KS, Dunn MS, Fenwick M, et al. A comparison of underwater bubble continuous positive airway pressure with ventilator-derived continuous positive airway pressure in premature neonates ready for extubation. Biol Neonate 1998;73:69–75.

7. Morley CJ, Lau R, De Paoli A, et al. Nasal continuous positive airway pressure: does bubbling improve gas exchange? Arch Dis Child Fetal Neonatal Ed 2005;90:F343–4.

8. Pillow JJ, Travadi JN. Bubble CPAP: is the noise important? An in vitro study. Pediatr Res 2005;57:826–30.

9. Pillow JJ, Hillman N, Moss TJ, et al. Bubble continuous positive airway pressure enhances lung volume and gas exchange in preterm lambs. Am J Respir Crit Care Med 2007;176:63–9.

10. Wu CS, Chou HC, Huang LT, et al. Bubble CPAP support after discontinuation of mechanical ventilation protects rat lungs with ventilator-induced lung injury. Respiration 2016;91:171–9.

11. Bailes SA, Firestone KS, Dunn DK, et al. Evaluating the effect of flow and interface type on pressures delivered with bubble CPAP in a simulated model. Respir Care 2016;61:333–9.

12. Murki S, Das RK, Sharma D, et al. A fixed flow is more effective than titrated flow during bubble nasal CPAP for respiratory distress in preterm neonates. Front Pediatr 2015;3:81.

13. Roberts CT, Kortekaas R, Dawson JA, et al. The effects of non-invasive respiratory support on oropharyngeal temperature and humidity: a neonatal manikin study. Arch Dis Child Fetal Neonatal Ed 2016;101:F248–52.

14. Tyagi P, Gupta N, Jain A, et al. Intra-gastric pressures in neonates receiving bubble CPAP. Indian J Pediatr 2015;82:131–5.

15. Davis P, Davies M, Faber B. A randomised controlled trial of two methods of delivering nasal continuous positive airway pressure after extubation to infants weighing less than 1000 g: binasal (Hudson) versus single nasal prongs. Arch Dis Child Fetal Neonatal Ed 2001;85:F82–5.

16. Bushell T, McHugh C, Meyer MP. A comparison of two nasal continuous positive airway pressure interfaces–a randomized crossover study. J Neonatal Perinatal Med 2013;6:53–9.

17. Kieran EA, Twomey AR, Molloy EJ, et al. Randomized trial of prongs or mask for nasal continuous positive airway pressure in preterm infants. Pediatrics 2012;130:e1170–6.

18. Youngquist TM, Richardson CP, Diblasi RM. Effects of condensate in the exhalation limb of neonatal circuits on airway pressure during bubble CPAP. Respir Care 2013;58:1840–6.

19. Wu CS, Lee CM, Yuh YS, et al. Influence of changing the diameter of the bubble generator bottle and expiratory limb on bubble CPAP: an in vitro study. Pediatr Neonatol 2012;53:359–65.

20. Diblasi RM, Zignego JC, Smith CV, et al. Effective gas exchange in paralyzed juvenile rabbits using simple, inexpensive respiratory support devices. Pediatr Res 2010;68:526–30.

21. Diblasi RM, Zignego JC, Tang DM, et al. Noninvasive respiratory support of juvenile rabbits by high-amplitude bubble continuous positive airway pressure. Pediatr Res 2010;67:624–9.

22. De Paoli AG, Lau R, Davis PG, et al. Pharyngeal pressure in preterm infants receiving nasal continuous positive airway pressure. Arch Dis Child Fetal Neonatal Ed 2005;90:F79–81.

23. Todd DA, Wright A, Broom M, et al. Methods of weaning preterm babies <30 weeks gestation off CPAP: a multicentre randomised controlled trial. Arch Dis Child Fetal Neonatal Ed 2012;97:F236–40.

24. Davis PG, Morley CJ, Owen LS. Non-invasive respiratory support of preterm neonates with respiratory distress: continuous positive airway pressure and nasal intermittent positive pressure ventilation. Semin Fetal Neonatal Med 2009;14:14–20.

25. Sandri F, Plavka R, Simeoni U. The CURPAP study: an international randomized controlled trial to evaluate the efficacy of combining prophylactic surfactant and early nasal continuous positive airway pressure in very preterm infants. Neonatology 2008;94:60–2.

26. Narendran V, Donovan EF, Hoath SB, et al. Early bubble CPAP and outcomes in ELBW preterm infants. J Perinatol 2003;23:195–9.

27. Pelligra P, Abdellatif M, Lee SK. Comparison of clinical outcomes between two modes of CPAP delivery: underwater bubble versus conventional ventilator-derived. E-PAS 2006;59:475.

28. Massaro AN, Abdel-Haq I, Aly HZ. Underwater seal bubble CPAP versus ventilator-derived CPAP: does mode of delivery make a difference in clinical outcome? PAS 2005;57:2053.

29. Mazzella M, Bellini C, Calevo MG, et al. A randomised control study comparing the Infant Flow Driver with nasal continuous positive airway pressure in preterm infants. Arch Dis Child Fetal Neonatal Ed 2001;85:F86–90.

30. McEvoy CT, Colaizy T, Crichton C, et al. Randomized trial of early bubble continuous positive airway pressure (BCPAP) versus conventional CPAP (CCPAP): effect on pulmonary function in preterm infants. PAS 2004;55:2988.

31. Tagare A, Kadam S, Vaidya U, et al. Bubble CPAP versus ventilator CPAP in preterm neonates with early onset respiratory distress–a randomized controlled trial. J Trop Pediatr 2013;59:113–9.

32. Hosseini MB, Heidarzadeh M, Balila M, et al. Randomized controlled trial of two methods of nasal continuous positive airway pressure (N-CPAP) in preterm infants with respiratory distress syndrome: underwater bubbly CPAP vs. Medijet system device. Turk J Pediatr 2012;54:632–40.

33. Yagui AC, Vale LA, Haddad LB, et al. Bubble CPAP versus CPAP with variable flow in newborns with respiratory distress: a randomized controlled trial. J Pediatr (Rio J) 2011;87:499–504.

34. Mazmanyan P, Mellor K, Dore CJ, et al. A randomised controlled trial of flow driver and bubble continuous positive airway pressure in preterm infants in a resource-limited setting. Arch Dis Child Fetal Neonatal Ed 2016;101:F16–20.

35. Bhatti A, Khan J, Murki S, et al. Nasal Jet-CPAP (variable flow) versus Bubble-CPAP in preterm infants with respiratory distress: an open label, randomized controlled trial. J Perinatol 2015;35:935–40.

36. Sadeghnia A, Barekateyn B, Badiei Z, et al. Analysis and comparison of the effects of N-BiPAP and Bubble-CPAP in treatment of preterm newborns with the weight of below 1500 grams affiliated with respiratory distress syndrome: a randomised clinical trial. Adv Biomed Res 2016;5:3.

37. Sun SC, Tien HC, Banabas S. Randomise controlled trial of two methods of nasal CPAP (NCPAP): flow driver vs onventional CPAP [abstract 1898]. Pediatr Res 1999;45:322A, 1999.vvbb.

38. Stefanescu BM, Murphy WP, Hansell BJ, et al. A randomized, controlled trial comparing two different continuous positive airway pressure systems for the

successful extubation of extremely low birth weight infants. Pediatrics 2003;112: 1031–8.

39. De Paoli AG, Davis PG, Faber B, et al. Devices and pressure sources for administration of nasal continuous positive airway pressure (NCPAP) in preterm neonates. Cochrane Database Syst Rev 2008;23:CD002977.
40. Gupta S, Sinha SK, Tin W, et al. A randomized controlled trial of post-extubation bubble continuous positive airway pressure versus Infant Flow Driver continuous positive airway pressure in preterm infants with respiratory distress syndrome. J Pediatr 2009;154(5):645–50.
41. Wilson BJ Jr, Becker MA, Linton ME, et al. Spontaneous minute ventilation predicts readiness for extubation in mechanically ventilated preterm infants. Journal of Perinatology 1998;18(6):436–9.

Continuous Positive Airway Pressure Strategies with Bubble Nasal Continuous Positive Airway Pressure

Not All Bubbling Is the Same: The Seattle Positive Airway Pressure System

Stephen E. Welty, MD

KEYWORDS

- CPAP • Continuous positive airway pressure • Bubbling • Seattle PAP system
- Premature infant • Bronchopulmonary dysplasia

KEY POINTS

- Evidence is accumulating that bubble nasal continuous positive airway pressure (CPAP) is preferred, and suggests that the bubbling provides support in addition to mere administration of CPAP.
- However, CPAP failure requiring intubation and mechanical ventilation is common. CPAP failure is associated increased morbidity (in developed countries) and mortality (in developing countries).
- More research to understand the effects of bubbling and CPAP on the developing respiratory system function and disease in premature infants is essential.
- The pilot work done on high-amplitude bubble nasal CPAP (Seattle PAP) has observed some encouraging results and additional trials of safety and efficacy are forthcoming.

INTRODUCTION

Neonatology is a relatively new field in pediatrics that was launched when information and practice about supportive therapies became available that improved survival in neonates that were afflicted with respiratory distress and/or prematurity. For example, understanding and addressing proper thermoregulation and humidity in premature infants in pioneering work from Silverman and coworkers[1,2] was

Disclosures: None.
Department of Pediatrics, Baylor College of Medicine, 6621 Fannin Street, W1604, Houston, TX 77030, USA
E-mail address: welty@bcm.edu

Clin Perinatol 43 (2016) 661–671
http://dx.doi.org/10.1016/j.clp.2016.07.004
0095-5108/16/© 2016 Elsevier Inc. All rights reserved.

associated with dramatic improvements in survival. Death from respiratory failure was also common and implementation of respiratory support strategies, including support with mechanical ventilation and supplemental oxygen, both improved survival, and created a "new" disease, termed bronchopulmonary dysplasia (BPD) in 1967.[3] Refining respiratory support strategies with positive pressure and supplemental oxygen have remained active areas of research and implementation at the same time that the population of premature infants have changed dramatically to markedly premature neonates poorly prepared developmentally for supportive therapeutics. Survival in markedly premature infants, as little as 22 to 23 weeks gestation, was possible, primarily through improvements in obstetric management in the perinatal period. The major improvements have been broad and have focused on the perinatal period, including the more widespread use of antenatal steroid administration to mothers likely to deliver a premature infant than before the consensus statement on antenatal steroids was published; the treatment of premature neonates with exogenous surfactant and less injurious forms of positive pressure support with nasal continuous positive airway pressure (CPAP) and other noninvasive modes of respiratory support.[4–6] Challenges remain in perinatal strategies, and one of the dominant challenges is how to improve success of noninvasive respiratory support in this challenging patient population until neonates mature to the extent that no respiratory support is needed.

CONTINUOUS POSITIVE AIRWAY PRESSURE IN PREMATURE INFANTS
Brief History of Nasal Continuous Positive Airway Pressure in Premature Neonates

Noninvasive respiratory support using nasal CPAP was first reported in 1973 by Kattwinkel and colleagues[7] and was demonstrated to be associated with a low incidence of BPD.[8] This report launched literally decades of work on implementation and research in improving nasal CPAP, which included evaluating nasal interfaces, and addressing different ways in which to generate CPAP.[9] Despite decades of experience in implementation of nasal CPAP and the strong data supporting its efficacy in improving outcomes in premature infants, other forms of noninvasive respiratory support including heated humidified high flow nasal cannula and nasal intermittent positive pressure have been studied and adopted widely despite a lack of evidence observing an improvement in outcomes or for that matter equivalent outcomes to routine utilization of nasal CPAP.[10–12] Reasons for investigation of alternatives to nasal CPAP include the difficulty of maintaining effective CPAP for a long period of time (literally weeks to months) that requires a highly qualified and trained bedside care team, and the reported failure rates for nasal CPAP when failure is defined as the need for intubation for more invasive support. In fact, in the 3 trials that have, in combination, shown that nasal CPAP administered immediately after delivery was associated with lower rates of death or BPD in infants between 24 and 29 weeks' gestation than in those supported with invasive ventilation (even when invasive ventilation was used only for administration of exogenous surfactant[13–15]), demonstrated failure rates of at least 50%. Thus, optimism from the improved outcomes as initial support and/or early support on nasal CPAP is tempered by the trial data, indicating that the need for intubation in these studies are high. In fact, in the SUPPORT trial (Surfactant, Positive Pressure, and Oxygenation Randomized Trial) the CPAP group had an intubation rate of 83% during the hospitalization.[15] Based on the data that early nasal CPAP improves outcomes and based on the high failure rates, efforts to lower the failure rate have been undertaken, and the mechanisms for high failure rates has not been resolved fully.

The primary possibilities for failure of nasal CPAP in premature infants include process failures for nasal CPAP. Nasal CPAP is an inherently complex process demanding consistent attention to the detail of managing effective nasal CPAP in the acute perinatal period and because of chest wall immaturity and apnea of prematurity nasal CPAP is probably necessary up to at least 32 weeks postmenstrual age. Long-term nasal CPAP support can be a daunting task in infants successfully transitioned to nasal CPAP at very early gestational ages. A lack of commitment of the culture of individual nursery systems to using nasal CPAP for noninvasive respiratory support, and the possibility that fundamentally nasal CPAP may simply not provide as much direct support needed for neonates at high risk for respiratory failure, are areas of open debate. These and other possible modes of failure are not mutually exclusive and all demand attention, investigation, and efforts to improve success rates for current forms of nasal CPAP are warranted. This article focuses on nasal CPAP as a tool to support the respiratory system in premature neonates and information available about how CPAP affects overall respiratory system function and how this tool may affect neonates susceptible to respiratory failure, from impaired gas exchange in the lung or from respiratory fatigue because of immature chest wall and immature muscles of respiration.

PHYSIOLOGY OF RESPIRATORY FAILURE IN PREMATURE INFANTS AND THE POSSIBLE ROLE FOR NASAL CONTINUOUS POSITIVE AIRWAY PRESSURE

Premature infants immediately after delivery frequently have reasonable muscle tone and respiratory effort and can be stabilized on noninvasive respiratory support without immediate tracheal intubation and mechanical ventilation. In neonates with respiratory effort, the primary respiratory problems independent of primary lung dysfunction include an exceedingly compliant chest wall and mixed apnea (both obstructive and central). The compliant chest wall means that, without some form of respiratory support usually with positive pressure, the functional residual capacity will be low and respiratory failure would otherwise ensue. Positive pressure respiratory support to maintain the functional residual capacity is needed. Nasal CPAP is a good tool to maintain functional residual capacity in this context, and administration of caffeine should be administered to address central apnea. After initial stabilization, respiratory failure in the first few days is commonly caused by progressive respiratory failure mediated by surfactant deficiency. Surfactant deficiency leads to alveolar collapse and stiff lungs, and this and the abnormal chest wall mechanics is such that the capacity of premature infant respiratory muscle function to support reasonable respiratory system function and gas exchange is not possible without mechanical ventilation. For the last 2 decades, the dramatic increase in the administration of maternal antenatal steroids has ensured that surfactant deficiency is less frequent and severe than previously, so that acute respiratory failure of "pure" hyaline membrane disease is less likely. Nasal CPAP is an excellent tool to maintain lung volume and air exchange to infants at risk of respiratory failure secondary to hyaline membrane disease, and a compliant chest wall. Respiratory failure in neonates with hyaline membrane disease in the first few days of life is characterized by increasing concentrations of supplemental oxygen needed to maintain arterial oxygenation in the range desired and respiratory muscle fatigue, which may present with hypoventilation and apnea. Well-applied nasal CPAP improves the ventilation to the low ventilation perfusion compartment of the lung and may prevent the progressive arterial hypoxemia by reducing the relative proportion of the low ventilation–perfusion lung compartment in the lung. Furthermore, respiratory muscle fatigue and failure is less likely, because keeping the respiratory system from losing volume increases lung compliance and reduces airway resistance. In contrast, low resting lung volumes are associated with high resistive and elastic loads to the respiratory system causing respiratory muscle fatigue and failure. Outside of the first few days of the neonatal period, respiratory failure is still common and should be minimized by effective administration of nasal CPAP, until the respiratory system is more mature and better prepared for function with no specific respiratory support.

Bubbling and 'Noisy' System of Continuous Positive Airway Pressure

Lung anatomy, physiology, and function is complex in patients with nonhomogenous diseases such as hyaline membrane disease,[16,17] as are the mechanics to accomplish air exchange in distal compartments of the lung. To deliver gas to air exchange units (identified as alveoli developmentally at 36 weeks gestation), there are literally thousands of airways delivering gas to air exchange units of different lengths radii in series and in parallel. Based on the complex mechanics underlying gas delivery and exchange in the air exchange units, the concept of introducing noise into respiratory support devices strategies to address "noisy" lung function has emerged.[18] In bubbling nasal CPAP, variable frequency and amplitude of pressure oscillations may open unrecruited lung units and enhance air exchange in lung units already open. Bubble CPAP is a "noisy" system addressing the stochastic properties of the lung. In an in vitro lung model Pillow and Travadi[18] observed that low compliance "lung units" were exposed to higher pressure fluctuations than in the lung units with greater compliance. The investigators speculated that parallel compartments in nonhomogeneous lung diseases with poorly recruited compartments would be exposed to different frequencies and higher pressures than well-ventilated and compliant lung units, which would be exposed to lower amplitude pressure waveforms. This modeling and the theoretic basis for parallel air exchange in nonhomogeneous lungs is difficult to test in vivo and there are few data to support or refute this possibility in neonates. Lee and colleagues[19] studied 10 premature infants who met criteria for extubation and they measured tidal volume, respiratory rate, minute ventilation, transcutaneous PCO_2 and oxygen saturation between bubble nasal CPAP and ventilator CPAP. They found that bulk tidal volumes, respiratory rates, and minute ventilation were lower when supported with bubble CPAP than when supported with ventilator nasal CPAP but with no differences in transcutaneous PCO_2 and/or oxygen saturation. These data suggest that the bubbling provided support for air exchange in excess of simply delivering CPAP and bulk flow ventilation, which supports the speculation that pressure oscillations provide enhanced air exchange in the lungs of premature infants. This suggests that CPAP delivered with bubbling is superior to CPAP delivered with ventilators, although data assessing relevant outcomes are not extensive. A recently published systematic review found that failure rates (defined as need for intubation for respiratory failure) were lower in neonates on bubble nasal CPAP than those on ventilator nasal CPAP with an odds ratio of 0.32 (95% confidence interval, 0.16–0.67).[20] However, the total number of infants assessed in this review was 194 and the studies were done in India and Iran, making it uncertain whether the data can be extrapolated broadly to developed countries. Nonetheless, the present evidence suggests that bubble nasal CPAP is probably the best or at least equal to the best form of noninvasive respiratory support in premature infants in developing and developed countries. Furthermore, recent studies report failure rates in neonates supported with bubble nasal CPAP between 24 and 29 weeks' gestation is very high. Innovations in bubble nasal CPAP with "noisy" pressure oscillations with different and variable pressure wave frequencies could provide better noninvasive respiratory support than current bubble CPAP systems.

THE PHYSICS AND PHYSIOLOGY OF BUBBLING

Lee and colleagues[19] studied premature neonates, measuring pressure waveforms at the airway on infants on bubble nasal CPAP delivered through a nasal endotracheal tube without leaks. A representative waveform is depicted in **Fig. 1**. Of note, the waveform amplitudes varied between 2 and 4 cm H_2O and the waveform frequency varied between 15 and 30 Hz. These measurements were made at system flows of 8 L/min. It should be noted that the amplitude and frequencies are likely to be different at different system flows. Subsequent studies used lung models in vitro to model the effect of system flow and compliance on the character of the bubbling. The pressure–time tracings suggest that system flows change the quality of the bubbling and pressures so generated, and interestingly that the lung in vitro (compliance) has an effect on the pressure delivered to the lung (**Fig. 2**).[18] If these findings are extrapolated to lungs in vivo, the findings suggest that the pressure amplitude and frequency to different parts of a nonhomogenous lung would be different, whereby the stiffer compartments of the lung may see higher pressure oscillations and at different pressure frequencies than the less diseased lung compartment(s). This speculation is made in the context of the greatest safety concern seen in some studies of nasal CPAP in neonates, that is, an increased incidence of air block in neonates supported with nasal CPAP. However, other factors in the various study designs may explain the development of air block in neonates on nasal CPAP. Most recent studies of nasal CPAP do not observe this complication at greater rates in neonates supported with this form of respiratory support.[13,15,21]

STUDIES WITH HIGH AMPLITUDE NASAL CONTINUOUS POSITIVE AIRWAY PRESSURE (SEATTLE POSITIVE AIRWAY PRESSURE SYSTEM)

When studying bubble nasal CPAP, the pressure amplitudes are relatively modest measured at the airway and proximal pressures delivered are probably higher than the pressures delivered to the terminal airways and alveoli/air exchange units.[22] Furthermore, the range of frequencies are distributed in a high range, typically greater than 10 Hz, whether measured in models in vitro or the few human studies in which frequencies were assessed. This high frequency is probably not as effective when delivered to the diseased lung than when the range of frequencies of the pressure oscillations are lower than 10 Hz and with a greater frequency range. Furthermore, a

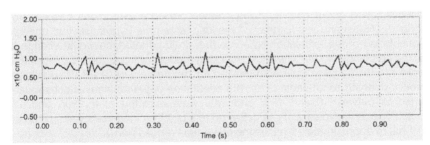

Fig. 1. Waveform produced at airway with bubble continuous positive airway pressure. Flow set at 8 L/min; amplitude of waveform 2 to 4 cm H_2O; waveform frequency approximately 15 to 30 Hz. (*From* Lee KS, Dunn MS, Fenwick M, et al. A comparison of underwater bubble continuous positive airway pressure with ventilator-derived continuous positive airway pressure in premature neonates ready for extubation. Biol Neonate 1998;73:70; with permission.)

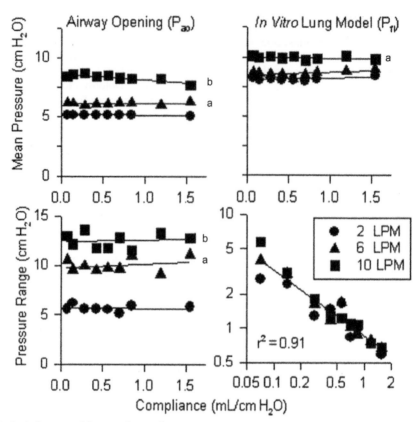

Fig. 2. Influence of flow and compliance on mean and oscillatory range of pressure during bubble continuous positive airway pressure (CPAP). (*Top*) Mean pressure. (*Bottom*) Range of oscillatory pressures in bubble CPAP pressure waveform. [a] $P<.05$ and [b] $P<.001$ versus 6 L/min (LPM). Duplicate measurements were obtained at each compliance and flow. (*From* Pillow JJ, Travadi JN. Bubble CPAP: is the noise important? An in vitro study. Pediatr Res 2005;57:827; with permission.)

detailed analysis about how bubbling creates pressure oscillations has not been described. DiBlasi and associates[23,24] recently tested the hypothesis that changing the orientation of the exhalation limb into the air liquid interface would change the pressure amplitudes at the airway and in a lung model in vitro. Bubble CPAP directed straight into the liquid to the depth desired for the delivery of CPAP as usually performed is denoted as an angle of 0°. The orientation of the tubing was subsequently oriented to between 0 and 180° and data were reported at 0°, 90°, and 135° (**Fig. 3**). Of note, the volume of gas delivered to a test lung increased from just greater than 1 mL to approximately 3 mL as the orientation ranged from 0° to 135° with no increase in volume at even greater angles (**Fig. 4**). In further assessments, pressure oscillations were greater at 135° than at 0° and the bandwidth of frequencies went from 9 to 20 Hz at 0° to between 2 and 5 Hz at 135° (**Fig. 5**). This study also showed that the amplitude of the oscillations at the airway and the volume delivered to the test lung went up as the bias flow went from 2 to 6 L/min with no effect at flows of greater than 6 L/min. These investigators also assessed how bubbling led to pressure

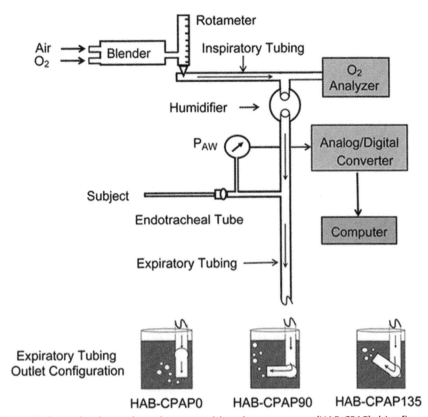

Fig. 3. High-amplitude nasal continuous positive airway pressure (HAB-CPAP): bias flow of air or O₂ was controlled with a rotameter connected to a semirigid circuit. A circuit "Y" connected the inspiratory tubing, expiratory tubing, airway pressure line, and endotracheal tube to the subject. The Fio₂ levels were verified with an O₂ analyzer. Airway pressure (P_{aw}) measurements were digitally processed and stored on a computer. Gas exited the system through the water seal with the bubbler angle set at 0° (HAB-CPAP0), 90° (HAB-CPAP90), or 135° (HAB-CPAP135). (*From* Diblasi RM, Zignego JC, Smith CV et al. Effective gas exchange in paralyzed juvenile rabbits using simple, inexpensive respiratory support devices. Pediatr Res 2010;68:527; with permission.)

oscillations using pressure tracings and high-speed videos. They noted a peak of pressure when a bubble was at the end of the straight portion of tubing entering the horizontal tubing before ascending at 135°. As the bubble ascended the tubing, the pressure decreased rapidly and was at its lowest as the bubble was about to exit the bubbler and then water rushed back into the bubbler and the cycle repeated as the water rushed in another bubble entered the system (see **Fig. 5**). These studies in vitro suggest that altering the angle of the exhalation limb provides a qualitatively and quantitatively different support than customary nasal CPAP. The pressure amplitudes generated by bubbling are greater and the frequencies of the oscillations are lower when oriented at 135° than when oriented straight into water. Whether these differences change the efficacy and safety of this kind of support to diseased lungs or to the lungs of premature neonate was studied in vivo. The investigators lavaged the lungs of juvenile rabbits to create a lung injury model with stiff, noncompliant lungs

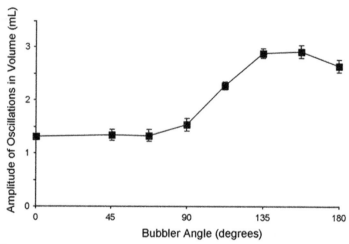

Fig. 4. Effect of bubbler angle on volumes delivered to test lung by high-amplitude nasal continuous positive airway pressure. Data are mean values ± standard error of the mean for 8 s of recorded data with bias flow of 6 L/min and no nasal interface or leak. Data were analyzed with 1-way analysis of variance, with Newman-Keuls post hoc. Data not sharing common symbols are different from each other, $P<.05$. (*From* Diblasi RM, Zignego JC, Tang DM, et al. Noninvasive respiratory support of juvenile rabbits by high-amplitude bubble continuous positive airway pressure. Pediatr Res 2010;67:625; with permission.)

to test the hypothesis that Seattle PAP (high-amplitude nasal CPAP) would provide a greater level of support than standard nasal CPAP as measured by an assessment of work of breathing. Work of breathing was assessed by calculating a pressure rate product (the change in intrathoracic pressure by esophageal catheter during

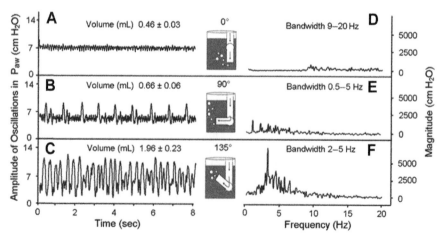

Fig. 5. Airway pressure (*A–C*) and power spectral analyses of airway pressure (*D–F*) while connected to the silastic test lung at a bias flow setting of 8 L/min recorded over 8 s. (*From* Diblasi RM, Zignego JC, Tang DM, et al. Noninvasive respiratory support of juvenile rabbits by high-amplitude bubble continuous positive airway pressure. Pediatr Res 2010;67:626; with permission.)

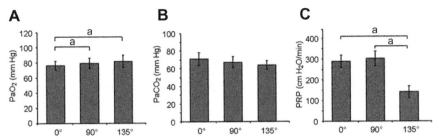

Fig. 6. Oxygenation (*A*), ventilation (*B*), and indices of work of breathing using pressure rate product (*C*) in lavaged rabbits supported by high-amplitude nasal continuous positive airway pressure. The mean arterial pressure and Fio_2 were held constant during the measurements of each animal. [a] $P<.05$. (*From* Diblasi RM, Zignego JC, Tang DM, et al. Noninvasive respiratory support of juvenile rabbits by high-amplitude bubble continuous positive airway pressure. Pediatr Res 2010;67:627; with permission.)

spontaneous breathing [ΔPes] multiplied by the respiratory rate). Animals were sedated and not paralyzed.[23] A slightly higher level of oxygenation was noted in the animals supported with high-amplitude nasal CPAP, but most strikingly the pressure rate product was essentially 50% lower in animals supported with high-amplitude nasal CPAP than with bubble nasal CPAP (0°; **Fig. 6**).

These promising findings in vitro and in vivo were followed by a pilot human study recently reported.[25] In this study, premature infants were studied at less than or equal to 32 weeks' gestation and between 6 and 72 hours of age. In this pilot study, eligible infants were stable as defined as being on 30% oxygen or less and having a CPAP of 8 cm H_2O or less. In this study, infants were assessed for 2 hours on standard bubble CPAP, followed by 2 hours on Seattle PAP, and 2 hours back on standard bubble CPAP. During this 6-hour time period, each infant had their pressure rate product assessed by measurements of esophageal pressure (ΔPes). The infants studied had a median gestational age of 29 weeks and a median weight of 1297 g. Forty patients completed the study, and no anticipated problems were observed. Furthermore, none of the infants developed BPD assessed at 36 weeks postmenstrual age. This study was different than the preclinical study in juvenile rabbits, in that the infants were stable and not sedated. Measuring assessments in periods of quiet breathing in human infants was challenging as opposed to the preclinical work, in which the subjects had diseased lungs and were sedated. Although patients in this study were not sick and not expected to develop respiratory failure we observed that on average the force per breath (ΔPes) was lower during the epoch in which Seattle PAP was assessed than it was during the other 2 epochs in which standard bubble CPAP was assessed. These findings are encouraging, but additional studies in smaller, sicker infants in which Seattle PAP is examined against standard CPAP for longer periods of time are needed. It is hoped that Seattle PAP would decrease the incidence of respiratory failure and morbidity in developed countries and respiratory failure, death, and morbidity in developing countries.

SUMMARY

Nasal CPAP is firmly established as the preferred respiratory support in premature infants.[26] Evidence is accumulating that bubble nasal CPAP is the preferred type of nasal CPAP, and suggests that the bubbling provides support in addition to mere administration of CPAP. Despite increased evidence for its use, CPAP failure requiring intubation and mechanical ventilation is common. In developed countries, CPAP failure is associated with increased morbidity, whereas in developing countries it is associated with increased mortality. Thus, more research to understand the effects of bubbling and CPAP on the developing respiratory system function and disease in premature infants is essential. The pilot work done on high-amplitude bubble nasal CPAP (Seattle PAP) has observed some encouraging results and additional trials of safety and efficacy are forthcoming.

REFERENCES

1. Silverman WA, Fertig JW, Berger AP. The influence of the thermal environment upon the survival of newly born premature infants. Pediatrics 1958;22:876–86.
2. Silverman WA, Balnc WA. The effect of humidity on survival of newly born premature infants. Pediatrics 1957;20:477–86.
3. Northway WH Jr, Rosan RC, Porter DY. Pulmonary disease following respirator therapy of hyaline-membrane disease. Bronchopulmonary dysplasia. N Engl J Med 1967;276:357–68.
4. National Institutes of Health Consensus Development Conference Statement. February 28-March 2, 1994.
5. Engle WA, American Academy of Pediatrics Committee on Fetus and Newborn. Surfactant-replacement therapy for respiratory distress in the preterm and term neonate. Pediatrics 2008;121:419–32.
6. Subramaniam P, Ho JJ, Davis PG. Prophylactic nasal continuous positive airway pressure for preventing morbidity and mortality in very preterm infants. Cochrane Database Syst Rev 2016;(6):CD001243.
7. Kattwinkel J, Fleming D, Cha CC, et al. A device for administration of continuous positive airway pressure by the nasal route. Pediatrics 1973;52:131–4.
8. Avery ME, Tooley WH, Keller JB, et al. Is chronic lung disease in low birth weight infants preventable? A survey of eight centers. Pediatrics 1987;79:26–30.
9. De Paoli AG, Davis PG, Faber B, et al. Devices and pressure sources for administration of nasal continuous positive airway pressure (NCPAP) in preterm neonates. Cochrane Database Syst Rev 2008;(1):CD002977.
10. Roberts CT, Owen LS, Manley BJ, et al. High-flow nasal cannulae as primary respiratory support for preterm infants – an international, multi-center, randomized, controlled, non-inferiority trial. Presented at the Pediatric Academic Societies. Baltimore, April 30, 2016.
11. Taha DK, Kornhauser M, Greenspan JS, et al. High flow nasal cannula use is associated with increased morbidity and length of hospitalization in extremely low birth weight infants. J Pediatr 2016;173:50–5.
12. Lemyre B, Davis PG, De Paoli AG, et al. Nasal intermittent positive pressure ventilation (NIPPV) versus nasal continuous positive airway pressure (NCPAP) for preterm neonates after extubation. Cochrane Database Syst Rev 2014;(9):CD003212.
13. Dunn MS, Kaempf J, de Klerk A, et al, Vermont Oxford Network DRM Study Group. Randomized trial comparing 3 approaches to the initial respiratory management of preterm neonates. Pediatrics 2011;128:e1069–1076.
14. Morley CJ, Davis PG, Doyle LW, et al, COIN Trial Investigators. Nasal CPAP or intubation at birth for very preterm infants. N Engl J Med 2008;358:700–8.
15. SUPPORT Study Group of the Eunice Kennedy Shriver NICHD Neonatal Research Network, Finer NN, Carlo WA, Walsh MC, et al. Early CPAP versus surfactant in extremely preterm infants. N Engl J Med 2010;362:1970–9.

16. Richardson P, Pace WR, Valdes E, et al. Time dependence of lung mechanics in preterm lambs. Pediatr Res 1992;31:276–9.
17. Richardson P, Jarriel S, Hansen TN. Mechanics of the respiratory system during passive exhalation in preterm lambs. Pediatr Res 1989;26:425–8.
18. Pillow JJ, Travadi JN. Bubble CPAP: is the noise important? An in vitro study. Pediatr Res 2005;57:826–30.
19. Lee KS, Dunn MS, Fenwick M, et al. A comparison of underwater bubble continuous positive airway pressure with ventilator-derived continuous positive airway pressure in premature neonates ready for extubation. Biol Neonate 1998;73:69–75.
20. Martin S, Duke T, Davis P. Efficacy and safety of bubble CPAP in neonatal care in low and middle income countries: a systematic review. Arch Dis Child Fetal Neonatal Ed 2014;99:F495–504.
21. Schmölzer GM, Kumar M, Pichler G, et al. Non-invasive versus invasive respiratory support in preterm infants at birth: systematic review and meta-analysis. BMJ 2013;347:f5980.
22. Poli JA, Richardson CP, DiBlasi RM. Volume oscillations delivered to a lung model using 4 different bubble CPAP systems. Respir Care 2015;60:371–81.
23. Diblasi RM, Zignego JC, Tang DM, et al. Noninvasive respiratory support of juvenile rabbits by high-amplitude bubble continuous positive airway pressure. Pediatr Res 2010;67:624–9.
24. Diblasi RM, Zignego JC, Smith CV, et al. Effective gas exchange in paralyzed juvenile rabbits using simple, inexpensive respiratory support devices. Pediatr Res 2010;68:526–30.
25. Welty SE, Rusin CR, Mandy GT, et al. Initial clinical evaluation of bubble nasal continuous positive airway pressure respiratory support using Seattle-PAP. Presented at the Pediatric Academic Societies. Baltimore, April 30, 2016.
26. Committee on Fetus and Newborn, American Academy of Pediatrics. Respiratory support in preterm infants at birth. Pediatrics 2014;133:171–4.

Nasal High-Flow Therapy for Preterm Infants

Review of Neonatal Trial Data

Brett J. Manley, PhD[a,b,*]

KEYWORDS

- Infant, premature • Intensive care, neonatal • Continuous positive airway pressure
- Respiratory distress syndrome, newborn

KEY POINTS

- There is insufficient evidence for nasal high-flow (HF) use as primary respiratory support for preterm infants.
- HF is equivalent to nasal continuous positive airway pressure (CPAP) as postextubation support for preterm infants, but there are limited data available in extremely preterm infants born less than 28 weeks' gestation.
- There is insufficient evidence to recommend using HF to wean from CPAP in preterm infants with evolving or established bronchopulmonary dysplasia.
- HF may prolong the duration of respiratory support for preterm infants when used in place of CPAP, but does not seem to increase the risk of bronchopulmonary dysplasia.
- HF use reduces rates of nasal trauma in preterm infants compared with CPAP, and does not increase the risk of pneumothorax.

INTRODUCTION

Nasal continuous positive airway pressure (CPAP) is a mainstay of noninvasive respiratory support for preterm infants, and has been well studied in clinical trials. Although its benefits are well recognized, effective application of CPAP in preterm infants requires highly skilled nursing care because of the bulky interfaces used and the need to minimize leak. CPAP use in preterm infants has been associated with pneumothorax,[1]

Disclosure Statement: B.J. Manley is an investigator on several clinical trials of nasal high-flow in newborn infants, both published and ongoing, and is a recipient of a research fellowship from the National Health and Medical Research Council (Australia). He is a coauthor of the recently published, updated *Cochrane Review* of nasal high-flow use in preterm infants (Wilkinson and colleagues 2016). He has no other conflicts of interest to declare.

[a] Neonatal Services, Newborn Research Centre, The Royal Women's Hospital, Level 7, 20 Flemington Road, Parkville, Victoria 3052, Australia; [b] Department of Obstetrics and Gynaecology, The University of Melbourne, Level 7, 20 Flemington Road, Parkville, Victoria 3052, Australia
* Newborn Research Centre, The Royal Women's Hospital, Level 7, 20 Flemington Road, Parkville, Victoria 3052, Australia.
E-mail address: brett.manley@thewomens.org.au

Clin Perinatol 43 (2016) 673–691
http://dx.doi.org/10.1016/j.clp.2016.07.005
0095-5108/16/© 2016 Elsevier Inc. All rights reserved.
perinatology.theclinics.com

gaseous abdominal distention,[2] and nasal injury.[3,4] Simpler, gentler alternatives are sought.

Heated, humidified, nasal high-flow (HF; **Fig. 1**) therapy has become a popular mode of noninvasive respiratory support for infants and children with respiratory illnesses.[5–7] In neonatology, HF use in developed countries has dramatically increased in the last 6 years.[8–11] The Australian and New Zealand Neonatal Network recently reported that more than half of very preterm infants born less than 30 weeks' gestation had received treatment with HF.[12] HF systems (**Fig. 2**) used in randomized trials in preterm infants, such as the Precision Flow (Vapotherm Inc, Exeter, NH) and Optiflow Junior (Fisher and Paykel Healthcare, Auckland, New Zealand) systems, heat and humidify the delivered gas, and are able to blend oxygen and air.

In addition to accumulating evidence of efficacy and safety, the increasing use of HF to treat preterm infants is also because of other perceived benefits over CPAP. These include the simpler interface, which is described as easier to apply than CPAP, and has been shown to be more comfortable for infants[13] and preferred by parents[14] and nurses.[15] Should HF be shown to be a safe and effective alternative to CPAP, particularly as primary respiratory support after admission to the nursery, it is a promising therapy for nontertiary settings and potentially in developing countries.

Although HF has become rapidly integrated into neonatal intensive care, it is only in the last few years that evidence from larger randomized clinical trials of HF has become available. This article discusses the evidence for HF use in preterm infants compared with other noninvasive supports from these trials for different clinical indications.

NASAL HIGH-FLOW AS EARLY RESPIRATORY SUPPORT FOR PRETERM INFANTS
Stabilization in the Delivery Room

There are no published randomized trials of HF use in the delivery room. However, Reynolds and colleagues[16] recently published a case series of 28 preterm infants born less than 30 weeks' gestation who were stabilized with HF. This was a single-center study in

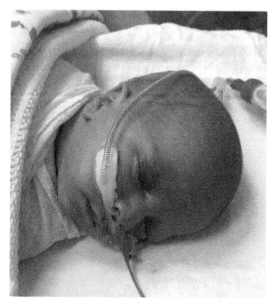

Fig. 1. A preterm infant treated with Optiflow Junior (Fisher and Paykel Healthcare, Auckland, New Zealand) nasal high-flow therapy.

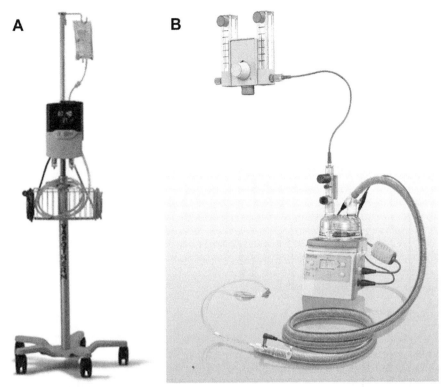

Fig. 2. Two commercial systems for delivering heated, humidified nasal high-flow therapy to infants. (*A*) Precision Flow. (*B*) Optiflow Junior. (*Courtesy of* [*A*] Vapotherm Inc, Exeter, NH, with permission; and [*B*] *Courtesy of* Fisher & Paykel Healthcare Pty Ltd, Melbourne, Australia; with permission.)

a center with extensive experience using HF as primary support. About 90% of infants were successfully stabilized and transferred to the neonatal intensive care unit on HF. Three of the four infants born at 23 or 24 weeks' gestation required intubation and ventilation in the delivery room. About half the infants that remained on HF went on to require surfactant treatment. A randomized trial is required before the use of HF for stabilization is recommended.

Nasal High-Flow as Primary Respiratory Support After Admission to the Neonatal Unit

Nasal high-flow versus continuous positive airway pressure

Three published trials[17–19] (**Table 1**) have compared HF with CPAP as primary support, enrolling a total of 372 preterm infants. In addition, the recently updated *Cochrane Review* on HF use in preterm infants[20] included a small unpublished study (Nair G, Karna P. Comparison of the effects of Vapotherm and nasal CPAP in respiratory distress. Pediatric Academic Societies 2005, Unpublished data; see **Table 1**) that randomized 67 preterm infants with respiratory distress on CPAP at 6 hours of age to continuing CPAP or changing to HF support, and was the only trial to include extremely preterm infants born less than 28 weeks' gestation. The evidence for HF use as primary support from these trials is inadequate: data are from a subgroup of a larger trial,[18] interim results of an ongoing trial,[19] trials that allowed surfactant therapy before treatment failure,[17,19] and an unpublished study (Nair G, Karna P.

Table 1
Details of randomized clinical studies of nasal HF as primary support included in this review

Study	Population	N	Intervention	Comparator	Primary Outcome	Key Results	Comments
Ciuffini et al,[19] 2014	Preterm infants 29–36 wk gestation with mild-moderate respiratory distress	177	HF 4–6 L/min (Precision Flow)	CPAP 4–6 cm H_2O (Infant Flow)	Need for intubation within 72 h of life (prespecified criteria); excluding brief intubation for surfactant (INSURE) treatment	More infants in the HF group were intubated, but this result did not reach statistical significance: 13% vs 5%; $P = .11$	Single-center Italian study, published in Italian Interim results from an ongoing trial (planned sample size 316) INSURE was not considered treatment failure, but unclear how many infants in each group got surfactant
Kugelman et al,[22] 2014	Preterm infants <35 wk gestation and birth weight >1000 g	76	HF 1 L/min, increasing up to 5 L/min (Precision Flow or 2000i)	Synchronized NIPPV (peak pressure, 14–22 cm H_2O, positive end-expiratory pressure 6 cm H_2O, 12–30 cycles per minute)	Treatment failure (prespecified criteria)	No difference in the primary outcome HF group spent longer on respiratory support (mean, 5.4 d vs 2.6 d; $P = .006$)	Single-center study in Israel Only study to compare HF with NIPPV HF group commenced on a lower gas flow than used in other studies

| Yoder et al,[18] 2013[a] | Preterm and term infants ≥28 wk gestation and ≥1000 g birth weight (N = 432) | 125 preterm infants in the primary support arm | HF 3–5 L/min (Vapotherm or ComfortFlo) | CPAP 5–6 cm H_2O (multiple devices) | Need for intubation within 72 h of commencing the allocated treatment, based on prespecified clinical criteria | Primary support arm: no difference in treatment failure or intubation rates Overall results: no difference in treatment failure or intubation, or in rates of BPD or pneumothorax HF group spent longer on the allocated respiratory support: median 4 vs 2 d; $P<.01$ HF group had less nasal trauma ($P = .047$) | Multicenter, international (United States and China) study Outcomes by treatment indication (primary vs postextubation) unpublished |

(continued on next page)

Table 1
(continued)

Study	Population	N	Intervention	Comparator	Primary Outcome	Key Results	Comments
Iranpour et al,[17] 2011	Preterm infants 30–35 wk gestation, enrolled at 24 h	70	HF 1.5–3 L/min	CPAP 6 cm H_2O	Not specified Multiple outcomes reported	No differences in the examined outcomes including death, duration of hospitalization, failure to treatment, BPD, and pneumothorax HF group had more normal examination of nasal mucosa	Single-center study, published in Persian Primary outcome unclear Used lower HF gas flows than in most studies, derived from a previous study[34] Infants who met prespecified criteria (before or after randomization) received surfactant via the INSURE technique
Nair, 2005 (unpublished data)	Preterm infants 27–34 wk gestation with respiratory distress in the first 6 h of life	67	HF with mean flow rates 5–6 L/min (Vapotherm 2000i)	CPAP (bubble)	Respiratory failure requiring reintubation based on prespecified criteria	No statistical difference in the primary outcome	Single-center, unpublished trial available in abstract form, which was included in the *Cochrane Review*[20] Ceased early because of a product recall of the Vapotherm HF system

Abbreviations: BPD, bronchopulmonary dysplasia; INSURE, intubation surfactant extubation technique; NIPPV, nasal intermittent positive pressure ventilation.
[a] The study by Yoder and coworkers had two study arms: primary support (n = 125 preterm infants) and postextubation support (n = 226 preterm infants).

Comparison of the effects of Vapotherm and nasal CPAP in respiratory distress. Pediatric Academic Societies 2005, Unpublished data). A meta-analysis of these four studies for the outcomes of treatment failure (based on trial definitions) (**Fig. 3**) and intubation within 7 days was performed in the *Cochrane Review*.[20] These two analyses were identical, and there were no statistical differences between HF and CPAP overall.

The results of the international, multicenter, noninferiority HIPSTER trial are awaited. This trial is comparing HF with CPAP as primary support after admission to the neonatal intensive care unit for preterm infants born greater than or equal to 28 weeks' gestation who have not been treated with exogenous surfactant. The primary outcome is treatment failure within 72 hours; detailed methodology is available in the published protocol.[21]

Nasal high-flow versus nasal intermittent positive pressure ventilation

One study that enrolled 76 infants has compared HF with synchronized nasal intermittent positive pressure ventilation (NIPPV) as primary respiratory support. Kugelman and coworkers[22] (see **Table 1**) had a primary outcome of treatment failure according to prespecified criteria, and found no difference between the groups. The HF group spent longer on respiratory support (mean, 5.4 vs 2.6 days; $P = .006$) but the durations of mechanical ventilation and hospitalization were similar.

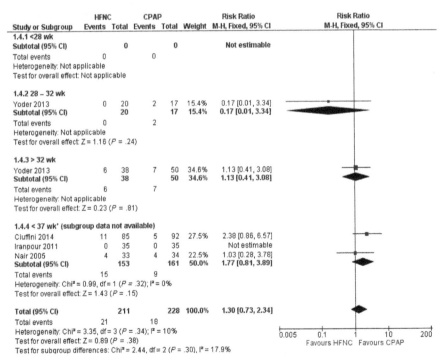

Fig. 3. Nasal HF versus CPAP as primary respiratory support in preterm infants: treatment failure within 7 days. Analysis for the outcome of intubation within 7 days was identical. In the figure, HF is described as HFNC. Results are presented as risk ratio (95% CI). CI, confidence interval; HFNC, high-flow nasal cannula. (*From* Wilkinson D, Andersen C, O'Donnell CPF, et al. High flow nasal cannula for respiratory support in preterm infants. Cochrane Database Syst Rev 2016; http://dx.doi.org/10.1002/14651858.CD006405.pub3; with permission.)

- Limited evidence suggests there are no differences in rates of treatment failure or intubation between HF and CPAP/NIPPV when used as primary respiratory support for preterm infants.
- No published studies of HF as primary support have included extremely preterm infants, or compared different HF devices.
- No randomized trials have compared HF with other noninvasive support modes for the stabilization of preterm infants in the delivery room.

NASAL HIGH-FLOW TO PREVENT EXTUBATION FAILURE IN PRETERM INFANTS
Nasal High-Flow Versus Continuous Positive Airway Pressure

Six randomized trials[18,23–27] (**Table 2**) comparing HF with CPAP as postextubation support have enrolled 936 preterm infants; these trials were mostly published in the last 2 years. Although gestational age subgroup data are not available from all trials, it seems less than 250 extremely preterm infants born less than 28 weeks' gestation were included, most in the two Australian studies.[24,25] In these two studies infants in the HF group could receive rescue CPAP/NIPPV when extubation failure criteria were satisfied. The *Cochrane Review*[20] performed meta-analyses for the outcomes of extubation failure (based on trial definitions) (**Fig. 4**; five studies included) and reintubation within 7 days (**Fig. 5**; six studies included). There were no statistically significant differences between HF and CPAP on pooled analysis overall for these outcomes, although there seemed to be a reduction in reintubation with HF in the subgroup of preterm infants 28 to 32 weeks' gestation.

Comparison of Different Nasal High-Flow Devices

One study by Miller and Dowd[28] compared the Vapotherm 2000i and Fisher and Paykel Optiflow systems (both now superseded by new models) as postextubation support in 40 very preterm infants (see **Table 2**). Eighteen percent of the Fisher and Paykel group and 9% of the Vapotherm group were reintubated within 72 hours ($P = .63$). Further trials are required to determine any differences in efficacy between available HF systems, as postextubation and early respiratory support.

When used as postextubation respiratory support:

- There is no difference in rates of treatment failure or reintubation between HF and CPAP, but limited data are available in extremely preterm infants.
- There is currently no evidence that any HF device is superior to another.

NASAL HIGH-FLOW TO WEAN PRETERM INFANTS FROM CONTINUOUS POSITIVE AIRWAY PRESSURE

Although it has been shown that the simplest way to successfully wean a preterm infant from CPAP is to cease the therapy outright, and reinstate it only if predetermined clinical criteria are met,[29,30] HF is being used as an interim support to aid weaning. There are two randomized studies of using HF to wean preterm infants from CPAP[31,32] (**Table 3**) with conflicting results. In the study by Abdel-Hady and coworkers[31] of 60 preterm infants greater than or equal to 28 weeks' gestation, the use of HF of 2 L/min to wean from CPAP resulted in more days on oxygen (median, 14 vs 5 days; $P<.001$) and respiratory support (18 vs 10.5 days; $P = .03$). There was no difference in success of CPAP weaning. The study by Badiee and coworkers[32] of 88 infants in a similar population found the opposite: the use of HF of 2 L/min to wean from CPAP significantly reduced the duration of supplemental oxygen (mean, 21 vs 50 hours; $P<.001$) and hospital stay (mean, 11 vs 15 days; $P = .04$).

Table 2
Details of randomized clinical studies of nasal high-flow to prevent extubation failure included in this review

Study	Population	N	Intervention	Comparator	Primary Outcome	Key Results	Comments
Mostafa-Gharehbaghi & Mojabi,[27] 2015	Preterm infants 30–34 wk gestation and birth weight 1250–2000 g Initially stabilized with CPAP and treated with INSURE before randomization	85	HF 6 L/min	CPAP 5–6 cm H_2O	Reintubation within 3 d of surfactant administration (according to prespecified criteria)	No difference in reintubation rate Nasal trauma less common in the HF group: 33% vs 63%; $P = .007$	Single-center study in Iran
Liu et al,[26] 2014	Preterm and term infants, <7 d old at extubation (N = 255)	150 preterm infants	HF 3–8 L/min depending on infant weight	CPAP, pressures set the same as pre-extubation	Included extubation failure (reintubation within 7 d), BPD, and death	No difference in these outcomes	Multicenter study in China, published in Chinese
Collins et al,[24] 2013	Preterm infants <32 wk gestation, first extubation	132	HF 8 L/min (Vapotherm)	CPAP 7–8 cm H_2O	Extubation failure within 7 d, objective failure criteria	Difference in extubation failure not significant: HF 22% vs CPAP 34%; $P = .14$ Treatment with HF significantly reduced the severity of nasal trauma ($P<.001$).	Single-center study in Australia Higher proportion of male infants in the CPAP group Some infants in both groups were rescued from reintubation by alternative noninvasive support modes (CPAP or nonsynchronized NIPPV) HF group commenced at 8 L/min, higher than in other studies

(continued on next page)

Table 2
(continued)

Study	Population	N	Intervention	Comparator	Primary Outcome	Key Results	Comments
Manley et al,[25] 2013	Preterm infants <32 wk gestation, being extubated for the first time	303	HF 5–7 L/min (Optiflow)	CPAP 7 cm H_2O (bubble or ventilator-generated)	Treatment failure within 72 h (objective criteria)	HF 'non-inferior' to CPAP by trial definition: risk difference (95% CI) 8.4% (−1.9% to 18.7%) Almost half the infants in whom HF treatment failed were rescued from reintubation by CPAP; no difference in reintubation rates Significantly less nasal trauma in the HF group ($P = .01$) No differences in death, BPD, or pneumothorax rates	Multicenter trial with a noninferiority design (margin of noninferiority 20%) Rescue CPAP allowed after treatment failure in the HF group Infants on CPAP could receive nonsynchronized NIPPV

Study	Population	N	HF	Comparison	Outcome	Results	Comments
Yoder et al,[18] 2013[a]	Preterm and term infants ≥28 wk gestation and ≥1000 g birth weight (N = 432)	226 preterm infants in the postextubation arm	HF 3–5 L/min (Vapotherm or ComfortFlo)	CPAP 5–6 cm H_2O	Need for intubation within 72 h of commencing the allocated treatment, based on prespecified clinical criteria	Postextubation arm: no difference in treatment failure or intubation rates. Overall results: no difference in treatment failure or intubation, or in rates of BPD or pneumothorax. HF group spent longer on the allocated respiratory support: median 4 d vs 2 d; $P<.01$. HF group had less nasal trauma ($P = .047$)	Multicenter, international (United States and China) study. Outcomes by treatment indication (primary vs postextubation) unpublished
Miller & Dowd,[28] 2010	Preterm infants 26–29 wk gestation	40	Optiflow HF 6 L/min	Vapotherm 2000i HF 6 L/min	Reintubation within 72 h, prespecified criteria	Reintubation occurred in 18% of the Fisher and Paykel group vs 9% of the Vapotherm group (not significant)	Single center, pilot study, funded by the two HF manufacturers. One infant died and was excluded from the analysis

(continued on next page)

Table 2
(continued)

Study	Population	N	Intervention	Comparator	Primary Outcome	Key Results	Comments
Campbell et al,[23] 2006	Preterm infants with birth weight ≤1250 g	40	Humidified, unheated HF, mean gas flow 1.6 L/min	CPAP 5–6 cm H_2O (Infant Flow)	Reintubation within 7 d	Significantly more infants in the HF group required reintubation (12/20 vs 3/20; $P = .003$) HF group had increased oxygen use and more apnea and bradycardia postextubation	Single-center Canadian study Used lower HF gas flows than in current clinical practice, derived from a previous study[34]

Abbreviations: BPD, bronchopulmonary dysplasia; INSURE, intubation surfactant extubation technique.

[a] The study by Yoder and coworkers had two study arms: primary support (n = 125 preterm infants), and postextubation support (n = 226 preterm infants).

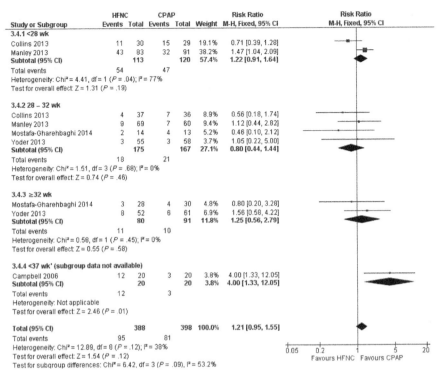

Fig. 4. Nasal HF versus CPAP after extubation in preterm infants: extubation failure within 7 days (five studies). In the figure, HF is presented as HFNC. Results are presented as risk ratio (95% CI). CI, confidence interval; HFNC, high-flow nasal cannula. (*From* Wilkinson D, Andersen C, O'Donnell CPF, et al. High flow nasal cannula for respiratory support in preterm infants. Cochrane Database Syst Rev 2016; http://dx.doi.org/10.1002/14651858.CD006405.pub3; with permission.)

When HF is used to wean from CPAP in preterm infants:

- There is no difference in weaning success.
- It is unclear how this practice effects durations of respiratory support, supplemental oxygen, and hospitalization.

NASAL HIGH-FLOW TO AID ESTABLISHMENT OF SUCK FEEDING IN PRETERM INFANTS

There are no randomized studies of HF with the primary outcome of suck feeding establishment in preterm infants. Despite this, HF is perceived to be of benefit in this role, and this seems to be a common reason for switching preterm infants with evolving or established bronchopulmonary dysplasia (BPD) from CPAP to HF while they convalesce.

A recent retrospective, single-center cohort study[33] compared two clinical eras: the first when CPAP was the main noninvasive support used in preterm infants with evolving BPD, and the second when infants on CPAP were routinely changed to HF subsequently (although the timing of this was not standardized). Feeds were trialed earlier in the second era, by about 4 days. There was no difference in the postmenstrual age when full oral feeds were achieved overall, but this was earlier in the second era in a subgroup of infants who remained on respiratory support at 34 weeks postmenstrual age. However, the difference in time to first and full feeds may be explained by a protocol that was in place not to suck feed infants receiving CPAP.

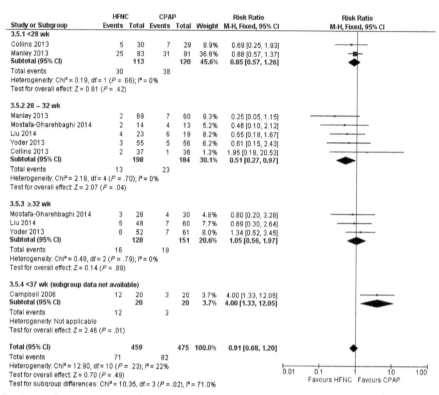

Fig. 5. Nasal HF versus CPAP after extubation in preterm infants: reintubation within 7 days (six studies). In the figure, HF is presented as HFNC. Results are presented as risk ratio (95% CI). CI, confidence interval; HFNC, high-flow nasal cannula. (*From* Wilkinson D, Andersen C, O'Donnell CPF, et al. High flow nasal cannula for respiratory support in preterm infants. Cochrane Database Syst Rev 2016; http://dx.doi.org/10.1002/14651858.CD006405.pub3; with permission.)

- No randomized trials have compared the effect of HF with other noninvasive supports on the establishment of suck feeding in preterm infants.

ADVERSE EVENTS

Adverse events including death, BPD, and pneumothorax were included outcomes in the *Cochrane Review*.[20] No differences were found in the combined outcome of death or BPD, or either of these outcomes individually, when HF was used for any studied clinical indication. Despite earlier concerns that unmonitored distending pressure generation in the lung with HF may increase the risk of air leak from the lung, pneumothorax rates are low in all randomized trials; in fact there was a nonsignificant reduction in rates of pneumothorax with HF use on pooled analysis in the *Cochrane Review*.

Although no differences in rates of BPD have been described with HF use, the trials used varying definitions, or did not define BPD clearly, and only one[26] included BPD as part of its primary outcome. Three studies have reported a longer duration of weaning from respiratory support or oxygen with HF use.[18,22,31] No HF trials have been powered sufficiently to demonstrate a difference in BPD rates, and none have reported

Table 3
Details of randomized clinical studies of nasal HF to wean from CPAP included in this review

Study	Population	N	Intervention	Comparator	Primary Outcome	Key Results	Comments
Badiee et al,[32] 2015	Preterm infants 28–36 wk gestation, stable on bubble CPAP 5 cm H_2O and F_{IO_2} <0.3 for ≥6 h	88	Changed to HF 2 L/min and F_{IO_2} 0.3, then oxygen weaned, followed by gradual weaning of HF gas flow	Continued on CPAP 5 cm H_2O, followed by weaning of oxygen, then CPAP ceased	Duration of supplemental oxygen requirement after randomization	Duration of oxygen supplementation was significantly less in the HF group (mean, 21 h vs 50 h; P<.001) The HF group also had a shorter hospital stay (mean, 11 d vs 15 d; P = .04)	Single-center study in Iran Used lower HF gas flows than in most other trials
Abdel-Hady et al,[31] 2011	Preterm infants ≥28 wk gestation, stable on CPAP 5 cm H_2O and F_{IO_2} <0.3	60	Changed to HF 2 L/min with F_{IO_2} 0.3, weaned from oxygen, then gradual weaning of HF gas flow	Continued on CPAP 5 cm H_2O, followed by weaning of oxygen, then CPAP ceased	Duration of supplemental oxygen	There was no difference in success of weaning from CPAP between groups The HF group had a longer duration of supplemental oxygen (median, 14 d vs 5 d; P<.001) and respiratory support (18 d vs 10.5 d; P = .03)	Single-center study in Egypt Used lower HF gas flows than in most other trials

Abbreviation: F_{IO_2}, fraction of inspired oxygen.

using an oxygen reduction test or grading the severity of BPD. Relatively few extremely preterm infants born less than 28 weeks' gestation, the population at highest risk of BPD, have been studied.

Trials have consistently reported lower rates of nasal trauma with HF compared with CPAP, and this reduction is confirmed with pooled analysis in the *Cochrane Review*.[20] It should be noted that none of the included trials blinded this outcome, and methods of screening for and grading nasal injury were variable.

When HF is used as respiratory support for preterm infants:

- It may prolong the duration of respiratory support or supplemental oxygen exposure compared with CPAP/NIPPV, but does not seem to increase rates of BPD.
- Rates of pneumothorax are low, and are not increased compared with CPAP (in fact, they may be reduced).
- It reduces rates of nasal trauma.

RECOMMENDATIONS

The following recommendations for HF use in preterm infants are based on a mix of evidence from clinical trials, opinion, and current clinical practice. Consider HF use

- As an alternative to CPAP as postextubation support in preterm infants, with caution recommended in extremely preterm infants.
- As an alternative to CPAP in stable preterm infants
  - Who are at risk of, or have established, nasal trauma or other pressure injuries attributed to the CPAP interface (eg, head molding).
  - Where HF may be preferred for neurodevelopmental reasons, such as with the aim of enhancing maternal contact or encouraging suck feeding.

There is insufficient evidence for HF use

- As primary support in the delivery room or neonatal unit, outside a clinical trial setting.
- To wean from CPAP.

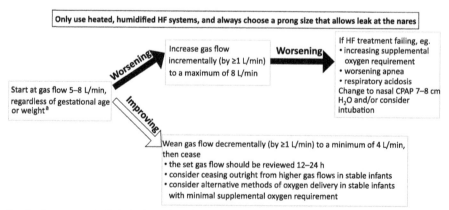

Fig. 6. A suggested clinical algorithm for nasal HF use in preterm infants. [a] If the infant is already receiving CPAP and changing to HF, choose an HF gas flow that is 1 to 2 L/min higher (numerically) than the set CPAP pressure. For example, if on CPAP 6 cm H_2O, start at an HF gas flow of 7 to 8 L/min.

Suggested Clinical Algorithm for High-Flow Use

A suggested algorithm for HF use in preterm infants is provided in **Fig. 6**. In the absence of an evidence-based HF weaning guideline, it is important to be diligent in weaning the gas flow as clinically indicated to avoid unnecessarily prolonging exposure to respiratory support. It is not recommended to prescribe gas flows higher than 8 L/min to preterm infants, unless in a clinical trial setting. When using HF to treat preterm infants, units should determine clear, objective failure criteria to expedite escalation of therapy when HF is failing.

Opportunities for Further High-Flow Research in Preterm Infants

Research into HF use in preterm infants is increasing, with many of the randomized clinical trials being published in the last few years. However, there are many questions remaining about how to best apply this therapy in preterm infants. Issues include the following:

- There is no evidence that any currently available HF device is superior to any other, yet different devices are favored in different parts of the world.
- None of the clinical trials have used HF gas flow rates higher than 8 L/min, and so it is unknown whether higher flows are more effective or safe.
- It is unknown whether HF is a better alternative for treating preterm infants with evolving BPD than supplemental oxygen alone.
- There is need for consensus on how to wean infants from HF most effectively.
- There are currently inadequate data on the use of HF in extremely preterm infants.
- No randomized trials have studied the use of HF to stabilize preterm (particularly extremely preterm) infants in the delivery room.
- It is unclear what the economic implications of increasing HF use are.

ACKNOWLEDGMENTS

Several figures used in this article were originally published in Wilkinson D, Andersen C, O'Donnell CPF, et al. High flow nasal cannula for respiratory support in preterm infants. *Cochrane Database Syst Rev* 2016;(2):CD006405. http://dx.doi.org/10.1002/14651858.CD006405.pub3 (http://dx.doi.org/10.1002/14651858.CD006405.pub3). Cochrane Reviews are regularly updated as new evidence emerges and in response to comments and criticisms, and the *Cochrane Database of Systematic Reviews* should be consulted for the most recent version of the Review.

The author thanks the following: colleagues in high-flow research in the Newborn Research Centre at The Royal Women's Hospital, Melbourne, Australia, particularly Louise Owen, Calum Roberts, and Peter Davis; Brad Yoder (University of Utah) for providing unpublished subgroup data for this review; coauthors on the previously mentioned *Cochrane Review*, Dominic Wilkinson (University of Oxford, Oxford, UK), Chad Andersen (Women's and Children's Hospital, North Adelaide, Australia), Colm O'Donnell (National Maternity Hospital, Dublin, Ireland), and Antonio De Paoli (Royal Hobart Hospital, Hobart, Australia); and Fisher and Paykel Healthcare and Vapotherm Inc for permission to use the included device images.

REFERENCES

1. Morley CJ, Davis PG, Doyle LW, et al. Nasal CPAP or intubation at birth for very preterm infants. N Engl J Med 2008;358(7):700–8.

2. Jaile JC, Levin T, Wung JT, et al. Benign gaseous distension of the bowel in premature infants treated with nasal continuous airway pressure: a study of contributing factors. Am J Roentgenol 1992;158:125–7.

3. Robertson NJ, McCarthy LS, Hamilton PA, et al. Nasal deformities resulting from flow driver continuous positive airway pressure. Arch Dis Child Fetal Neonatal Ed 1996;75(3):F209–12.

4. Shanmugananda K, Rawal J. Nasal trauma due to nasal continuous positive airway pressure in newborns. Arch Dis Child Fetal Neonatal Ed 2007;92(1):F18.

5. Spentzas T, Minarik M, Patters AB, et al. Children with respiratory distress treated with high-flow nasal cannula. J Intensive Care Med 2009;24(5):323–8.

6. McKiernan C, Chua LC, Visintainer PF, et al. High flow nasal cannulae therapy in infants with bronchiolitis. J Pediatr 2010;156(4):634–8.

7. Schibler A, Pham TM, Dunster KR, et al. Reduced intubation rates for infants after introduction of high-flow nasal prong oxygen delivery. Intensive Care Med 2011; 37(5):847–52.

8. Hough JL, Shearman AD, Jardine LA, et al. Humidified high flow nasal cannulae: current practice in Australasian nurseries, a survey. J Paediatr Child Health 2012; 48(2):106–13.

9. Hochwald O, Osiovich H. The use of high flow nasal cannulae in neonatal intensive care units: is clinical practice consistent with the evidence? J Neonatal Perinatal Med 2010;3(3):187–91.

10. Nath P, Ponnusamy V, Willis K, et al. Current practices of high and low flow oxygen therapy and humidification in UK neonatal units. Pediatr Int 2010;52:893–4.

11. Ojha S, Gridley E, Dorling J. Use of heated humidified high-flow nasal cannula oxygen in neonates: a UK wide survey. Acta Paediatr 2013;102(3):249–53.

12. Chow SSW, Le Marsney R, Hossein S, et al. Report of the Australian and New Zealand Neonatal Network 2013. Sydney (Australia): ANZNN; 2015.

13. Osman M, Elsharkawy A, Abdel-Hady H. Assessment of pain during application of nasal-continuous positive airway pressure and heated, humidified high-flow nasal cannulae in preterm infants. J Perinatol 2015;35(4):263–7.

14. Klingenberg C, Pettersen M, Hansen EA, et al. Patient comfort during treatment with heated humidified high flow nasal cannulae versus nasal continuous positive airway pressure: a randomised cross-over trial. Arch Dis Child Fetal Neonatal Ed 2014;99(2):F134–7.

15. Roberts CT, Manley BJ, Dawson JA, et al. Nursing perceptions of high-flow nasal cannulae treatment for very preterm infants. J Paediatr Child Health 2014;50(10): 806–10.

16. Reynolds P, Leontiadi S, Lawson T, et al. Stabilisation of premature infants in the delivery room with nasal high flow. Arch Dis Child Fetal Neonatal Ed 2016;101(4): F284–7.

17. Iranpour R, Sadeghnia A, Hesaraki M. High-flow nasal cannula versus nasal continuous positive airway pressure in the management of respiratory distress syndrome. Journal of Isfahan Medical School 2011;29(143):761–71.

18. Yoder BA, Stoddard RA, Li M, et al. Heated, humidified high-flow nasal cannula versus nasal CPAP for respiratory support in neonates. Pediatrics 2013;131(5): e1482–90.

19. Ciuffini F, Pietrasanta C, Lavizzari A, et al. Comparison between two different modes of non-invasive ventilatory support in preterm newborn infants with respiratory distress syndrome mild to moderate: preliminary data. Pediatr Med Chir 2014;36(4):88.

20. Wilkinson D, Andersen C, O'Donnell CPF, et al. High flow nasal cannula for respiratory support in preterm infants. Cochrane Database Syst Rev 2016;(2):CD00640.
21. Roberts CT, Owen LS, Manley BJ, et al. A multicentre, randomised controlled, non-inferiority trial, comparing high flow therapy with nasal continuous positive airway pressure as primary support for preterm infants with respiratory distress (the HIPSTER trial): study protocol. BMJ Open 2015;5(6):e008483.
22. Kugelman A, Riskin A, Said W, et al. A randomized pilot study comparing heated humidified high-flow nasal cannulae with NIPPV for RDS. Pediatr Pulmonol 2014; 50(6):576–83.
23. Campbell DM, Shah PS, Shah V, et al. Nasal continuous positive airway pressure from high flow cannula versus infant flow for preterm infants. J Perinatol 2006; 26(9):546–9.
24. Collins CL, Holberton JR, Barfield C, et al. A randomized controlled trial to compare heated humidified high-flow nasal cannulae with nasal continuous positive airway pressure postextubation in premature infants. J Pediatr 2013;162(5): 949–54.e1.
25. Manley BJ, Owen LS, Doyle LW, et al. High-flow nasal cannulae in very preterm infants after extubation. N Engl J Med 2013;369(15):1425–33.
26. The Collaborative Group for the Multicenter Study on Heated Humidified High flow Nasal Cannula Ventilation. Efficacy and safety of heated humidified high·flow nasal cannula for prevention of extubation failure in neonates. Zhonghua Er Ke Za Zhi 2014;52(4):271–6.
27. Mostafa-Gharehbaghi M, Mojabi H. Comparing the effectiveness of nasal continuous positive airway pressure (NCPAP) and high flow nasal cannula (HFNC) in prevention of post extubation assisted ventilation. Zahedan J Res Med Sci 2015;17(6):e984.
28. Miller SM, Dowd SA. High-flow nasal cannula and extubation success in the premature infant: a comparison of two modalities. J Perinatol 2010;30(12):805–8.
29. Todd DA, Wright A, Broom M, et al. Methods of weaning preterm babies <30 weeks gestation off CPAP: a multicentre randomised controlled trial. Arch Dis Child Fetal Neonatal Ed 2012;97(4):F236–40.
30. O'Donnell SM, Curry SJ, Buggy NA, et al. The NOFLO trial: low-flow nasal prongs therapy in weaning nasal continuous positive airway pressure in preterm infants. J Pediatr 2013;163(1):79–83.
31. Abdel-Hady H, Shouman B, Aly H. Early weaning from CPAP to high flow nasal cannula in preterm infants is associated with prolonged oxygen requirement: a randomized controlled trial. Early Hum Dev 2011;87(3):205–8.
32. Badiee Z, Eshghi A, Mohammadizadeh M. High flow nasal cannula as a method for rapid weaning from nasal continuous positive airway pressure. Int J Prev Med 2015;6:33.
33. Shetty S, Hunt K, Douthwaite A, et al. High-flow nasal cannula oxygen and nasal continuous positive airway pressure and full oral feeding in infants with bronchopulmonary dysplasia. Arch Dis Child Fetal Neonatal Ed 2016. http://dx.doi.org/10.1136/archdischild-2015-309683.
34. Sreenan C, Lemke RP, Hudson-Mason A, et al. High-flow nasal cannulae in the management of apnea of prematurity: a comparison with conventional nasal continuous positive airway pressure. Pediatrics 2001;107(5):1081–3.

Evidence Support and Guidelines for Using Heated, Humidified, High-Flow Nasal Cannulae in Neonatology

Oxford Nasal High-Flow Therapy Meeting, 2015

Charles C. Roehr, MD, PhD[a,b,*], Bradley A. Yoder, MD[c],
Peter G. Davis, MD[d], Kevin Ives, MD[a]

KEYWORDS

- Preterm • Nasal high-flow • Therapy • Cannula

KEY POINTS

- Current evidence suggests that nasal high-flow therapy (nHFT) at flows between 2 and 8 L/min is safe and efficacious for term and most preterm infants.
- When applying nHFT, allow for generous egress of gas by ensuring that the prong diameter is no more than half that of the nostril.
- The gas should be heated to between 34°C to 37°C and optimally humidified.
- A clear unit protocol for use of nHFT needs to be in place to ensure safe management of infants treated with nHFT.

Continued

Financial Disclosure: No authors have financial relationships relevant to this review to disclose. Conflict of Interest: The authors have no perceived conflicts of interest. K. Ives and C.C. Roehr have both received unconditional financial support from Vapotherm (Exeter, New Hampshire USA) and Fisher & Paykel (Auckland, New Zealand) for attending scientific meetings. Dr B.A. Yoder acted as consultant for Fisher & Paykel, Vapotherm and Dräger Medical (Lübeck, Germany). The meeting was supported by Fisher and Paykel Healthcare.
Contributors Statement: All authors contributed to writing of this review article.

[a] Newborn Services, John Radcliffe Hospital, Oxford University Hospitals, NHS Foundation Trust, Headley Way, Oxford OX3 9DU, UK; [b] Department of Neonatology, Charité University Medical School, Charitéplatz 1, Berlin 10117, Germany; [c] Division of Neonatology, University of Utah School of Medicine, Williams Building 295, Chipeta Way, Salt Lake City, UT 84108, USA; [d] Neonatal Research, The Royal Women's Hospital, Locked Bag 300, Cnr Grattan Street & Flemington Road, Parkville, Victoria 3052, Australia
* Corresponding author. Newborn Services, John Radcliffe Hospital, Oxford University Hospitals, NHS Foundation Trust, Headley Way, Oxford OX3 9DU, United Kingdom.
E-mail address: charles.roehr@ouh.nhs.uk

Clin Perinatol 43 (2016) 693–705
http://dx.doi.org/10.1016/j.clp.2016.07.006
0095-5108/16/© 2016 Elsevier Inc. All rights reserved.

Continued

- The use of nHFT during initial resuscitation or stabilization needs further study.
- Additional large randomized controlled clinical trials are needed to evaluate nHFT use in extremely low birth weight infants, to compare different flows, cannulae and devices, and to investigate nHFT during neonatal transport.

This article reports on an international meeting of experts to discuss nasal high-flow therapy (nHFT) in neonatology, held in Oxford, June 2015. The aim of the meeting was to establish consensus among leading researchers and clinicians on the current best understanding of the mechanism of action and the clinical indications for heated, humidified, high-flow nasal cannula (HHHFNC) therapy for newborn infants. This article presents a summary of discussions from the meeting together with treatment recommendations based on the latest available evidence from randomized clinical trials and the collective experience of the attendees.

WHY WAS THE MEETING HELD?

As the use of nHFT increases it is important that guidelines are developed to ensure that it is used safely and in accordance with the accumulating evidence. The term nasal high-flow therapy was proposed to emphasize that it refers to a specific treatment of infants and young children using a conditioned (heated and humidified), high-velocity gas flow. Having clear guidelines has been shown to improve patient care and assists in identifying areas in which further research is needed.[1] Clear recommendations are needed on when to initiate nHFT, for which indications, and at what settings clinicians should start nHFT. Guidance is also necessary on how to wean and when to stop nHFT.[2]

DEVELOPING TREATMENT RECOMMENDATIONS: WHO WAS INVOLVED?

A group of 24 international experts with a particular interest in neonatal and pediatric nHFT gathered to discuss the present state of research into the respiratory management of newborn infants and young children. The group comprised neonatal and pediatric clinicians with first-hand experience in the use of nHFT, clinical trialists, and primary investigators of the major studies of nHFT in infants and children. Further, respiratory physiologists, epidemiologists, authors of main reviews on nHFT, as well as policy makers attended the meeting (see Appendix 1 for participants). The meeting was held at Jesus College, Oxford, and was supported by an unconditional grant from Fisher and Paykel Healthcare (Auckland, New Zealand).

THE EVOLUTION OF NONINVASIVE RESPIRATORY SUPPORT IN NEONATES: FROM NASAL CONTINUOUS POSITIVE AIRWAY PRESSURE TO NASAL HIGH-FLOW THERAPY

Historically, the management of newborn infants with respiratory distress included the use of mechanical ventilation (MV). However, soon after its introduction to neonatal medicine, MV was recognized as an independent risk factor for chronic lung disease or bronchopulmonary dysplasia (BPD), particularly in preterm infants.[3] As an alternative to MV, noninvasive respiratory support was introduced as a treatment option.[4] The beneficial effects of noninvasive ventilation (NIV) include an increase in tidal volume and minute ventilation, a decrease in oxygen requirement, better surfactant preservation, a more stable thorax, and less frequent extubation failure.[5] The application of nasal respiratory support, specifically continuous positive airway pressure (CPAP), evolved quickly from Gregory's head-encasing box,[4] to the use of cut-down endotracheal tubes used as single nasopharyngeal prongs,[6] to short binasal prongs.[7] However, the choice of device used to deliver nasal CPAP (nCPAP) varies across centers.[8] In the presurfactant era, Avery and colleagues[9] showed that nCPAP significantly reduced the incidence of BPD. However, it took until the early years of this century to establish that newborn infants, in particular very low birth weight infants (VLBWI), can be successfully supported with nCPAP from birth.[10–15] Recognizing the benefits of nCPAP versus MV (ie, improved rates of survival free from BPD; number needed to treat 25–35),[16,17] the American Academy of Pediatrics recommends the use of nCPAP from birth.[18] Different forms of nasally applied, noninvasive respiratory support have been studied with good results to support infants extubated from MV and for those with significant apnea-bradycardia syndrome.[19–21] Although the initiation of nCPAP as primary respiratory support is efficacious in a large proportion of newborns with respiratory distress, an inverse relationship between gestational age and sustained success of nCPAP in the VLBWI subgroup of neonates has been noted.[22–24] Investigators of the CPAP or INtubation (COIN) Trial, a large randomized controlled clinical trial (RCT) comparing MV or nCPAP for breathing VLBWI (25–28 + 6/40) at birth, found that 42% of the 303 infants in the nCPAP group were never intubated. Other trials have shown similar results.[11,13] However, nCPAP delivery systems are prone to cause nasal trauma. Fischer and colleagues[25] suggest that this occurs in as many as 40% of neonates receiving this form of respiratory support. The development of nHFT has provided what seems to be a better tolerated and equally effective nasal respiratory support for several groups of newborn infants, as recently reported by various investigators[26–37] and reviewed by Manley and colleagues.[2]

One of the most recent developments in neonatal noninvasive respiratory support is the use of high-velocity gas jets, applied via small nasal cannulae.[38] The various proposed mechanisms of action of nHFT, as previously summarized by Dysart and colleagues,[39] were extensively discussed at the meeting. Briefly, the cannula's high velocity air jet leads to very effective nasopharyngeal carbon dioxide wash-out. It also causes a reduction of inspiratory resistance in the upper airways and, consequentially, a reduction in the work of breathing (WOB), comparable to the nCPAP effect.[40] It has further been proposed that heating and humidification of the breathing gases minimizes the metabolic WOB and is thought to improve the respiratory conductance and pulmonary compliance. All of these result in improvements in the physiologic variables such as respiratory rate, peripheral oxygen saturation (SpO_2), and fraction of inspired oxygen (Fio_2) in neonates and small children.[41]

The application of heated and humidified gas at defined gas flow rates and Fio_2 has gained rapid popularity throughout many neonatal intensive care units (NICUs) in the industrialized world[42–46] (Fig. 1). According to Hochwald and Osiovich,[42] around 69% of US-American academic NICUs were applying nHFT to preterm infants, and around 77% of surveyed NICUs in the UK reported the use of HHHFNC in a telephone survey performed by Ojha and colleagues.[44] Roberts and colleagues[46] report an increase of nHFT use in Australasian NICUs from 15% in 2009% to 35% in 2012. With respect to the aims of the Oxford meeting on nHFT, it was of particular interest that the use of nHFT had dramatically expanded despite the absence of high-quality evidence to support its use.[2,47,48] This expert symposium was staged with the intention of forming a better understanding of this promising form of NIV and to foster international collaboration for further research into its clinical use. The practice guidelines (see later discussion) for applying nHFT in the neonatal setting were prepared as consensus recommendations.

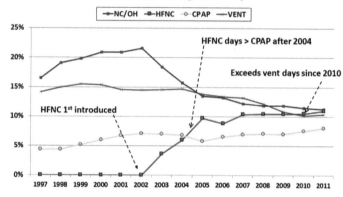

Fig. 1. Increasing use of nHFT among US-American NICUs. HFNC, high-flow nasal cannula. (*Courtesy of* B Yoder, R Clark, personal communication, University of Utah, Salt Lake City, Utah, USA.)

CURRENT STATE OF CLINICAL EVIDENCE

The meeting was held in June 2015, by which time 4 RCTs had been published, presenting data from more than 1100 preterm infants.[49–52] These trials primarily investigated nHFT in the context of postextubation use. These trials showed that infants treated with nHFT had failure rates that were similar to those managed with nCPAP. Infants managed with nHFT did not have increased adverse events, in particular there was no increase in air leaks, and they did not have longer durations of oxygen use or hospital stay (only limited data are available for infants born <27 weeks gestational age).[49–51] One additional trial, comparing the efficacy of nHFT to nasal intermittent positive airway pressure (NIPPV) as initial support of moderate preterm infants diagnosed with respiratory distress syndrome (RDS), found no significant differences in failure (defined as need for subsequent intubation) between the 2 modalities.[53] Two trials have investigated the perceptions of nHFT by nurses, patients, and parents.[54,55] Klingenberg and colleagues[55] studied the patient and parental responses to nCPAP and nHFT in newborn infants with mild respiratory distress in an open, randomized crossover trial. The investigators found that babies had comparable comfort scores while on nHFT and nCPAP but significantly lower respiratory rates when on nHFT. Parents had a preference for nHFT versus nCPAP because their babies seemed calmer and caring for their child was easier when on nHFT. Roberts and colleagues[54] reported that nursing staff preferred nHFT to nCPAP as postextubation support for preterm infants 28 weeks or older gestational age. Most nurses strongly agreed that nHFT was more comfortable for infants and was the parents' preferred mode.

INDICATIONS FOR NASAL HIGH-FLOW THERAPY IN THE NEONATAL CARE SETTING

At present, the highest quality evidence addresses the use of nHFT for postextubation support, which may be preferred for a variety of reasons, including the ease of care, perceived benefits for neurodevelopmental care, or pressure relief for nasal trauma acquired while on nCPAP.[56,57] At the time of the symposium, the use of nHFT as primary respiratory support for RDS or other acute neonatal respiratory disorders had been addressed by only 1 trial.[53] One other had been reported in abstract form[58] and 2 trials were reported as ongoing.[59,60] In the first trial, Kugelman and colleagues[53] randomized 76 infants to either nHFT or NIPPV. The investigators found no statistically significant difference in intubation rate. There were no statistically significant differences in other pulmonary and nonpulmonary outcomes. However, the investigators reported that subjects in the nHFT group remained longer on respiratory support (*P*<.006). Lavizzari and colleagues[58] randomized 316 premature infants (29 + 0 to 36 + 6 weeks of gestation) with a requirement for respiratory support at birth. The investigators compared nHFT of 4 to 6 L/min with nCPAP (or bilevel positive airway pressure) of 4 to 6 cm H_2O. The primary outcome was the need for intubation within 72 hours of life, defined as infants having severe apnea, needing increased Fio_2 or refractory hypercarbia (Pco_2 >70 mm Hg) and pH less than 7.20. Surfactant was given to infants with an oxygen requirement of Fio_2 greater than 0.35 (to reach target SpO_2 between 86% and 93%) by Intubate-Surfactant-Extubate (INSURE) technique in both groups, followed by the studied interventions. There were no significant differences in intubation rates or other secondary outcomes. The investigators concluded that, for preterm infants from 29 + 0 to 36 + 6 weeks of gestation, nHFT seemed to have similar efficacy and safety as nCPAP as primary treatment of mild to moderate RDS.[58] Reynolds presented video footage of VLBWIs being stabilized on nHFT immediately after birth. Data from this pilot study (n = 28) have subsequently been published.[59] Davis briefly reported on an ongoing, large RCT comparing nHFT to nCPAP from a few hours after birth, which aimed to recruit over 700 preterm babies.[60] This trial was orally presented at the Pediatric Academic Societies (PAS) 2016 meeting.[61] Roberts and colleagues[60] randomized 564 preterm infants older than 28 weeks' gestation, who had not previously received intubation or surfactant, to receive nHFT (6–8 L/min) or nCPAP (6–8 cm H_2O) as primary respiratory support after birth. Failure criteria for nHFT were defined as (1) sustained increase in oxygen requirement higher than 40% or more to maintain oxygen saturation in the target range for that center; (2) frequent apnea, 6 or more apneas requiring intervention in a 6-hour period, or 2 or more apneas requiring facemask positive pressure ventilation in a 24-hour period; or (3) respiratory acidosis, blood pH 7.20 or less and carbon dioxide greater than 60 mm Hg on capillary or arterial blood gas. The investigators found significantly higher rates of treatment failure in infants treated with nHFT (25.5% vs 13.3%; risk difference 12.3%, 95% CI 5.8–18.7, *P*<.001). Infants managed with nHFT who reached failure criteria were offered rescue nCPAP. Subsequently, intubation rates did not differ between groups (15.5% vs 11.5%; risk difference 3.9%, 95% CI -1.7 to 9.6, *P* = .17).[61] Further large scale RCTs are required to determine the role of nHFT in the primary treatment of RDS.

SYNTHETIZING THE EVIDENCE ON NASAL HIGH-FLOW THERAPY USE IN PRETERM INFANTS

A recent update on the Cochrane Review on "High-flow nasal cannula for respiratory support in preterm infants" was kindly made available to the group by the authors.[62] They concluded that nHFT, compared with other forms of noninvasive respiratory support, seems to have similar rates of efficacy in preterm infants for preventing treatment failure, death, and BPD. The largest proportion of evidence was available for the use of nHFT for respiratory support following extubation. Here, nHFT was clearly associated with reduced rates of nasal trauma when compared with nCPAP. There may also be a reduced incidence of pneumothorax.

They concluded that good quality evidence comparing nHFT with other forms of noninvasive respiratory support from birth and for weaning from noninvasive support was lacking. Further studies are required to evaluate the safety and efficacy of nHFT in the extremely preterm and near-term infant, and for comparing different nHFT devices.[62] Roberts and colleagues[46] pointed out that little is known about the optimal settings for gas flow during nHFT because trials have investigated the efficacy of nHFT at a maximum settings of between 6 and 8 L/min and only for a limited selection of nasal cannulae and delivery devices. The Oxford meeting established that hardly any evidence is available to guide clinicians on cannula-to-nares ratio to allow adequate gas egress, ideal temperature and percentage of gas humidity, starting flow rate, increment and decrement regimes for escalating and weaning flow, use of nasogastric or orogastric feeding tubes, or the question of safety of oral feeding while on nHFT.

GUIDELINES: OXFORD BEST PRACTICE RECOMMENDATIONS FOR USING NASAL HIGH-FLOW THERAPY IN NEONATES

Led by Yoder and Davis, the group agreed on the following best practices for using nHFT in preterm infants.

WHEN TO CONSIDER USING NASAL HIGH-FLOW THERAPY

nHFT can be considered for most infants in whom nCPAP would have traditionally been applied. Consider using nHFT in preterm infants who show signs of respiratory distress with tachypnoea, increased WOB, oxygen requirement, and the need for ongoing respiratory support. The same level of monitoring and nursing observations should be adopted as would be in place for a baby receiving nCPAP. Any patient with nasal trauma from nCPAP should be considered a candidate for rescue with nHFT. There may be a role for use of objective scoring systems (for instance the Silverman and Anderson[63] score) if these are already in practice for determining nCPAP requirement.

PATIENTS AND SITUATIONS FOR WHICH NOT TO CONSIDER NASAL HIGH-FLOW THERAPY

Infants with signs of severe RDS ($Fio_2 > 0.7$), severe apnea, significant active air leak, or craniofacial or airway anomalies should not be considered for nHFT.

CHOICE OF CANNULA SIZE

During nCPAP, optimal pressure delivery is achieved by minimizing leak through the use of well-fitted nasal prongs (de Paoli 2002).[7] However, nasal leak and gas egress is vital to ensure patient safety when using nHFT. Because cannula dimensions and flow resistance may vary, nHFT cannulae need to be carefully chosen and used only as recommended by the manufacturers. Mixing components from circuits of different manufacturers is not advisable. Sivieri and colleagues[37] have investigated the influence of leak on delivered pressure in an in vitro study. The investigators concluded that safe and effective use of nHFT requires selection of an appropriate nasal prong-to-nares ratio, even with an integrated pressure relief valve. Clinicians should ensure that the cannula occupies less than 50% of the area of the aperture of the nares to allow for ample egress of gas.

HOW TO CONDITION THE GASES

Gases should always be heated and humidified. The temperature of the warmed gas mixture is set optimally at 37°C. If there is rainout in the delivery tubing and cannula it may be necessary to reduce this to 34°C to 35°C, at flow rates of less than 4 L/min.

WHICH INITIAL GAS FLOWS SHOULD BE USED

Start with an initial gas flow of 4 to 6 L/min for preterm infants, although it is acknowledged that in 1 trial flows were commenced at 8 L/min and were weaned down.[50] When stepping-down from MV, some clinicians use the mean airway pressure to offer guidance on likely flow requirement. Increments in flow rate by 1 L/min up to a maximum of 8 L/min should be made in response to increased WOB, tachypnea, increased oxygen requirement, and respiratory acidosis. Using a reproducible RDS score or radiographic changes may be helpful. The guide for initiating nHFT and altering flow and Fio_2 based on birth weight, respiratory rate, and WOB, used by the NICU team at the University of Utah's Medical Center, is provided (**Table 1**).

WHEN TO ESCALATE FROM NASAL HIGH-FLOW THERAPY TO OTHER FORMS OF RESPIRATORY SUPPORT

Do not use nHFT at flow rates outside the manufacturers' recommendations. Consider escalating to other forms of NIV if the infant continues to have increased WOB, increased rates of apnea or bradycardia, or an oxygen demand exceeding Fio_2 greater than 0.5 to maintain normal SpO_2 levels, or when respiratory acidosis persists in the absence of reversible lung disease (pneumothorax).

WEANING NASAL HIGH-FLOW THERAPY

Consider weaning the level of nHFT in infants who are stable for 12 to 24 hours. Tips for weaning from nHFT include wean Fio_2 first and then wean flow rate. Weaning is more likely to be successful in infants with a Fio_2 requirement less than 0.3. Wean by 1 L/min every 12 hours, guided by the WOB of the infant. Consider discontinuing nHFT at flow rates between 2 and 4 L/min (the lowest flow rate will be device specific and any benefits of maintaining infants on flow rates of 3 L/min or less need further study).

Table 1
Consented guide to the initiation and alteration of nasal high flow therapy in neonates

Current Weight	Initiation of Flow	Escalation of Flow	Weaning Flow	Discontinuing nHFT
<1500 g	4–6 lpm	Fio_2 >35% or ↑ RR, WOB	↓ by 0.5 lpm Q 12–24 h	Typically at flow = weight (kg)
1500–3000 g	5–7 lpm	Fio_2 >35% or ↑ RR, WOB	↓ by 0.5–1 lpm Q 6–12 h	Typically at 2 lpm
> 3000 g	6–8 lpm	Fio_2 >35% or ↑ RR, WOB	↓ by 0.5–1 lpm as indicated	Typically at 2 lpm
Comments	Max flow 8 lpm	↑ by 1–2 lpm Q 15–20 min PRN	Typically slower wean with BPD	—

SUMMARY

Surveys confirm that nHFT is widely used throughout neonatal units worldwide. A growing body of evidence from RCTs confirms that nHFT can be considered safe and efficacious as supportive therapy for preterm infants following extubation. The safety and efficacy of nHFT as primary respiratory support is currently being further investigated. Also to be further investigated is the safety and efficacy of nHFT for the group of extremely low birth weight infants (ELBWIs) and specifically infants with a gestation at birth at less than 26 weeks. Additional research is needed to define appropriate minimum and maximum flow rates for infants of all gestational ages. Comparative studies, looking at the effectiveness of different nHFT delivery devices are required, as well as studies on safe weaning strategies from nHFT.

Best practices

What is the current practice?

Current evidence supports the use safety and efficacy of nHFT at flow rates between 2 and 8 L/min in term and most preterm infants. No more than 50% of the area of the aperture of the nares should be occluded. Gas conditioning with warmth and humidity is important.

Care path objective

Additional large RCTs are needed

- To further evaluate nHFT use in ELBWIs and those less than 26/40 gestation
- To compare nHFT with nCPAP during initial stabilization or resuscitation
- To establish safe use of nHFT during neonatal transport
- To define effective and safe minimum and maximum flow rates
- To evaluate nHFT for specific respiratory conditions
- To compare different nHFT devices
- To evaluate different approaches to delivering nHFT
- To assess the economic impact of nHFT

What changes in current practice are likely to improve outcomes?

Neonatal units using nHFT should have a clear treatment guideline for the initiation, weaning, and discontinuation of support.

Rating of Evidence: Bibliographic Sources

Cochrane review: High flow nasal cannula for respiratory support in preterm infants. http://dx. doi.org/10.1002/14651858.CD006405.pub3.[62]

Summary Statement

A growing body of evidence from randomized clinical trials supports previous observations that nHFT can be considered safe and efficacious as supportive therapy following extubation for term and most preterm infants. Further study on its efficacy and safety in ELBWI and/or less than 26 weeks gestation infants and as first-line treatment for RDS is required.

ACKNOWLEDGMENTS

We acknowledge the generous support from very many individuals and institutions, without which the meeting would not have been possible. Our thanks go to all the participants for actively contributing to the meeting. Special thanks to Kirpalani, MD for helping with the recruitment of participants; to Michelle Muir and the staff of Fisher and Paykel Healthcare for logistical and financial support; to Georg Holländer for helping organize the venue (Jesus College, Oxford); to Dr Eleri Adams, Clinical Director Newborn Services, Oxford University Hospitals NHS Foundation Trust for her on-going support for the meeting; and to Dr Faith Emery for photography and note keeping.

REFERENCES

1. Soll RF. Evaluating the medical evidence for quality improvement. Clin Perinatol 2010;37:11–28.
2. Manley BJ, Dold SK, Davis PG, et al. High-flow nasal cannulae for respiratory support of preterm infants: a review of the evidence. Neonatology 2012;102:300–8.
3. Jobe AH, Bancalari E. Bronchopulmonary dysplasia. Am J Respir Crit Care Med 2001;163:1723–9.
4. Gregory GA, Kitterman JA, Phibbs RH, et al. Treatment of the idiopathic respiratory-distress syndrome with continuous positive airway pressure. N Engl J Med 1971;284:1333–40.
5. Polin R, Sahni R. Continuous positive airway pressure: old questions and new controversies. J Neonatal Perinat Med 2008;1:1–10.
6. Dunn PM, Thearle MJ, Parsons AC, et al. Respiratory distress syndrome and continuous positive airway pressure. Lancet 1971;2:971, 7.
7. De Paoli AG, Davis PG, Faber B, et al. Devices and pressure sources for administration of nasal continuous positive airway pressure (NCPAP) in preterm neonates. Cochrane Database Syst Rev 2002;(4):CD002977.
8. Roehr CC, Schmalisch G, Khakban A, et al. Use of continuous positive airway pressure (CPAP) in neonatal units–a survey of current preferences and practice in Germany. Eur J Med Res 2007;12:139–44.
9. Avery ME, Tooley WH, Keller JB, et al. Is chronic lung disease in low birth weight infants preventable? A survey of eight centers. Pediatrics 1987;79:26–30.
10. Morley CJ, Davis PG, Doyle LW, et al. COIN Trial Investigators. Nasal CPAP or intubation at birth for very preterm infants. N Engl J Med 2008;358:700–8.
11. Finer NN, Carlo WA, Walsh MC, et al. SUPPORT Study Group of the Eunice Kennedy Shriver NICHD Neonatal Research Network. Early CPAP versus surfactant in extremely preterm infants. N Engl J Med 2010;362:1970–9.
12. Sandri F, Plavka R, Ancora G, et al. CURPAP Study Group. Prophylactic or early selective surfactant combined with nCPAP in very preterm infants. Pediatrics 2010;125:e1402–9.
13. Dunn MS, Kaempf J, de Klerk A, et al. Vermont Oxford Network DRM Study Group. Randomized trial comparing 3 approaches to the initial respiratory management of preterm neonates. Pediatrics 2011;128:e1069–76.
14. Göpel W, Kribs A, Ziegler A, et al. German Neonatal Network. Avoidance of mechanical ventilation by surfactant treatment of spontaneously breathing preterm infants (AMV): an open-label, randomised, controlled trial. Lancet 2011;378:1627–34.
15. Kanmaz HG, Erdeve O, Canpolat FE, et al. Surfactant administration via thin catheter during spontaneous breathing: randomized controlled trial. Pediatrics 2013;131:e502–9.
16. Schmölzer GM, Kumar M, Pichler G, et al. Non-invasive versus invasive respiratory support in preterm infants at birth: systematic review and meta-analysis. BMJ 2013;347:f5980.
17. Fischer HS, Bührer C. Avoiding endotracheal ventilation to prevent bronchopulmonary dysplasia: a meta-analysis. Pediatrics 2013;132:e1351–60.

18. Committee on Fetus and Newborn, American Academy of Pediatrics. Respiratory support in preterm infants at birth. Pediatrics 2014;133:171–4.

19. Davis PG, Morley CJ, Owen LS. Non-invasive respiratory support of preterm neonates with respiratory distress: continuous positive airway pressure and nasal intermittent positive pressure ventilation 2009;14:14–20.

20. Roehr CC, Proquitté H, Hammer H, et al. Positive effects of early continuous positive airway pressure on pulmonary function in extremely premature infants: results of a subgroup analysis of the COIN trial. Arch Dis Child Fetal Neonatal Ed 2011;96:F371–3.

21. Lista G, Castoldi F, Fontana P, et al. Nasal continuous positive airway pressure (CPAP) versus bi-level nasal CPAP in preterm babies with respiratory distress syndrome: a randomised control trial. Arch Dis Child Fetal Neonatal Ed 2010; 95:F85–9, 19.

22. Ammari A, Suri M, Milisavljevic V, et al. Variables associated with the early failure of nasal CPAP in very low birth weight infants. J Pediatr 2005;147:341–7.

23. Fuchs H, Lindner W, Leiprecht A, et al. Predictors of early nasal CPAP failure and effects of various intubation criteria on the rate of mechanical ventilation in preterm infants of <29 weeks gestational age. Arch Dis Child Fetal Neonatal Ed 2011;96:F343–7.

24. Dargaville PA, Aiyappan A, De Paoli AG, et al. Continuous positive airway pressure failure in preterm infants: incidence, predictors and consequences. Neonatology 2013;104:8–14.

25. Fischer C, Bertelle V, Hohlfeld J, et al. Nasal trauma due to continuous positive airway pressure in neonates. Arch Dis Child Fetal Neonatal Ed 2010;95:F447–51.

26. Sreenan C, Lemke RP, Hudson-Mason A, et al. High-flow nasal cannulae in the management of apnea of prematurity: a comparison with conventional nasal continuous positive airway pressure. Pediatrics 2001;107:1081–3.

27. Campbell DM, Shah PS, Shah V, et al. Nasal continuous positive airway pressure from high flow cannula versus Infant Flow for Preterm infants. J Perinatol 2006;26: 546–9.

28. Woodhead DD, Lambert DK, Clark JM, et al. Comparing two methods of delivering high-flow gas therapy by nasal cannula following endotracheal extubation: a prospective, randomized, masked, crossover trial. J Perinatol 2006;26:481–5.

29. Saslow JG, Aghai ZH, Nakhla TA, et al. Work of breathing using high-flow nasal cannula in preterm infants. J Perinatol 2006;26:476–80.

30. Shoemaker MT, Pierce MR, Yoder BA, et al. High flow nasal cannula versus nasal CPAP for neonatal respiratory disease: a retrospective study. J Perinatol 2007;27: 85–91.

31. Holleman-Duray D, Kaupie D, Weiss MG. Heated humidified high-flow nasal cannula: use and a neonatal early extubation protocol. J Perinatol 2007;27:776–81.

32. Spence KL, Murphy D, Kilian C, et al. High-flow nasal cannula as a device to provide continuous positive airway pressure in infants. J Perinatol 2007;27:772–5.

33. Kubicka ZJ, Limauro J, Darnall RA. Heated, humidified high-flow nasal cannula therapy: yet another way to deliver continuous positive airway pressure? Pediatrics 2008;121:82–8.

34. Wilkinson DJ, Andersen CC, Smith K, et al. Pharyngeal pressure with high-flow nasal cannulae in premature infants. J Perinatol 2008;28:42–7.

35. Lampland AL, Plumm B, Meyers PA, et al. Observational study of humidified high-flow nasal cannula compared with nasal continuous positive airway pressure. J Pediatr 2009;154:177–82.

36. Miller SM, Dowd SA. High-flow nasal cannula and extubation success in the premature infant: a comparison of two modalities. J Perinatol 2010;30:805–8.

37. Sivieri EM, Gerdes JS, Abbasi S. Effect of HFNC flow rate, cannula size, and nares diameter on generated airway pressures: an in vitro study. Pediatr Pulmonol 2013;48:506–14.

38. Dani C, Pratesi S, Migliori C, et al. High flow nasal cannula therapy as respiratory support in the preterm infant. Pediatr Pulmonol 2009;44:629–34.

39. Dysart K, Miller TL, Wolfson MR, et al. Research in high flow therapy: mechanisms of action. Respir Med 2009;103:1400–5.

40. Lavizzari A, Veneroni C, Colnaghi M, et al. Respiratory mechanics during NCPAP and HHHFNC at equal distending pressures. Arch Dis Child Fetal Neonatal Ed 2014;99:F315–20.

41. Hough JL, Pham TM, Schibler A. Physiologic effect of high-flow nasal cannula in infants with bronchiolitis. Pediatr Crit Care Med 2014;15:e214–9.

42. Hochwald O, Osiovich H. The use of high flow nasal cannulae in neonatal intensive care units: is clinical practice consistent with the evidence? J Neonatal Perinat Med 2010;3:187–91.

43. Nath P, Ponnusamy V, Willis K, et al. Current practices of high and low flow oxygen therapy and humidification in UK neonatal units. Pediatr Int 2010;52:893–4.

44. Ojha S, Gridley E, Dorling J. Use of heated humidified high-flow nasal cannula oxygen in neonates: a UK wide survey. Acta Paediatr 2013;102:249–53.

45. Manley BJ, Owen L, Doyle LW, et al. High-flow nasal cannulae and nasal continuous positive airway pressure use in non-tertiary special care nurseries in Australia and New Zealand. J Paediatr Child Health 2012;48:16–21.

46. Roberts CT, Owen LS, Manley BJ, et al. Network (ANZNN). High-flow support in very preterm infants in Australia and New Zealand. Arch Dis Child Fetal Neonatal Ed 2015. http://dx.doi.org/10.1136/archdischild-2015-309328.

47. Finer NN. Nasal cannula use in the preterm infant: oxygen or pressure? Pediatrics 2005;116:1216–7.

48. Finer NN, Mannino FL. High-flow nasal cannula: a kinder, gentler CPAP? J Pediatr 2009;154:160–2.

49. Yoder BA, Stoddard RA, Li M, et al. Heated, humidified high-flow nasal cannula versus nasal CPAP for respiratory support in neonates. Pediatrics 2013;131:e1482–90.

50. Collins CL, Holberton JR, Barfield C, et al. A randomized controlled trial to compare heated humidified high-flow nasal cannulae with nasal continuous positive airway pressure postextubation in premature infants. J Pediatr 2013;162:949–54.e1.

51. Manley BJ, Owen LS, Doyle LW, et al. High-flow nasal cannulae in very preterm infants after extubation. N Engl J Med 2013;369:1425–33.

52. Collaborative Group for the Multicenter Study on Heated Humidified High-flow Nasal Cannula Ventilation. Efficacy and safety of heated humidified high-flow nasal cannula for prevention of extubation failure in neonates. Zhonghua Er Ke Za Zhi 2014;52:271–6 [in Chinese].

53. Kugelman A, Riskin A, Said W, et al. A randomized pilot study comparing heated humidified high-flow nasal cannulae with NIPPV for RDS. Pediatr Pulmonol 2015;50:576–83.

54. Roberts CT, Manley BJ, Dawson JA, et al. Nursing perceptions of high-flow nasal cannulae treatment for very preterm infants. J Paediatr Child Health 2014;50:806–10.

55. Klingenberg C, Pettersen M, Hansen EA, et al. Patient comfort during treatment with heated humidified high flow nasal cannulae versus nasal continuous positive airway pressure: a randomised cross-over trial. Arch Dis Child Fetal Neonatal Ed 2014;99:F134–7.

56. Daish H, Badurdeen S. Humidified heated high flow nasal cannula versus nasal continuous positive airway pressure for providing respiratory support following extubation in preterm newborns. Arch Dis Child 2014;99:880–2.

57. Kotecha SJ, Adappa R, Gupta N, et al. Safety and efficacy of high-flow nasal cannula therapy in preterm infants: a meta-analysis. Pediatrics 2015;136:542–53.

58. Lavizzari A, Colnaghi M, Ciuffini F, et al. Heated, humidified high-flow nasal cannula vs nasal continuous positive airway pressure for respiratory distress syndrome of prematurity: a randomized clinical noninferiority trial. JAMA Pediatr 2016. [Epub ahead of print].

59. Reynolds P, Leontiadi S, Lawson T, et al. Stabilisation of premature infants in the delivery room with nasal high flow. Arch Dis Child Fetal Neonatal Ed 2016. http://dx.doi.org/10.1136/archdischild-2015-309442.

60. Roberts CT, Owen LS, Manley BJ, et al. A multicentre, randomised controlled, non-inferiority trial, comparing high flow therapy with nasal continuous positive airway pressure as primary support for preterm infants with respiratory distress (the HIPSTER trial): study protocol. BMJ Open 2015;5:e0084.

61. Roberts CT, Owen LS, Manley BJ, et al. Nasal high-flow therapy for primary respiratory support in preterm infants. N Engl J Med 2016;375:1142–51.

62. Wilkinson D, Andersen C, O'Donnell CPF, et al. High flow nasal cannula for respiratory support in preterm infants. Cochrane Database Syst Rev 2016;(2):CD006405.

63. Silverman WA, Andersen DH. A controlled clinical trial of effects of water mist on obstructive respiratory signs, death rate and necropsy findings among premature infants. Pediatrics 1956;17:1–10.

FURTHER READING

Committee on Fetus and Newborn, American Academy of Pediatrics. Respiratory support in preterm infants at birth. Pediatrics 2014;133:171–4.

Davis PG, Morley CJ, Owen LS. Non-invasive respiratory support of preterm neonates with respiratory distress: continuous positive airway pressure and nasal intermittent positive pressure ventilation. Semin Fetal Neonatal Med 2009;14:14–20.

Dysart K, Miller TL, Wolfson MR, et al. Research in high flow therapy: mechanisms of action. Respir Med 2009;103:1400–5.

Kotecha SJ, Adappa R, Gupta N, et al. Safety and efficacy of high-flow nasal cannula therapy in preterm infants: a meta-analysis. Pediatrics 2015;136:542–53.

Manley BJ, Dold SK, Davis PG, et al. High-flow nasal cannulae for respiratory support of preterm infants: a review of the evidence. Neonatology 2012;102:300–8.

Polin R, Sahni R. Continuous positive airway pressure: old questions and new controversies. J Neonatal Perinat Med 2008;1:1–10.

Wilkinson DJ, Andersen CC, Smith K, et al. Pharyngeal pressure with high-flow nasal cannulae in premature infants. J Perinatol 2008;28:42–7.

Wilkinson D, Andersen C, O'Donnell CPF, et al. High flow nasal cannula for respiratory support in preterm infants. Cochrane Database Syst Rev 2016;(2):CD006405.

APPENDIX 1: PARTICIPANTS

Amir Kugelman	Haifa	Israel
Anna Lavizzari	Milan	Italy
Andy Schibler	Brisbane	Australia
Amit Gupta	Oxford	UK
Brad Yoder	Salt Lake City	USA
Charles C Roehr	Oxford	UK
Claus Klingenberg	Tromsø	Norway
Ed Juszczak	Oxford	UK
Elane Boyle	Leicester	UK
Eleri Adams	Oxford	UK
Emidio Silvieri	Philadelphia	USA
Faith Emery	Bristol	UK
Gianluca Lista	Milan	Italy
Haresh Kirpilani	Philadelphia	USA
Kevin Ives	Oxford	UK
Martin Keszler	Providence	USA
Michelle Muir	Auckland	NZ
Paolo Tagliabue	Monza	Italy
Peter Davis	Melbourne	Australia
Peter Reynolds	Chertsey	UK
Richard Polin	New York City	USA
Roland Wauer	Berlin	Germany
Roland Hentschel	Freiburg	Germany
Soraya Abbasi	Philadelphia	USA

Neurally Adjusted Ventilatory Assist for Noninvasive Support in Neonates

CrossMark

Kimberly S. Firestone, MSc, RRT[a], Jennifer Beck, PhD[b,c], Howard Stein, MD[d,e,*]

KEYWORDS

- Noninvasive ventilation • Premature infant • Neural trigger
- Neurally adjusted ventilatory assist (NAVA) • Patient-ventilator interaction
- Synchrony • Respiratory distress syndrome

KEY POINTS

- Neurally adjusted ventilatory assist (NAVA) and noninvasive ventilation (NIV)-NAVA allow both the timing and degree of ventilatory assist to be controlled by the patient.
- NIV-NAVA delivers synchronized ventilation independent of leaks.
- NIV-NAVA results in improved patient-ventilator interaction, reliable respiratory monitoring, and effective ventilation at levels determined by the patient.
- NIV-NAVA has great potential as a mode of respiratory support in neonates to prevent endotracheal intubation, allow early extubation, and as a novel way to deliver continuous positive airway pressure.

Disclosure Statement: Dr J. Beck has made inventions related to neural control of mechanical ventilation that are patented. The patents are assigned to the academic institution(s) in which inventions were made. The license for these patents belongs to Maquet Critical Care. Future commercial uses of this technology may provide financial benefit to Dr J. Beck through royalties. Dr J. Beck and her spouse, Dr C. Sinderby, each own 50% of Neurovent Research Inc (NVR). NVR is a research and development company that builds the equipment and catheters for research studies. NVR has a consulting agreement with Maquet Critical Care. Dr H. Stein and Ms K.S. Firestone are members of the Speakers Bureau for Maquet Critical Care.
Funding Sources: None.

[a] Neonatal Respiratory Outreach Clinical Liaison, Neonatal Intensive Care Unit, Neonatology Department, Akron Children's Hospital, One Perkins Square, Akron, OH 44308, USA; [b] Keenan Research Centre for Biomedical Science, St. Michael's Hospital, Department of Pediatrics, University of Toronto, 30 Bond Street, Toronto, ON M5B 1W8, Canada; [c] Institute for Biomedical Engineering and Science Technology (iBEST), Ryerson University and St. Michael's Hospital, Department of Chemistry and Biology, 350 Victoria Street, Toronto, ON M5B 2K3, Canada; [d] Neonatal Intensive Care Unit, Promedica Toledo Children's Hospital, Department of Pediatrics, 2142 North Cove Boulevard, Toledo, OH 43606, USA; [e] University of Toledo, Department of Pediatrics, University of Toledo Health Science Campus, 3000 Arlington Avenue, Toledo, OH 43614, USA
* Corresponding author. Department of Pediatrics, Promedica Toledo Children's Hospital, 2142 North Cove Boulevard, Toledo, OH 43606.
E-mail address: Howardstein@bex.net

INTRODUCTION

The prolonged use of an endotracheal tube and mechanical ventilation may cause upper airway damage and predispose the neonate to the development of chronic lung disease (CLD) or bronchopulmonary dysplasia.[1] Respiratory support without endotracheal intubation has become a primary mode of management to avoid intubation or as postextubation treatment for spontaneously breathing respiratory deficient infants. This often can be accomplished through the use of noninvasive respiratory support delivered via nasal mask or prongs. The options of nasal continuous positive airway pressure (nCPAP) or nasal intermittent positive pressure ventilation (NIPPV) are predominant selections of choice for this support. Recently a Cochrane review compared available literature for NIPPV versus nCPAP in preterm infants after extubation and showed that NIPPV may be more effective than nCPAP in reducing extubation failure.[2]

The goal of NIPPV, similar to invasive ventilation, is to provide respiratory muscle unloading and adequate ventilation while maintaining lung volume through the application of positive end-expiratory pressure (PEEP) while also preserving normal physiologic functions, decreasing airway injury, and preventing respiratory tract infections. This method of noninvasive support has been used by many neonatologists; recent data from more than 900 neonatal intensive care units (NICUs) in the Vermont Oxford Network showed that 28% to 31% of very low birth weight neonates received support with NIPPV at some point during their hospitalization. However, failure can occur, with approximately 30% of these infants requiring reintubation.[2]

Although noninvasive ventilation (NIV) may be clinically effective without synchronization, it may be important in delivering effective NIPPV for many reasons. Nonsynchronized NIV is time-cycled, pressure-controlled ventilation with or without a preset constant flow and can be unresponsive to the patient's spontaneous breathing pattern. Alternatively, synchronized NIPPV has been delivered using pneumatic controller signals, such as pressure, flow, or abdominal displacement. However, in the presence of leaks, rapid respiratory rates, and small tidal volumes, achieving good communication between the patient and the ventilator remains a challenge.[3] The matter of appropriate cycling-off is not addressed, and most conventional NIPPV modes are pressure targeted, which provides no accountability for the variable respiratory demand observed in preterm newborns.[4] Asynchrony during ventilation has the potential for adverse effects that can lead to upper airway constrictor muscle activation,[5,6] diversion of ventilator breaths into the stomach,[7] increased mean airway pressure and fraction of inspired oxygen (Fio_2), and fluctuations in blood pressure and intracranial pressure.[8] Nonsynchronized ventilation may deliver high pressures during spontaneous exhalation, increasing the risk of barotrauma to the airways and airleak.[8] Often ignored, during NIPPV, monitoring the patient's respiration is problematic, as the parameters used to evaluate respiratory metrics are also affected by leaks.

One newer method of delivering assisted ventilation has the potential to overcome these challenges. The neural trigger uses the electrical activity of the diaphragm (Edi) to trigger and control the ventilator. This type of ventilation is known as neurally adjusted ventilatory assist (NAVA). The ventilator delivers mechanical breaths that are synchronized to initiation, size, and termination with each patient's breath and is controlled by the patient.[9,10] This Edi signal is obtained from a specialized indwelling nasogastric feeding tube with embedded sensing electrodes (NAVA catheter). When it is properly positioned, it can accurately and reliably trigger and cycle the ventilator breath, independent of airway leaks.[11] This makes it possible to use nasal interfaces that cannot achieve a tight seal. Conceptually, these characteristics may make

NIV-NAVA an ideal mode to provide effective, appropriate noninvasive respiratory support to newborns with respiratory insufficiency.

The authors recently published a review on noninvasive NAVA (NIV-NAVA),[12] and this article reviews the major points and adds some newer literature.

NONINVASIVE NEURALLY ADJUSTED VENTILATORY ASSIST

NIV-NAVA is a mode of mechanical ventilation intended for use in spontaneously breathing patients. In theory, it is the ideal noninvasive ventilatory mode because it is synchronized for breath initiation, size, and termination with an ongoing, breath-by-breath basis. The patient's individual Edi waveform is used to trigger-on and cycle-off each assisted breath, and also controls the amount of pressure delivered, therefore providing truly synchronized and proportional assist.[10] A standard-sized nasogastric or orogastric feeding tube with small electrodes embedded within is positioned in the lower esophagus at the level of the crural diaphragm to measure the Edi signal. This provides the Edi waveform when positioned correctly and connected to a Servo ventilator (Maquet Critical Care, AB, Solna, Sweden) that is equipped to provide NAVA ventilation to the patient. This catheter is well tolerated, easy to place, and is not affected by the act of feeding or handling of the infant or the infant's movements.[13,14]

The Electrical Activity of the Diaphragm Waveform Physiologic Foundation

The infant's neural respiratory drive is measured by the Edi waveform, and because it is an electrical signal, is independent of pneumatic influences. The respiratory centers in the brainstem continuously receive afferent information about diaphragmatic firing, lung de-recruitment, CO_2 response, lung stretch, respiratory muscle loading, and other reactions. The output of the respiratory centers, which represents all respiratory reflexes and responses, moves down the phrenic nerves and electrically activates the diaphragm motor units. The Edi waveform is a representation of this neural initiation (motor unit recruitment and firing rate). During NIV-NAVA, the same physiologic responses driving the patient's diaphragm are also simultaneously driving the ventilator throughout each breath.[15]

The Edi waveform in infants is highly variable as compared with adults (**Fig. 1**[16]); it can be measured breath-by-breath for its peak (Edi_{peak}, representing tidal inspiratory effort) and its minimum (Edi_{min}, representing the effort to prevent de-recruitment) values. The infant's neural recruitment maneuvers for sighs (large neural inspiratory effort) and central apneas (flat Edi waveform, not shown) can be distinguished, as well as other respiratory metrics, such as the neural respiratory rate, and can be measured, even in the presence of leaks.[11]

Noninvasive Neurally Adjusted Ventilatory Assist and Patient-Ventilator Interaction

Edi and ventilator pressure tracings for a newborn breathing on NIV-NAVA are denoted in **Fig. 2**. The precise synchrony between the Edi (patient) and airway pressure (ventilator), in terms of timing and proportionality is displayed. The Edi signal triggers inspiration for each breath once a threshold change in Edi has been exceeded. After the initial trigger, the pressure delivered follows the Edi waveform in a proportional fashion. The level of support for the patient can be adjusted by changing the NAVA level. The supported breath increases until the onset of neural exhalation, when the ventilator will cycle off when the Edi has decreased by 30% from the peak. Once it cycles off, the assist returns to the set PEEP level. This type of ventilation provides the patient control of his or her own ventilator initiation, rate, and level of assist with every breath. Upper pressure limits can be set by the clinician, along with a backup ventilation for the occurrence of apnea or accidental catheter removal.[10]

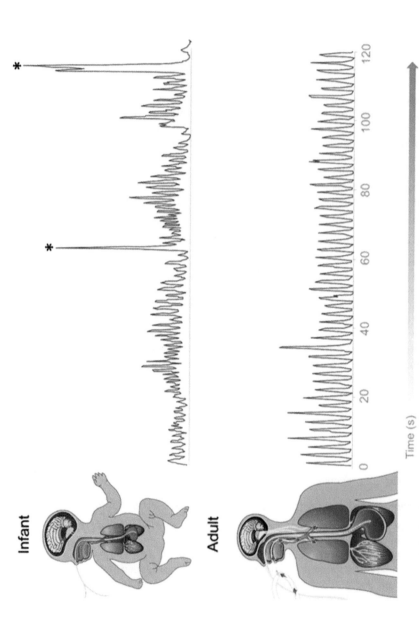

Fig. 1. Edi waveform in preterm infant and adult patients. *Top panel:* Processed Edi waveform obtained in a nonintubated premature infant. *Bottom panel:* Processed Edi waveform obtained in an intubated adult. The Edi waveform in infants can be characterized by larger variability in timing and amplitude, with a distinct amount of changes in the baseline, so-called "tonic" activity of the diaphragm. The Edi waveform in adults is generally less variable with minimal tonic Edi. Note the presence of "sighs" (ie, recruiting breaths, in the neonate breathing pattern), as indicated by stars. (*Adapted from* Sinderby C, Beck J. Neurally adjusted ventilatory assist. Principles and practice of mechanical ventilation. McGraw Hill; 2012; with permission.)

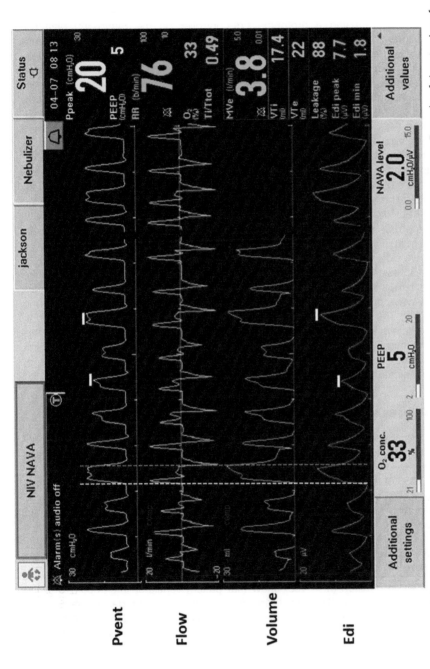

Fig. 2. Ventilator and diaphragm electrical activity waveforms during noninvasive NAVA in a premature neonate. Example of time tracings for ventilator pressure (*top, yellow*), flow (*green*), volume (*blue*), and Edi (*bottom, dark green*). Note the synchrony and proportionality between Edi and ventilator pressure, despite a leak (88%). The onset of diaphragm activity and the onset of ventilator pressure coincide (*white vertical dashed line*), as do the early decrease in Edi and ventilator pressure (*orange vertical dashed line*). Proportionality is maintained: for small breaths, less pressure is delivered than larger breaths (indicated by *thick horizontal white bars*).

EARLY STUDY TESTING OF NONINVASIVE NEURALLY ADJUSTED VENTILATORY ASSIST

Beck and colleagues[17] first showed that NIV-NAVA was an optimal ventilator mode that could improve patient-ventilator synchrony in an animal model with hypoxemic respiratory failure using a prototype Edi-controller on the Servo-300 platform. Three-kilogram rabbits with experimental lung injury were used to demonstrate ventilation via a single nasal prong (75% leak). The subjects were unable to trigger conventional NIV with pressure support but when NIV-NAVA was activated, synchronized proportional assist could be delivered with improved ventilation. Subsequently, there was no significant difference in trigger delays, or cycling-off delays between invasive (leak-free NAVA), and NIV-NAVA. Of paramount interest, despite the extreme leak (75%) and the 50% reduction in lung compliance, these lung-injured animals were effectively ventilated without complications, or gastric distension, even when peak inspiratory pressures with nasal prongs reached up to 40 cm H_2O.

Mirabella and colleagues[18] examined lung injury markers using the same animal model after 6 hours of volume control ventilation with a lung protective strategy using 6 mL/kg with PEEP. This was compared with 6 hours of NIV-NAVA and spontaneous breathing and no PEEP finding a lower lung injury score and plasma interleukin-8 for the NIV-NAVA group. Of note, even with no PEEP being applied during NIV-NAVA, the upper airways were able to support in the maintenance of the functional residual capacity.

A known side effect of NIV is gastric insufflation into the esophagus and stomach. Moreau-Brussiere and colleagues[5] demonstrated in spontaneously breathing, awake newborn lambs the activation of the thyroarytenoid (a glottal constrictor) at high levels of noninvasive pressure support, which was not observed in any of the lambs during NIV-NAVA.[6] The neural coordination of upper airway dilation and neural inspiration likely explain these advantageous outcomes during NIV-NAVA. When using this same prototype, Beck and colleagues[11] were able to exhibit in a small pilot of low birth weight infants that NIV-NAVA was feasible and not affected by leaks, in terms of patient-ventilator interaction.

INVASIVE NEURALLY ADJUSTED VENTILATORY ASSIST IN NEONATES

Over the past decade, the literature available on the topic of NAVA has considerably expanded. A total of 235 peer-reviewed articles have been published, with 54 of these pertaining to children (age 0–18 years, including premature infants), which is approximately 25% of the publications. Most of these publications address the use of invasive NAVA. A systemic review on the topic of NAVA in infants is provided for the reader for these summaries.[15] A relevant study review on invasive NAVA is provided later in this article.

Neurally Adjusted Ventilatory Assist Studies Show Improvement in Patient-Ventilator Interaction

The studies in children (n = 163) show that patient-ventilator interaction explicitly improved from 12% to 29% asynchrony during conventional modes, to 0% to 11% during NAVA.[19–27] Longhini and colleagues[27] studied 14 intubated preterm infants with gestational age range of 27 to 35 weeks, with a crossover trial of 12 hours of ventilation using pressure-regulated volume control (PRVC) compared with 12 hours of NAVA. In PRVC, they found distinct differences between ventilator and patient respiratory rates as much as 5 times that of the patient, signifying auto-triggering or backup ventilation. Central apneas, shown by flat Edi waveforms, were significantly reduced with the use of NAVA.

Invasive Neurally Adjusted Ventilatory Assist Limits Peak Inspiratory Pressures and Tidal Volume

A total of 318 infants studied during spontaneous breathing on NAVA manifested lower peak inspiratory pressures (PIP) and tidal volume (VT) compared with conventional ventilation (targeted by the clinician).[21,28–35] The Hering-Breuer reflex and improved comfort due to improved synchrony could be explanations for this downregulation of the Edi resulting in lower pressures and tidal volumes. In animal experimentation, evidence points to reflex lung protection, which is vagally mediated.[36–38] NAVA is neurally integrated with these essential lung protective reflexes. As lung inflation progresses, vagally mediated stretch receptors in the lungs sense an adequate level of lung distension and turn off inspiration. For the infant on NAVA, the ventilator breath will be cycled-off when neural exhalation begins.

Specific evidence for functional lung reflexes in premature infants comes from the work by Firestone and colleagues,[39] who carried out NAVA level titrations in 21 premature neonates (mean weight at study was 795 g, range 500–1441 g). Starting at a NAVA level of 0.5 cm $H_2O/\mu V$, systematic increases in the NAVA level were performed every 3 minutes until they reached 4 cm $H_2O/\mu V$. This supported the same responses in Edi and ventilator pressure previously described in animals[36–38] and adults.[40] At first, PIP and VT increased with increasing NAVA levels, followed by a plateau phase in which the PIP and VT did not increase further, due to downregulation of Edi. The investigators termed this NAVA level, the "breakpoint."[39]

To summarize the literature for invasive ventilation, 19 studies in 457 infant patients have compared NAVA with conventional ventilation. For those who report the variables, ventilation parameters adopted by the patient are consistent with current understanding of respiratory physiology in newborns: VT: 6.4 ± 1.7 mL/kg; respiratory rate: 45.4 ± 9.8 breaths per minute; PIP: 13.9 ± 2.7 cm H_2O; NAVA level: 1.4 ± 0.4 cm $H_2O/\mu V$; Edi peak: 8.6 ± 2.3 μV.

CLINICAL STUDIES ABOUT NONINVASIVE NEURALLY ADJUSTED VENTILATORY ASSIST IN NEONATES

Improved patient-ventilator interaction with reliable respiratory monitoring and self-regulation for lower PIPs and VTs is evident with NIV-NAVA compared with conventional modes.

Patient-Ventilator Interaction

NIPPV in the neonate is often delivered unsynchronized due to the intrinsic complications in producing a sensitive and reliable triggering method. Conventional methods of providing synchronous NIPPV are also characteristically flawed when leaks are present because either the controller signal may fail to trigger (wasted effort) or can auto-trigger.

Ventilator screen shots from preterm newborns breathing on 2 conventional NIPPV modes demonstrate the asynchrony between the patient (Edi waveform), and the ventilator (pressure waveform). **Fig. 3** (*Panel A*) clearly displays complete failure of the ventilator to trigger and auto-triggering ("asynchrony") in pressure control (PC) mode. **Fig. 3** (*Panel B*) demonstrates similar asynchronies with NIV pressure support ventilation (PSV), including timing errors for triggering, and for cycling-off each breath. These figures illustrate the importance of monitoring the Edi waveform. In its absence, the ventilator pressure waveform seems appropriate. These figures also show how the patient's Edi amplitude can vary

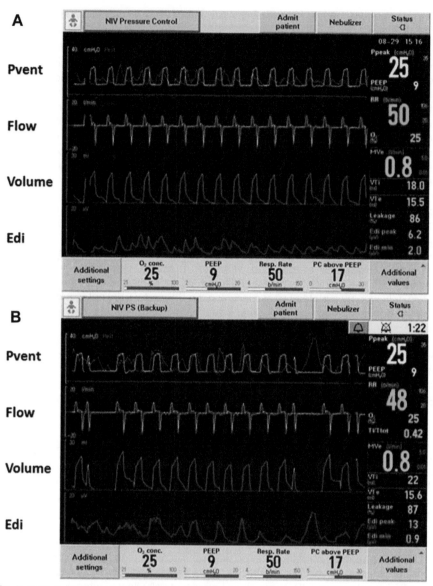

Fig. 3. Patient-ventilator asynchrony and dyssynchrony in 2 preterm infants breathing with noninvasive PC and noninvasive pressure support. Example of ventilator waveforms (*yellow*, ventilator pressure; *green*, flow: *blue*, volume), and diaphragm electrical activity (*bottom*, *pale green* AND *white* tracing in upper tracing overlaid on top of ventilator pressure). Panels A and B, show similar tracings, but in 2 neonates breathing on NIV-PC (*Panel A*) and NIV-PSV (*Panel B*). In each panel severe asynchrony is demonstrated both in terms of timing, and proportionality, as well as wasted efforts (Edi waveform without ventilator being triggered).

breath-by-breath, but the NIV-PC and NIV-PSV deliver the same pressure regardless of the patient's needs. **Fig. 4** demonstrates the synchrony during NIV-NAVA, for both timing and proportionality, despite the large leak (88%) when spontaneous breathing is present.

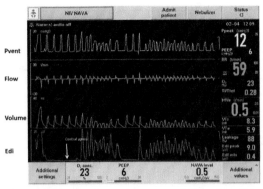

Fig. 4. Patient-ventilator synchrony in one preterm infant breathing with NIV-NAVA. Example of ventilator waveforms (*yellow*, ventilator pressure; *green*, flow: *blue*, volume), and diaphragm electrical activity (*bottom, pale green*). Note the time scale has been extended to show longer time tracings. Note the synchrony in terms of both timing and proportionality. Note also, at the beginning of the tracings, the central apnea period (flat Edi waveform, *vertical gray arrow*), and subsequent initiation of backup ventilation. On resolution of central apnea, there is an automatic re-initiation of NIV-NAVA.

Only one study in preterm neonates has evaluated the improved patient-ventilator interaction during NAVA (with the commercially available Servo-I ventilator) compared with conventional NIPPV (NIV-PS). Lee and colleagues,[41] in a crossover randomized study, looked at trigger delays, excessive delivery of assist, wasted efforts and auto-triggering, in a group of 15 preterm neonates (gestational age [GA] 27 [26–28] weeks; birth weight 790 [675–1215] g). There was more than a threefold improvement in patient-ventilator interaction during NIV-NAVA, mainly due to the reduced occurrence of wasted efforts (Edi breath is present but ventilator does not respond). As previously shown with invasive NAVA, PIPs and peak Edi values were lower during NIV-NAVA, indicating much more efficient ventilation.

Recently, Longhini and colleagues[42] analyzed physiologic and ventilator variables in 10 term infants (mean weight 3 kg) breathing for 2 hours while intubated on NAVA and then extubated to NIV-NAVA, with the same ventilator settings. The investigators found no differences in terms of gas exchange or breathing pattern between the 2 ventilation periods. Of note, there were no differences in patient-ventilator interaction, sedation requirements, or vital signs for invasive or NIV-NAVA.

Noninvasive Neurally Adjusted Ventilatory Assist Limits Peak Inspiratory Pressures and Tidal Volume

The breakpoint described by Firestone and colleagues[39] with invasive ventilation is still observed during NIV-NAVA level titrations, despite the large leak. They showed in infants as young as 24 weeks that low NIV-NAVA levels increase the Edi, and as the NAVA level increases, there is a certain level at which the infants de-activate their diaphragms (downregulate their Edi). **Fig. 5** shows a representative premature infant titration during NIV-NAVA.

It should be noted that depending on the leak around and compliance of the interface, the PIP displayed and measured by the ventilator is not necessarily the pressure reaching the lung. As shown by De Paoli and colleagues,[43] in the presence of leaks, CPAP-delivered pressures may be an overestimation of the actual pharyngeal pressure. The advantage of NIV-NAVA is that the inherent lung-distending reflexes

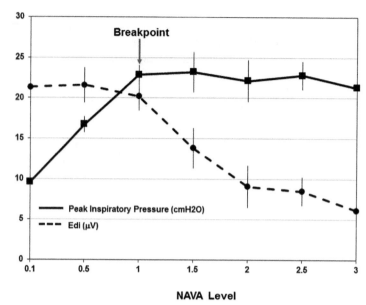

Fig. 5. Physiologic response to increasing NAVA levels in a preterm infant. Electrical activity of the diaphragm (Edi) and peak inspiratory pressure data from a premature neonate on NIV-NAVA, as the NAVA level is increased from 0.1 to 3.0 cm $H_2O/\mu V$. The first response is evident by increases in peak inspiratory pressure as the NAVA level increases from 0.1 to 1.0 cm $H_2O/\mu V$. At a level of 1 cm $H_2O/\mu V$, the peak pressure no longer increases, and the Edi peak begins to decrease with additional increases in NAVA level. The breakpoint (or point of optimal respiratory muscle unloading) would be determined as a NAVA level of 1 cm $H_2O/\mu V$.

"switch-off" neural inspiration, and then cycle-off the ventilator, when an appropriate volume/pressure has been reached.

Monitoring Electrical Activity of the Diaphragm in the Preterm Neonate

The Edi signal in preterms can be characterized as a cyclic waveform, with distinct inspiratory peak and end-expiratory minimum values.[16] Infants demonstrate postinspiratory activity, or "tonic Edi."[4,44,45] Although not occurring often, pure "tonic bursts" may appear.[4] Often, large neural inspiratory efforts can be observed ("sighs"), as well as periods of flat Edi, so-called "central apnea" (see **Figs. 1** and **4**). Compared with adults, the Edi signal in children demonstrates a high variability,[4,46] with elevated tonic Edi in nonventilated preterms[4] and in intubated term infants.[44] The reader is referred to the review by Ducharme-Crevier and colleagues[47] for an in-depth analysis of Edi monitoring in children.

Soukka and colleagues[48] were the first to report valid Edi measurements in preterm infants with and without Kangaroo Care (when an infant is positioned skin-to-skin with a parent, shown to improve hospital stay). Seventeen neonates were studied during NIV-NAVA (mean birth weight 900 g, mean GA 28 weeks) while in the incubator, or during Kangaroo Care. Edi_{min} values were lower during Kangaroo Care, with a tendency for lower Edi_{peak} values, indicating less energy expenditure of the diaphragm.

Regarding Edi monitoring during high flow nasal cannula (HFNC), Nasef and colleagues[49] compared neural breathing pattern during nasal CPAP and HFNC matched to target the same mean airway pressure, in 10 preterm infants (<1500 g). They found that HFNC was associated with higher Edi peak, and increased neural inspiratory time, compared with nasal CPAP. As well, they observed a discrepancy between the respiratory rate of the patient determined from the Edi, and the respiratory rate noted by readings from the plethysmograph.

Clinical Experience with Noninvasive Neurally Adjusted Ventilatory Assist

Evidenced-based management guidelines on the use of NIV-NAVA have not been developed to date; therefore, the authors provide experience-based clinical strategies. The NICU at Toledo Children's Hospital treated 129 (60%) of 216 neonates 23 to 28 weeks' GA from July 1, 2010, to December 31, 2014, with NIV-NAVA at some point during their NICU stay.[12] Ninety-two percent of those treated with NIV-NAVA were initially intubated, treated with surfactant, and then extubated to NIV-NAVA; 74% of those were successful extubations and were maintained on NIV-NAVA a median of 8 days until they were transitioned to nasal CPAP. Eight percent of the neonates were never intubated, and treated with NIV-NAVA only. Many of these neonates were also on conventional modes for varying amounts of time, so outcomes specifically attributed to NIV-NAVA could not be determined. Of importance, no adverse outcomes (including pneumothorax, feeding intolerance, intraventricular hemorrhage, or pulmonary hemorrhage) attributed to NIV-NAVA were noted.

APPLYING NONINVASIVE NEURALLY ADJUSTED VENTILATORY ASSIST IN THE NEONATE

There are multiple parameters to set when placing neonates on NIV-NAVA. PEEP and Fio_2, are set similarly to any type of NIV. Other parameters require an advanced understanding of how NIV-NAVA works. The assist, or NAVA level, determines the proportionality between the Edi and the ventilator pressure, and allows the work of breathing to be unloaded from the patient to the ventilator. The apnea time is the time the infant can be apneic before going into backup and determines the minimum rate. The peak pressure limit, the maximum pressure the ventilator will deliver, must be set high enough to allow recruiting breaths to prevent atelectasis (the assist will be limited at 5 cm H_2O below the number dialed). Although the Edi trigger is adjustable, the default setting of 0.5 µV is suitable for most neonates. The cycling-off criteria are fixed at 70% of the peak Edi.

Patient safety is enhanced with backup ventilation that is provided in the case of no Edi (central apnea or accidental catheter removal). Backup settings need to be selected carefully, as the infant may decompensate if appropriate support is not provided during these episodes. Undersupport can result in desaturation and bradycardia, and oversupport can result in hypocapnea and continued absence of the Edi.

For a more detailed description and recommendations on how to set up NAVA for both invasive ventilation and NIV, the reader is referred to Stein and Firestone.[50]

Determining and Adjusting the Noninvasive Neurally Adjusted Ventilatory Assist Level

The NAVA level determines the degree of respiratory unloading from the infant to the ventilator. Insufficient unloading, or undersupport, results in increased work of breathing; oversupport results in depression of the respiratory drive. Several methods have been proposed for adjusting the NAVA level. NIV-NAVA titrations can be used to determine an adequate NAVA level.[39] This procedure is based on the physiologic responses of the infant during stepwise increases in the NAVA level (by a fixed amount [eg, 0.5 cm $H_2O/µV$] at regular time intervals [eg, every 5–10 seconds]). At some specific NAVA level, the infant will downregulate his or her respiratory drive to prevent further increases in assist or VT. This "breakpoint" would be considered the appropriate NAVA level for that infant, as has been shown in animal studies.[36,38]

Another method is to increase the NAVA support until the Edi peak is within the "normal" range (5–15 μV)[13,51] and the patient looks comfortable with minimal work of breathing. Clinical experience with more than 260 infants (all GAs) at Toledo Children's NICU suggests that starting at a NAVA level of 2 cm $H_2O/\mu V$ is appropriate for most patients. If retractions persist or peak Edi remains greater than 15 to 20 μV, the NAVA level can be increased in steps of 0.5 cm $H2O/\mu V$ until the patient is adequately unloaded (looks comfortable and peak Edi <15 μV) to a maximum of 4 cm $H_2O/\mu V$.[12] Alternate ventilator modes should be considered if the patient continues to have increased work of breathing. Despite looking comfortable with low Edi, many of these infants remain tachypneic and respiratory rate alone does not seem to be a useful guide to measure the effectiveness of this noninvasive support.

The manufacturers have provided an "overlay window," which displays an "estimated" or "ghost" waveform that would be obtained if the patient were in the NIV-NAVA mode simultaneously with the airway pressure waveform during conventional ventilation. Although breathing on conventional NIPPV, the clinician is able to adjust the NIV-NAVA level, in an attempt to match the desired peak pressure. Although this may have some value when the infant is intubated, large and variable air leaks, with noninvasive interfaces, result in limited reliability of this method to achieve an adequate NAVA level. In addition, this assumes that the assist provided during conventional NIPPV is the appropriate level.

Weaning Noninvasive Neurally Adjusted Ventilatory Assist

As soon as the neonate is comfortably stable with acceptable blood gases, weaning the NIV-NAVA level should be attempted. With an acute lung process (eg, respiratory distress syndrome), weaning can be done in increments of 0.5 cm $H_2O/\mu V$ until at an NIV-NAVA level of 1 cm $H_2O/\mu V$, and then a trial of CPAP can be undertaken. This NAVA level decrease can be done as often as 1 to 3 times per day as tolerated. If neonates fail a CPAP trial, and especially in those less than 25 weeks' gestation, it may be reasonable to stay on NIV-NAVA of 1 cm $H_2O/\mu V$ for a few days to weeks until ready to try CPAP again. In infants with CLD, a slower wean consisting of decreasing the NAVA level by smaller increments of 0.1 to 0.3 cm $H_2O/\mu V$ every 1 to 2 days may be better tolerated.[12]

POTENTIAL LIMITATIONS IN PRETERM NEONATES OF NONINVASIVE NEURALLY ADJUSTED VENTILATORY ASSIST

There are currently 2 known potential limitations to the use of NIV-NAVA in preterm infants.

Loss or Absence of Electrical Activity of the Diaphragm Signal

A functional NAVA catheter (a conventional feeding tube with embedded, miniaturized sensors for detecting Edi) is necessary and should be positioned appropriately at the level of the crural diaphragm. Catheter positioning is straightforward and has been validated using the catheter positioning screen on the ventilator.[28,52] If the catheter is accidently removed or disconnected, no Edi signal will be present, and, after an apnea time set by the clinician, the ventilator provides backup ventilation with nonsynchronous NIPPV at peak pressures and rates determined by the clinician.

If the catheter is well positioned and functioning, absence of an Edi signal usually indicates central apnea. If this is detected by the ventilator, after an apnea time set by the clinician, backup ventilation will begin. It should be noted that all modes of NIPPV that attempt synchronization are limited by central apnea and should also deliver mandatory backup breaths if there is no effort detected.

Erratic or Inappropriate Respiratory Drive or Responses

It has been shown that infants as young as 24 weeks have an appropriate physiologic response to unloading so that removing the assist (lowering the NAVA level) increases respiratory drive, and adding assist (increasing the NAVA level) downregulates respiratory drive.[39] If this de-activation of the diaphragm with added inspiratory assist does not occur, that pathophysiology should be investigated. If acceptable ventilation and/or gas exchange are not achieved during NIV-NAVA, application of another mode should be considered. Respiratory rates greater than 90 on NIV-NAVA can occasionally be confused with heart rate by the ventilator and, to prevent ventilation in synchrony with the heart rate, the ventilator goes into backup despite the presence of an Edi signal. One alternative is to provoke a reduction in respiratory rate temporarily by manipulating PEEP. Should this occur (the ventilator alarms with "HR-RR coupling") it is best to place the infant in an alternate ventilator mode until the respiratory rate decreases. However, monitoring of the Edi during alternate modes may still provide vital information, such as respiratory drive and timing, and could be used to determine clinical response and optimize synchrony and assist delivery.

WHEN TO USE NONINVASIVE NEURALLY ADJUSTED VENTILATORY ASSIST
Noninvasive Neurally Adjusted Ventilatory Assist for Nasal Intermittent Positive Pressure Ventilation

The use of NIV-NAVA in neonates has promise as a primary mode of ventilation to aid in the prevention of intubation. In those neonates who require surfactant treatment, NIV-NAVA may allow for optimal success with minimally invasive surfactant delivery techniques by providing, synchronized noninvasive positive pressure to aid in the dispersion of the surfactant to the lung while maintaining adequate ventilation.

Early extubation may be enhanced with NIV-NAVA of those neonates requiring intubation for numerous reasons. A vigorous Edi in a ventilated patient confirms the presence of good spontaneous respiration, suggesting that the infant may tolerate liberation from the endotracheal tube. Positive pressure from the ventilator may better support the underdeveloped pharynx of the neonate than CPAP alone. The ability to provide synchronous NIV allows clinicians the opportunity to extubate infants earlier with increased confidence than with previous post extubation support.

Noninvasive Neurally Adjusted Ventilatory Assist with Nasal Continuous Positive Airway Pressure

A major challenge of using CPAP in neonates is frequent apnea. During these apneic events, neonates can deteriorate clinically and may even require reintubation. A novel approach for use of NIV-NAVA is setting the NAVA level at zero, which results in the patient receiving minimal ventilatory support above PEEP when there is an Edi signal present.[12] If the patient becomes apneic for a predetermined amount of time, backup ventilation is initiated and the patient is ventilated with PC until breathing and an Edi signal resumes. The patient is returned to CPAP at this point. **Fig. 6** shows how NIV-NAVA can work as a CPAP mode with backup.

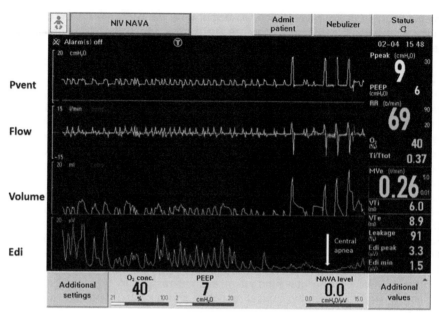

Fig. 6. NIV-NAVA as a CPAP mode. Example of ventilator waveforms (*yellow*, ventilator pressure; *green*, flow: *blue*, volume), and diaphragm electrical activity (*bottom, pale green*) for an infant breathing on a zero NAVA level with spontaneous breathing. When central apnea occurs (flat Edi), the pressure control backup kicks in, until Edi resumes.

This allows sufficient support during episodes of apnea so that clinical decompensation is prevented.

SUMMARY

NIV-NAVA provides patients, including premature neonates, the ability to use physiologic feedback to control their ventilation by synchronizing the delivery or noninvasive support on a breath-by-breath basis. It uses all aspects of physiologic respiratory control to provide the ideal ventilation based on the patient's ever-changing needs. The Edi signal provides the caregiver the ability to access information and details about the central respiratory drive that was not available previously. This signal is a valuable respiratory vital sign for weaning and diagnostics, providing the clinician direction to the patient's respiratory status both with timing and depth of his or her breathing pattern.

An increasing body of literature demonstrates that NIV-NAVA works well, even in very preterm neonates and in the face of large air leaks. Although this mode of ventilation shows promise for the neonatal patient, at this time there is not enough evidence to recommend NIV-NAVA as the primary mode for NIV. Clinical experience combined with recent studies suggests that NIV-NAVA is a viable mode that can be used as option in the neonatologist's NIV resource. NIV-NAVA may be used as a primary mode to prevent intubation, to facilitate extubation, or as a rescue therapy for infants failing CPAP or other forms of NIV.

Future studies with multicenter, randomized, adequately powered trials are required to determine if NIV-NAVA is more effective than other modes of NIV in preventing intubation, facilitating extubation with enhanced post extubation support, decreasing time of ventilation, reducing the incidence of CLD, decreasing length of stay, or improving overall long-term outcome in preterm neonates.

Best practice

Best practices are evolving for ventilating the premature infant with respiratory compromise. Noninvasive ventilation (NIV) has been proven to be a modality used in the NICU to avoid intubation or as post extubation support for these infants with a spontaneous respiratory drive. In the ideal situation, the ventilator providing NIV should precisely follow the patient's neural output from the respiratory center, as denoted by the neural activity of the phrenic nerves. This technology provided by neurally adjusted ventilatory assist (NAVA), significantly decreases dyssynchronies, which can contribute to higher inspiratory pressures, patient agitation, and significant cause of NIV failure. Air leaks that are universal during NIV do not affect the pressures delivered by NIV-NAVA because pneumatic triggering is not involved.

This article reviews the literature comprehensively to support the use of NIV-NAVA with the most recent neonatal studies. Clinical experience is provided along with recommendations for management guidelines. Although it is recommended that multicenter, randomized, adequately powered trials are required to support the efficacy of NIV-NAVA, it shows to be a promising mode of ventilation for the respiratory compromised neonatal patient.

REFERENCES

1. Jobe AH, Ikegami M. Prevention of bronchopulmonary dysplasia. Curr Opin Pediatr 2001;13(2):124–9.
2. Lemyre B, Davis PG, De Paoli AG, et al. Nasal intermittent positive pressure ventilation (NIPPV) versus nasal continuous positive airway pressure (NCPAP) for preterm neonates after extubation. Cochrane Database Syst Rev 2014;(9):CD003212.
3. Keszler M. State of the art in conventional mechanical ventilation. J Perinatol 2009;29(4):262–75.
4. Beck J, Reilly M, Grasselli G, et al. Characcterization of neural breathing pattern in spontaneously breathing preterm infants. Pediatr Res 2011;70(6):607–13.
5. Moreau-Bussière F, Samson N, St-Hilaire M, et al. Laryngeal response to nasal ventilation in nonsedated newborn lambs. J Appl Physiol 2007;102(6):2149–57.
6. Hadj-Ahmed M, Samson N, Bussières M, et al. Absence of inspiratory laryngeal constrictor muscle activity during nasal neurally adjusted ventilatory assist in newborn lambs. J Appl Physiol 2012;113(1):63–70.
7. Garland J, Nelson D, Rice T, et al. Increased risk of gastrointestinal perforation in neonates mechanically ventilated with either face mask or nasal prongs. Pediatrics 1985;76:406–10.
8. DiBlasi RM. Neonatal noninvasive ventilation techniques: do we really need to intubate? Respir Care 2011;56(9):1273–97.
9. Sinderby C, Navalesi P, Beck J, et al. Neural control of mechanical ventilation in respiratory failure. Nat Med 1999;5(12):1433–6.
10. Sinderby C, Spahija J, Beck J. Neurally-adjusted ventilatory assist. In: Vincent J-L, Slutsky AS, Brochard L, editors. Mechanical ventilation. Heidelberg (Germany): Springer Berlin Heidelberg; 2005. p. 125–34.

11. Beck J, Reilly M, Grasselli G, et al. Patient-ventilator interaction during neurally adjusted ventilatory assist in low birth weight infants. Pediatr Res 2009;65(6): 663–8.

12. Stein H, Beck J, Dunn M. Non-invasive ventilation with neurally adjusted ventilatory assist in newborns. Semin Fetal Neonatal Med 2016;21(3):154–61.

13. Stein H, Hall R, Davis K, et al. Electrical activity of the diaphragm (Edi) values and Edi catheter placement in non-ventilated preterm neonates. J Perinatol 2013; 33(9):707–11.

14. Barwing J, Pedroni C, Quintel M, et al. Influence of body position, PEEP and intra-abdominal pressure on the catheter positioning for neurally adjusted ventilatory assist. Intensive Care Med 2011;37(12):2041–5.

15. Beck J, Emeriaud G, Liu Y, et al. Neurally adjusted ventilatory assist (NAVA) in children: a systematic review. Minerva Anestesiol 2016;82(8):874–83.

16. Sinderby C, Beck J. Neurally adjusted ventilatory assist. Principles and practice of mechanical ventilation. New York: McGraw Hill; 2012.

17. Beck J, Brander L, Slutsky AS, et al. Non-invasive neurally adjusted ventilatory assist in rabbits with acute lung injury. Intensive Care Med 2008;34(2):316–23.

18. Mirabella L, Grasselli G, Haitsma J, et al. Lung protection during non-invasive synchronized assist versus volume control in rabbits. Crit Care 2014;18(1):R22.

19. Clement K, Thurman T, Holt S, et al. Neurally triggered breaths reduce trigger delay and improve ventilator response times in ventilated infants with bronchiolitis. Intensive Care Med 2011;37(1826–1832):1826.

20. Bengtsson JA, Edberg KE. Neurally adjusted ventilatory assist in children: an observational study. Pediatr Crit Care Med 2010;11:253–7.

21. Zhu L, Shi Z, Ji G, et al. Application of neurally adjusted ventilatory assist in infants who underwent cardiac surgery for congenital heart disease. Zhongguo Dang Dai Er Ke Za Zhi 2009;11(6):433–6 [in Chinese].

22. de la Oliva P, Schüffelmann C, Gómez-Zamora A, et al. Asynchrony, neural drive, ventilatory variability and COMFORT: NAVA versus pressure support in pediatric patients. A non-randomized cross-over trial. Intensive Care Med 2012;38(5): 838–46.

23. Alander M, Peltoniemi O, Pokka T, et al. Comparison of pressure-, flow-, and NAVA-triggering in pediatric and neonatal ventilatory care. Pediatr Pulmonol 2012;47:76–83.

24. Vignaux L, Grazioli S, Piquilloud L, et al. Optimizing patient-ventilator synchrony during invasive ventilator assist in children and infants remains a difficult task. Pediatr Crit Care Med 2013;14(7):e316–25.

25. Breatnach C, Conlon NP, Stack M, et al. A prospective crossover comparison of neurally adjusted ventilatory assist and pressure-support ventilation in a pediatric and neonatal intensive care unit population. Pediatr Crit Care Med 2010; 11(1):7–11.

26. Bordessoule A, Emeriaud G, Morneau S, et al. Neurally Adjusted Venitlatory Assist (NAVA) improves patient-ventilator interaction in infants compared to conventional ventilation. Pediatr Res 2012;72(2):194–202.

27. Longhini F, Ferrero F, De Luca D, et al. Neurally adjusted ventilatory assist in preterm neonates with acute respiratory failure. Neonatology 2014;107(1):60–7.

28. Duyndam A, Bol B, Kroon A, et al. Neurally adjusted ventilatory assist: assessing the comfort and feasibility of use in neonates and children. Nurs Crit Care 2013; 18(2):86–92.

29. Piastra M, De Luca D, Costa R, et al. Neurally adjusted ventilatory assist vs pressure support ventilation in infants recovering from severe acute respiratory distress syndrome: nested study. J Crit Care 2014;29(2):312.e1-5.

30. Lee J, Kim H, Sohn J, et al. Randomized crossover study of neurally adjusted ventilatory assist in preterm infants. J Pediatr 2012;161(5):808–13.

31. Stein HM, Alosh H, Ethington P, et al. Prospective crossover comparison between NAVA and pressure control ventilation in premature neonates less than 1500 grams. J Perinatol 2013;33(6):452–6.

32. Stein HM, Howard D. Neurally adjusted ventilatory assist (NAVA) in neonates less than 1500 grams: a retrospective analysis. J Pediatr 2012;160(5):786–9.

33. Kallio M, Peltoniemi O, Anttila E, et al. Neurally adjusted ventilatory assist (NAVA) in pediatric intensive care - a randomized controlled trial. Pediatr Pulmonol 2015; 50(1):55–62.

34. Liet J, Dejode J, Joram N, et al. Respiratory support by neurally adjusted ventilatory assist (NAVA) in severe RSV-related bronchiolitis: a case series report. BMC Pediatr 2011;11:92.

35. Gentili A, Masciopinto F, Mondardini M, et al. Neurally adjusted ventilatory assist in weaning of neonates affected by congenital diaphragmatic hernia. J Matern Fetal Neonatal Med 2013;26(6):598–602.

36. Allo JC, Beck JC, Brander L, et al. Influence of neurally adjusted ventilatory assist and positive end-expiratory pressure on breathing pattern in rabbits with acute lung injury. Crit Care Med 2006;34(12):2997–3004.

37. Brander L, Sinderby C, Lecomte F, et al. Neurally adjusted ventilatory assist decreases ventilator-induced lung injury and non-pulmonary organ dysfunction in rabbits with acute lung injury. Intensive Care Med 2009;35(11):1979–89.

38. Lecomte F, Brander L, Jalde F, et al. Physiological response to increasing levels of neurally adjusted ventilatory assist (NAVA). Respir Physiol Neurobiol 2009; 166(2):117–24.

39. Firestone KS, Fisher S, Reddy S, et al. Effect of changing NAVA levels on peak inspiratory pressures and electrical activity of the diaphragm in premature neonates. J Perinatol 2015;35(8):612–6.

40. Brander L, Leong-Poi H, Beck J, et al. Titration and implementation of neurally adjusted ventilatory assist in critically ill patients. Chest 2009;135(3):695–703.

41. Lee J, Kim H, Jung Y, et al. Non-invasive neurally adjusted ventilatory assist in preterm infants: a randomised phase II crossover trial. Arch Dis Child Fetal Neonatal Ed 2015;100(6):F507–13.

42. Longhini F, Scarlino S, Gallina M, et al. Comparison of neurally adjusted ventilator assist in infants before and after extubation. Minerva Pediatr 2015. [Epub ahead of print].

43. De Paoli A, Lau R, Davis P, et al. Pharyngeal pressure in preterm infants receiving nasal continuous positive airway pressure. Arch Dis Child Fetal Neonatal Ed 2005;90:F79–81.

44. Emeriaud G, Beck J, Tucci M, et al. Diaphragm electrical activity during expiration in mechanically ventilated infants. Pediatr Res 2006;59(5):705–10.

45. Larouche A, Massicotte E, Constantin G, et al. Tonic diaphragmatic activity in critically ill children with and without ventilatory support. Pediatr Pulmonol 2015; 50(12):1304–12.

46. Baudin F, Wu H, Bordessoule A, et al. Impact of ventilatory modes on the breathing variability in mechanically ventilated infants. Front Pediatr 2014;25(2):13.

47. Ducharme-Crevier L, Du Pont-Thibodeau G, Emeriaud G. Interest of monitoring diaphragmatic electrical activity in the paediatric intensive care unit. Crit Care Res Pract 2013;2013:1–7.

48. Soukka H, Grönroos L, Leppäsalo J, et al. The effects of skin-to-skin care on the diaphragmatic electrical activity in preterm infants. Early Hum Dev 2014;90(9): 531–4.

49. Nasef N, El-Gouhary E, Schurr P, et al. High-flow nasal cannulae are associated with increased diaphragm activation compared with nasal continuous positive airway pressure in preterm infants. Acta Paediatr 2015;104(8):e337–43.

50. Stein HM, Firestone KS. NAVA ventilation in neonates: clinical guidelines and management strategies. Neonatology Today 2012;7(4):1–8.

51. Stein HM, Wilmoth J, Burton J. Electrical activity of the diaphragm in a small cohort of term neonates. Respir Care 2012;57(9):1483–7.

52. Barwing J, Ambold M, Linden N, et al. Evaluation of the catheter positioning for neurally adjusted ventilatory assist. Intensive Care Med 2009;35(10):1809–14.

High-Frequency Ventilation as a Mode of Noninvasive Respiratory Support

Amit Mukerji, MD, FRCP(C)[a],*, Michael Dunn, MD, FRCP(C)[b,c]

KEYWORDS

- Noninvasive high-frequency ventilation • Ventilator-induced lung injury
- Bronchopulmonary dysplasia • Nasal intermittent positive pressure ventilation
- Ventilation efficacy • Postextubation prophylaxis • Alveolar development

KEY POINTS

- In recent decades, use of noninvasive respiratory support in preterm neonates has increased in an effort to minimize ventilator-induced lung injury.
- A variety of noninvasive modes exist but despite extensive research, the optimal modality, interface, and settings remain unknown.
- Noninvasive high-frequency ventilation (NIHFV) is a relatively new mode that aims to combine the efficacy of high-frequency ventilation with the gentleness of noninvasive support.
- Current evidence suggests that NIHFV may be superior to other noninvasive modes in terms of supporting alveolar ventilation and preventing need for endotracheal mechanical ventilation.
- Large, adequately powered comparative trials are warranted to establish the superiority as well as indications, optimal settings, and safety of noninvasive high-frequency ventilation.

INTRODUCTION

The use of noninvasive respiratory support (NRS) in neonatal intensive care has increased in recent decades as a means to reduce ventilator-induced lung injury (VILI).[1–3] Various modes of NRS available and in common use include nasal continuous positive airway pressure (nCPAP), bilevel (or biphasic) nCPAP, nasal intermittent positive airway pressure (NIPPV), and heated humidified high flow nasal cannula.[2]

---

[a] Division of Neonatology, Department of Pediatrics, McMaster Children's Hospital, McMaster University, 1280 Main Street West, HSC-4F1E, Hamilton, Ontario L8S 4K1, Canada; [b] Department of Pediatrics, University of Toronto, Toronto, Ontario, Canada; [c] Department of Newborn and Developmental Pediatrics, Sunnybrook Health Sciences Centre, Room M4-222, 2075 Bayview Avenue, Toronto, Ontario M4N 3M5, Canada
* Corresponding author.
E-mail address: mukerji@mcmaster.ca

Clin Perinatol 43 (2016) 725–740
http://dx.doi.org/10.1016/j.clp.2016.07.008
0095-5108/16/© 2016 Elsevier Inc. All rights reserved.

A relatively new form of NRS gaining popularity is noninvasive high-frequency venti-lation (NIHFV).[4,5] This modality aims to combine the proficiency of high-frequency ventilation with the gentleness of NRS. Even though its clinical use was first described almost 2 decades ago,[6] evidence for its efficacy and safety in comparison to other NRS modes remains limited. In this article, we present the rationale for the use of NIHFV, review the existing evidence, and highlight key knowledge gaps that warrant further investigation.

NONINVASIVE RESPIRATORY SUPPORT

Endotracheal positive pressure ventilation (PPV) has been strongly implicated in the causation of VILI in preterm neonates.[7–11] Studies have revealed that endotracheal PPV is associated with a number of adverse outcomes, including bronchopulmonary dysplasia (BPD), subglottic stenosis, infection, and air leak syndromes.[12–15] These ob-servations have prompted a number of clinicians to move toward the preferential use of nCPAP as a primary mode of respiratory support.[3,16] Although it might be argued that the uptake has been slow and variable, it is now recommended that nCPAP be used whenever possible to minimize the exposure of preterm infants to the harmful ef-fects of endotracheal PPV.[17]

Although CPAP is very effective in stabilizing the compliant chest wall, splinting the upper airways, helping with the maintenance of FRC, and reducing work of breath-ing,[16,18] many preterm infants cannot be adequately maintained on nCPAP and require higher levels of support.[19] In some cases, this is a consequence of severe lung disease that necessitates intubation and mechanical ventilation, but in many cases, infants fail because their spontaneous respiratory drive is insufficient to provide adequate alveolar ventilation. Impending respiratory failure is often heralded by increasing oxygen requirements, increased work of breathing, increased frequency or severity of apneas, and CO_2 retention with respiratory acidosis.[20]

Rather than moving directly to intubation and mechanical ventilation in infants who are failing nCPAP, clinicians have used other methods of NRS in an attempt to enhance the level of support and thereby stabilize the infant.[21,22] Because all minute ventilation must be provided through the spontaneous efforts of an infant on nCPAP, noninvasive modes that can provide a degree of ventilation in addition to the stabiliz-ing effects of CPAP are desirable. Several have been developed and tested; in partic-ular, NIPPV and NIHFV show promise.[2,23,24]

NIPPV can be used as an alternative mode of primary NRS instead of nCPAP or as a mode to "rescue" infants failing nCPAP. Previous trials comparing use of NIPPV to nCPAP either as initial respiratory support or after extubation suggested superior-ity,[22,25,26] but a recent large multicentre randomized controlled trial did not show any benefit with use of NIPPV over nCPAP.[27] The use of traditional unsynchronized NIPPV to support tidal ventilation is limited because the timing and magnitude of deliv-ered breaths are unrelated to the baby's spontaneous efforts, leading to a large pro-portion of delivered breaths being ineffective.[21] This problem may be ameliorated by the application of newer ventilators with effective triggering in noninvasive modes. Noninvasive neurally adjusted ventilator assist for the delivery of synchronized and proportional NIPPV is highly promising and currently under investigation.[28] NIHFV has a theoretic advantage over NIPPV in that it does not depend on synchronization for effective ventilation.[24,29] In addition, it may be a more powerful ventilation tool, potentially making it a more effective noninvasive mode for rescue after nCPAP failure.

Avery and coworkers[30] published one of the first reports illustrating the possible benefits of liberal use of nCPAP rather than invasive mechanical ventilation. Clinicians from the center with the lowest rate of BPD avoided elective intubation and mechanical ventilation while using nCPAP produced by continuous gas flow to an underwater seal. Lee and colleagues[31] observed that the vigorous bubbling produced at the outlet with bubble CPAP led to noticeable vibration of the chests of treated infants. They found that low-amplitude airway oscillations were produced by the bubbling and that CO_2 elimination could be facilitated (**Fig. 1**). Although the relative advantages of bubble compared with other CPAP generators remains inconclusive,[32–34] this observation raised the possibility that HFV could be applied noninvasively and used to facilitate CO_2 removal in preterm neonates, especially if deliberately applied using ventilators designed to deliver HFV. More recently, bench, animal, and clinical studies using high-frequency ventilators have been done to assess the effectiveness of NIHFV.

HIGH-FREQUENCY VENTILATION

High-frequency ventilation (HFV) allows for adequate ventilation despite using tidal volumes below dead space. Several different devices have been used to deliver HFV, including those that deliver high-frequency oscillations, flow interrupters, or the Bunnell Life Pulse (Bunnell, Inc, Salt Lake City, UT) high-frequency jet ventilator.[35] Although there are some differences in the way each of these devices accomplishes effective gas exchange, mechanisms include convective transport of gases resulting from asymmetric velocity profiles during inspiration and expiration, pendelluft owing to inhomogeneity of time constants in neighboring alveoli, Taylor-type dispersion, cardiogenic mixing, and molecular diffusion in addition to direct alveolar ventilation by bulk convection as in conventional ventilation.[36,37] The use of low tidal volumes in combination with optimal continuous distending pressure results in minimization of both volutrauma and atelectrauma, thereby minimizing VILI.[38] Indeed, numerous animal studies have demonstrated the superiority of HFV over conventional ventilation with respect to short-term physiology, pressure exposure, and lung pathology. HFV has been shown to work at lower proximal airway pressures than conventional ventilation, reduce lung inflammatory markers, minimize oxygen exposure, and reduce VILI.[39–45]

In human trials with neonates, however, the use of HFV has not consistently resulted in improved clinical outcomes. A systematic review and metaanalysis from 2010 examining individual patient data from 10 randomized controlled trials failed to reveal an advantage to the use of elective HFV versus conventional ventilation with regards to mortality and/or BPD.[46] A more recent Cochrane review of elective HFV comprising 19 studies found no difference in mortality rates.[47] Although BPD rates were reduced with use of HFV, this was highly inconsistent across the studies, likely owing to differences in application of the method. Interestingly, a recent long-term follow-up study arising from 1 HFV trial suggests some benefit with regard to pulmonary outcome, even though there were no short-term benefits in the original study.[48] Despite the lack of apparent benefit in most trials and inconsistent results in synthesis of the evidence, HFV is considered a valuable mode of assisted ventilation and is often used clinically as a rescue mode when conventional ventilation has failed, or as the primary ventilation mode of choice as a lung protective strategy in units that are well-versed in its application.[49,50]

NONINVASIVE HIGH-FREQUENCY VENTILATION

The widespread adoption of HFV by many neonatologists accompanied by a renewed interest in the use of NRS has spawned interest in the possible application of NIHFV as

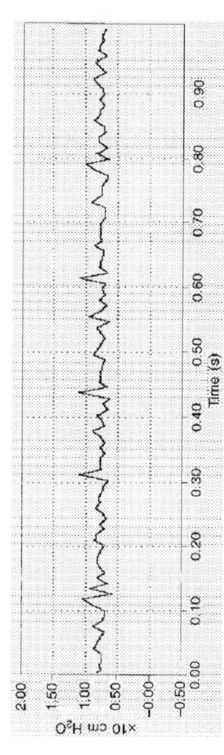

Fig. 1. Use of bubble continuous positive airway pressure producing a waveform at airway with an amplitude of 2 to 4 cm H_2O and frequency of approximately 15 to 30 Hz. (*Adapted from* Lee KS, Dunn MS, Fenwick M, et al. A comparison of underwater bubble continuous positive airway pressure with ventilator-derived continuous positive airway pressure in premature neonates ready for extubation. Biol Neonate 1998;73(2):69–75.)

a mode of respiratory support in neonates. Despite a paucity of data, this mode is being used by a considerable number of clinicians in Europe and elsewhere. In a recent survey by Fischer and colleagues,[4] clinicians at 30 of 172 (17%) European NICUs surveyed indicated that they used NIHFV, most frequently in premature infants who were failing on nCPAP. A recent survey of 28 Canadian NICUs revealed NIHFV use in 5 units (18%).[5] NIHFV is a mode of NRS that has considerable potential and a small number of investigators have examined the physiologic effects and clinical usefulness.

Bench and Animal Studies

De Luca and colleagues[51,52] tested the usefulness of NIHFV using a variety of parameters and interfaces in 2 bench studies. In both experimental setups, a closed system was created with short, soft binasal prongs of 2 different sizes (although with the same internal diameter), with a flow sensor juxtaposed between the prongs and an artificial lung. In the control setup, the ventilator tubing was connected directly to the lung (no interface). In the first study,[51] a range of frequencies was used and the 2 prong sets were compared with the control setup with regards to delivered tidal volume and pressure (measured in the distal lung). As compared with the open control circuit, there was a progressive decrease in tidal volume ($56.3 \pm 7.5\%$ and $26.1 \pm 4.8\%$) and lung pressure ($83.2 \pm 8.5\%$ and $78.9 \pm 9.4\%$) when moving from the larger to the smaller prongs, suggesting that significant dampening of the oscillations occurred especially with small diameter prongs. In their second study, inspiratory time and amplitude were varied.[52] The experimental circuits with the prongs achieved 83% of the tidal volume attained with the control circuit, while the oscillation pressure ratio ([oscillation] measured in the distal lung]/[oscillation in the proximal circuit]) was reduced to 40% of control value. This pattern was consistent for both inspiratory times (33% and 50%), and did not differ between the 2 nasal prongs. However, an inspiratory time of 50% led to significantly higher tidal volume compared with 33%.

In another bench study, Mukerji and colleagues[53] evaluated efficacy of NIHFV as it relates to CO_2 elimination from artificial lungs in comparison with CPAP and NIPPV. In contrast with the experimental setup of De Luca and coworkers, their model attempted to more closely mimic everyday clinical systems with the use of an anatomically appropriate mannequin with artificial lungs. An end-tidal CO_2 detector placed in the posterior pharynx was used to determine rate of CO_2 clearance after a fixed amount was infused directly into the lungs. NIHFV was much more effective in CO_2 elimination than either CPAP (no CO_2 clearance) or NIPPV (3 times lower), despite a significant decrease in measured pressure to the distal lung (**Fig. 2**).

A number of animal studies have evaluated the extended use of NIHFV. These challenging experiments were performed by using a "Lamb Intensive Care Unit" in which preterm lambs could be supported around the clock by trained attendants for prolonged periods of time. Null and colleagues[54] conducted a study on NIHFV (with superimposed positive pressure breaths) versus endotracheal ventilation in preterm lambs to assess efficacy of ventilation and oxygenation as well as alveolar development. At both 3 and 21 days, oxygen and ventilatory requirements to maintain predetermined Pao_2 and $Paco_2$ levels were significantly lower with NIHFV. In addition, the use of NIHFV was associated with improved alveolarization at both time points (**Fig. 3**). In the same preterm lamb model, Rehan and colleagues[55] compared 21 days of NIHFV versus endotracheal ventilation on alveolar parathyroid hormone-related protein-peroxisome proliferator-activated receptor-γ signaling, which is known to be critically important in alveolar formation. There was a decrease in key homeostatic alveolar epithelial–mesenchymal markers with endotracheal ventilation, whereas they were increased in the NIHFV group. Hadj-Ahmed and colleagues[56] studied the effect of NIHFV versus

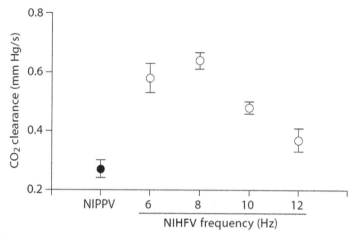

Fig. 2. Elimination of CO_2 was significantly greater with use of noninvasive high-frequency ventilation (NIHFV) as compared with nasal intermittent positive airway pressure (NIPPV), and appeared to be most effective at frequencies of 6 to 10 Hz. (*Adapted from* Mukerji A, Finelli M, Belik J. Nasal high-frequency oscillation for lung carbon dioxide clearance in the newborn. Neonatology 2013;103(3):161–5.)

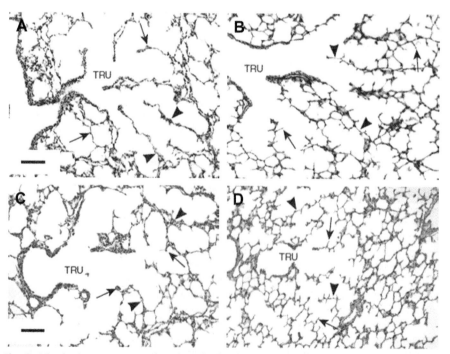

Fig. 3. Histologic appearance of preterm lambs show more uniform distal airspaces, thinner distal airspace walls (*arrowheads*), and more and thinner alveolar secondary septa (*arrows*) at terminal respiratory units (TRU) with noninvasive high-frequency ventilation versus endotracheal ventilation at 3 days (*B* vs *A*) and 21 days (*D* vs *C*). (*Adapted from* Null DM, Alvord J, Leavitt W, et al. High-frequency nasal ventilation for 21 d maintains gas exchange with lower respiratory pressures and promotes alveolarization in preterm lambs. Pediatr Res 2014;75(4):507–16.)

NIPPV on laryngeal muscle activity in newborn lambs. Increased glottal constriction was noted with increasing peak inspiratory pressures on NIPPV, an occurrence not observed with NIHFV. Interestingly, there were more episodes of central apnea (without overt hypocapnia) with the use of 4 Hz compared with 8 Hz on NIHFV, purported to be as a result of increase in vagal pulmonary stretch receptor activity (resulting from increased volumes), as well as increased thoracic wall afferent activity.

These bench and animal experiments, although limited in number, point to the feasibility of NIHFV use with evidence of effective and superior ventilation compared with other NRS modes. Data on improved alveolar development[54,55] with NIHFV compared with endotracheal ventilation are particularly intriguing. If replicated in future studies, this would provide strong physiologic rationale in favor of NIHFV use over endotracheal ventilation. It would also be interesting to evaluate alveolar growth and development with NIHFV compared with other NRS modes. A distinct advantage of NIHFV use is suggested by lack of glottis constriction, which is demonstrated with high peak pressures on NIPPV.[56] This phenomenon, along with asynchrony of breaths, may contribute to gastric distension during NIPPV use. Whether this is reduced with NIHFV at equivalent airway pressures is unknown, but merits investigation.

Clinical Evidence from Human Studies

The first clinical study (all results presented as median [20th–80th %ile]) of NIHFV use in human neonates was by van der Hoeven and colleagues.[6] In this observational study, 21 preterm and term neonates with a wide range of respiratory conditions managed with nCPAP of 6 cm H_2O (range, 5–7) were switched to NIHFV owing to CO_2 retention (16 infants) or increasing oxygen requirements (5 infants). The Infant Star ventilator (Infrasonics, San Diego, CA) was used to administer NIHFV. The mean airway pressure was raised as deemed necessary, the amplitude was adjusted to achieve visible chest vibrations, and frequency maintained at 10 Hz (**Table 1**). Fifteen infants were placed on NIHFV early in their course of respiratory illness at 17 hours (range, 2–36), with the remainder initiated at age 9 days (range, 6–21). The duration of NIHFV use in the 2 groups was 35 hours (range, 2–144) and 40 hours (range, 17–126), respectively. Only 5 patients (24%) were intubated after NIHFV use after 6.5 hours (range, 2–8.5). Arterial or capillary blood gases drawn before and after NIHFV initiation showed a decline in P_{CO_2} levels from 8.3 kPa (range, 7.4–9.1) to 7.2 kPa (range, 6.6–8.3).

Hoehn and colleagues[57] reported successful use of NIHFV in a 24 weeks' gestation male infant whose clinical course had been complicated by posthemorrhagic hydrocephalus and bowel perforation. On day 24 of life, he developed CO_2 retention after extubation from HFV to nCPAP. Given that the endotracheal mode was HFV, NIHFV was applied using a Babylog 8000 (Drager, Lubeck, Germany). Shortly after NIHFV initiation, the CO_2 level (measured transcutaneously after confirmation of calibration with arterial blood gas) decreased from 92 mm Hg to between 63 and 67 mm Hg. It remained in this range for 24 hours, after which nCPAP was resumed.

In 2008, Colaizy and colleagues[58] conducted an experimental study in which 14 preterm neonates on nCPAP with stable respiratory status were placed on NIHFV for 2 hours. NIHFV was delivered with an Infant Star ventilator (Mallinckrodt, St Louis, MO, USA). The mean airway pressure for NIHFV was chosen to be the same as the nasal CPAP pressure, the amplitude was adjusted to achieve visible neck or chest vibration and the frequency was fixed at 10 Hz (see **Table 1**). A number of physiologic parameters such as heart rate, respiratory rate, oxygen saturation and transcutaneous CO_2 levels were monitored during NIHFV use with provisions to discontinue if transcutaneous CO_2 levels reached either less than 30 torr or greater than 80 torr. After

Table 1
Summary of human studies on NIHFV

Author, Year	Population	Indication(s)	Interface	NIHFV Settings			Key Findings
				MAP (cm H_2O)	Amp (cm H_2O)	Freq (Hz)	
Van der Hoeven et al,[6] 1998	21 preterm and term infants with respiratory disease	CO_2 retention, increasing oxygen requirement	NPT	7 (6–8.6)[a]	37 (29–46)[a]	10	5 of 21 infants required intubation In a pre- and post-comparison, CO_2 levels decreased after NIHFV used
Hoehn & Krause,[57] 2000	1 preterm infant with CO_2 retention after extubation	CO_2 retention on nasal CPAP after extubation from HFV	NPT	7 (mbar)	100[f]	n/a	Decrease in CO_2 level after NIHFV initiation
Colaizy et al,[58] 2008	14 preterm infants with stable respiratory status on nCPAP	Experimental 2-h trial of NIHFV	NPT	5 (4–7)[b]	50 (29–30)[c]	10	Decrease in CO_2 levels after 2 h of NIHFV Downward trend in heart rate and no evidence of air trapping with NIHFV use
De La Roque et al,[59] 2011	40 term infants with TTN and low oxygen saturation	Experimental – randomized controlled trial (NIHFV vs nasal CPAP)	Heated, humidified nasal probe	5	33	5	Significantly reduced duration of TTN and level of oxygen supplementation with NIHFV

Study	Population	Indication	Interface	Freq	MAP	Amp	Outcomes
Czernik et al,[60] 2012	20 preterm infants at high risk of extubation failure	After extubation ("prophylactic")	NPT	8[d]	20[d]	10[d]	6 out of the 20 infants required reintubation CO_2 levels were statistically lower after 32 h of NIHFV use No side effects (air trapping or NEC) were reported
Mukerji et al,[62] 2015	52 preterm infants trialed on NIHFV on 79 occasions	"Rescue" after failure of another NRS mode or "prophylactic" after extubation	Short soft binasal prongs or nasal masks	8–24[e]	20–60[e] (20–100)[f]	6–14[e]	Prevention of intubation in the majority of patients with NIHFV use Decrease in spells, Fio_2 requirements and CO_2 levels after NIHFV use
Aktas et al,[61] 2016	3 preterm neonates	After extubation after previous extubation failures (n = 2) and avoidance of intubation after NIPPV (n = 1)	RAM cannula (NeoTECH)	9–13[e]	70–100[f]	n/a	2 out of the 3 cases were maintained on NRS after NIHFV use No consistent decline in CO_2 levels with NIHFV use

Abbreviations: Amp, amplitude; CPAP, continuous positive airway pressure; Fio_2, fraction of inspired oxygen; Freq, frequency; HFV, high-frequency ventilating; MAP, mean airway pressure; nCPAP, nasal continuous positive airway pressure; NEC, necrotizing enterocolitis; NIHFV, noninvasive high-frequency ventilation; NIPPV, nasal intermittent positive pressure ventilation; NRS, noninvasive respiratory support; TTN, transient tachypnea of the newborn.

[a] Median (20th–80th percentiles reported).
[b] Mean (range).
[c] Median (range).
[d] Starting parameters.
[e] Range.
[f] Amplitude in percent (on Babylog 8000).

2 hours, a capillary gas was drawn and patients resumed on nCPAP with prestudy settings. The level of capillary Pco_2 decreased from (mean) 50 torr to 45 torr ($P = .01$) with a concomitant rise in pH from 7.37 to 7.40 ($P = .04$) with NIHFV use (**Fig. 4**). There were no changes in respiratory rate or oxygen saturations during NIHFV use, but the heart rate showed a downward trend during NIHFV use (176 bpm before NIHFV to 166 2 hours after NIHFV; $P = .084$). A chest radiograph taken 1 hour after NIHFV showed no evidence of air trapping in any patient.

In the only published randomized trial to date, Dumas De La Roque and colleagues[59] randomized 46 term infants with transient tachypnea of the newborn to receive support with either NIHFV or nCPAP. NIHFV was delivered with a high-frequency percussive ventilator VDR3 (Percussionaire Corp, Sagle, ID). The airway pressures oscillated between 2 and 35 cm H_2O and the mean airway pressure and frequency were set (and unchanged) at 5 cm H_2O and 5 Hz, respectively. The duration of respiratory illness, as assessed by an independent unblinded observer, was decreased significantly in the NIHFV group (105 ± 20 minutes vs 377 ± 150 minutes; $P<.001$). Duration of oxygen supplementation was significantly decreased in the NIHFV group (6.3 ± 3.3 minutes vs 19.1 ± 8.1 minutes; $P<.001$) and the level of oxygen administration, defined as ([Fio_2 − 0.21]/time of O_2 therapy), was also lower with NIHFV (0.29 ± 0.16 min^{-1} vs 0.46 ± 0.50 min^{-1}; $P<.001$). None of the randomized patients required any escalation of respiratory support.

To prevent reintubation in a sequential cohort of 20 preterm infants (gestational age of <30 weeks) deemed to be at high risk of extubation failure, NIHFV was used "prophylactically" after extubation by Czernik and colleagues.[60] Most (19 of the 20) had a primary diagnosis of respiratory distress syndrome and hydrocortisone was given to 14 infants (70%) to facilitate extubation. The estimated high risk of extubation failure was based on a previous failed extubation (9 infants) or at least one of the after at time of extubation: mean airway pressure of greater than 8 cm H_2O on conventional mechanical ventilation or greater than 10 cm H_2O on HFV; Pco_2 of greater than 65 mm Hg or Fio_2 of greater than 0.4. A Leoni Plus (Heinen & Lowenstein, Bad Ems, Germany) ventilator was used for NIHFV. The initial parameters on NIHFV were as follows: mean airway pressure of 8 cm H_2O, amplitude of 20 cm H_2O, and frequency of 10 Hz. The median duration of NIHFV was 136.5 hours (range, 7.0–456.0). Six infants (30%) required reintubation; extubation success was higher among those without a previous failed extubation (91% vs 44%; $P = .0498$). There were no differences in SaO_2 and Pao_2 values before and after NIHFV initiation, but a significant decrease in $Paco_2$

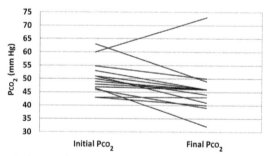

Fig. 4. Levels of CO_2 before and 2 hours after noninvasive high-frequency ventilation use in 14 stable preterm neonates. In 1 patient with am increase in CO_2 levels, the nasal tube was found to be plugged with secretions at the end of study period. (*Adapted from* Colaizy TT, Younis UM, Bell EF, et al. Nasal high-frequency ventilation for premature infants. Acta Paediatr 2008;97(11):1518–22.)

was noted at the 32-hour mark after NIHFV initiation (50.7 vs 59.8 mm Hg; $P<.01$). No side effects (air-trapping or necrotizing enterocolitis), feeding intolerance, or skin lesions were reported as a result of NIHFV use.

Aktas and colleagues[61] reported 3 cases, in 2 of which NIHFV was used after extubation and in the third after NIPPV to prevent intubation. NIHFV was delivered by a Babylog 8000 (Drager). One of the postextubation patients on NIHFV required reintubation owing to persistent apneas secondary to sepsis, whereas in the other case the patient was transitioned to another NRS mode without requiring reintubation. In the third case of NIHFV trial after NIPPV failure owing to increased work of breathing and oxygen requirements, intubation was prevented and the patient was transitioned after 42 hours to another NRS mode. A decline in P_{CO_2} levels was only noted (53, 47.5, and 45.7 mm Hg at 0, 4, and 24 hours, respectively) in one of the cases.

In the largest report of NIHFV use to date, Mukerji and colleagues[62] performed a retrospective review of NIHFV use in 4 large tertiary Canadian neonatal intensive care units between July 2010 and September 2012. During this period, 52 infants were placed on NIHFV on 79 occasions at a median postmenstrual age of 28 weeks (range, 24–46). The indications for NIHFV were "rescue" in 58 of 79 (73%) and postextubation "prophylaxis" in the remainder. The most common indication for "rescue" NIHFV was an increase in "spells"—defined as apneas, bradycardias, or desaturation episodes (31 cases, 39% of all NIHFV use). NIHFV was administered using the Babylog 8000, Drager VN 500 (both Drager) or Leoni Plus (Heinen &Lowenstein). There was a wide range of settings used, as shown in **Table 1**. Intubation was prevented in 58% of cases along with decreases in the following parameters after NIHFV initiation: "spells" (3.2 [0.4] to 1.2 [0.3] per hour), Fio_2 (48% [3] to 40% [2]), and CO_2 levels (74 mm Hg [6] to 62 mm Hg [4]). No adverse events attributable to NIHFV were reported.

These clinical studies have small sample sizes, are largely observational, and use a wide range of NIHFV ventilators, interfaces, and settings. Nevertheless, they do suggest that NIHFV is a feasible mode of NRS that may have superior ventilation capability compared with other NRS modes.[6,58,62] A few of the studies and cases described also suggest that NIHFV as a rescue mode after failure of other NRS modes may prevent need for endotracheal intubation and ventilation.[6,61,62] Finally, use of NIHFV as a postextubation prophylaxis mode has also shown promise in those infants deemed to be at a high risk of extubation failure in uncontrolled studies.[60] The only comparative randomized trial performed has been in term infants[59] and is thus not directly relevant to the population of preterm infants who are of most interest. The faster recovery from transient tachypnea of the newborn with NIHFV in this study is intriguing but because the study was unblinded, it is difficult to speculate to what extent the results are influenced by observer bias versus there being a true beneficial effect of NIHFV on disease pathophysiology. A pilot randomized controlled trial comparing NIHFV versus biphasic nCPAP in preterm infants after nCPAP failure (clinicantrials.gov: NCT02051491) has recently been completed at Mount Sinai Hospital, Toronto, and final data analysis and publication are awaited. Although the studies were not powered to clearly establish safety, none have reported any major short-term adverse effects related to NIHFV use. However, a recent survey of NIHFV use in 5 European countries reported abdominal distension, upper airway obstruction owing to secretions, and highly viscous secretions as commonly observed side effects,[4] but whether this relationship is directly causal is unclear.

RECOMMENDATIONS

Based on the limited literature available, routine and widespread use of NIHFV cannot be recommended. There are currently no data to support use of NIHFV as the primary

NRS mode for preterm infants with respiratory disease. However, NIHFV may be considered as a "rescue" mode after failure of other NRS modes to prevent intubation. It may also be considered "prophylactically" postextubation in specific cases where multiple previous extubations have failed, or when extubation is being performed from high pressures and settings on either high frequency or conventional ventilation. There are few data regarding optimal settings on NIHFV, but an initial mean airway pressure equal to or 1 to 2 cm H_2O above the previous NRS mode as needed would seem appropriate. The safe upper limit of mean airway pressure remains unknown. Most effective frequency seems to be 6 to 10 Hz and amplitude should be adjusted to achieve visible or palpable chest vibrations with close monitoring of oxygenation and ventilation. The choice of interfaces includes nasopharyngeal tubes, nasal masks, or short binasal prongs. At this time, there is not enough evidence to support use of nasal cannulas such as the RAM cannula with NIHFV. It is emphasized that all of these recommendations are derived largely from clinical experience and uncontrolled observational studies.

FUTURE DIRECTIONS

Despite suggestions that NIHFV may be a highly effective mode of NRS, significant knowledge gaps remain. Adequately powered comparative trials are needed to establish its superiority in preventing invasive mechanical ventilation compared with other NRS modes. Such trials may evaluate NIHFV versus other NRS modes as primary therapy of respiratory disease of prematurity, or as postextubation prophylaxis in a predefined high-risk population. Studies directly comparing NIPPV and NIHFV after failure of nCPAP failure are also needed. Such trials should comparatively evaluate effectiveness of NIHFV against other NRS modes, while also assessing short- and long-term safety. Further studies are also required to determine optimal settings and interfaces as well as choice of ventilator to provide NIHFV. In most cases, oscillators or flow interrupters have been used to deliver NIHFV and whether either is to be preferred is unclear. To date, no studies with noninvasive high-frequency jet ventilation have been published, although this mode of NIHFV may have considerable potential. Finally, a combined approach with NIPPV and NIHFV delivered together to achieve augmented CO_2 elimination and lung recruitment warrants further exploration.

SUMMARY

NIHFV holds promise as a mode of NRS, although current knowledge on its use in preterm neonates remains limited and is based on relatively few observational studies. Nevertheless, emerging evidence from bench, animal, and human studies suggests that HFV applied noninvasively retains ventilation efficacy while potentially reducing VILI and optimizing alveolar growth. By allowing for improved CO_2 elimination as compared with other NRS modes, NIHFV may allow spontaneously breathing infants to achieve physiologic blood gases with reduced work of breathing. It has been used to successfully prevent intubation in cases when other NRS modes failed, as well as successfully support infants without the need for invasive ventilation when used "prophylactically" in high-risk cases. However, whether this strategy confers any long-term advantages with respect to clinical outcomes in human neonates remains unknown. In addition, the long-term safety consequences of NIHFV such as brain injury and neurodevelopmental outcomes, particularly if used early in the course of a preterm neonate, are not known. Some oscillatory vibrations will be transmitted to the infant's head, and it is unclear as of yet whether this may have a negative impact on brain development or hearing.

REFERENCES

1. Bhandari V. The potential of non-invasive ventilation to decrease BPD. Semin Perinatol 2013;37(2):108–14.
2. Mahmoud RA, Roehr CC, Schmalisch G. Current methods of non-invasive ventilatory support for neonates. Paediatr Respir Rev 2011;12(3):196–205.
3. Roberts CL, Badgery-Parker T, Algert CS, et al. Trends in use of neonatal CPAP: a population-based study. BMC Pediatr 2011;11:89.
4. Fischer HS, Bohlin K, Buhrer C, et al. Nasal high-frequency oscillation ventilation in neonates: a survey in five European countries. Eur J Pediatr 2015;174(4): 465–71.
5. Mukerji A, Shah PS, Shivananda S, et al. Survey of non-invasive respiratory support practices in Canadian neonatal intensive care units. Pediatr Acad Societies 2016;1533:709.
6. van der Hoeven M, Brouwer E, Blanco CE. Nasal high frequency ventilation in neonates with moderate respiratory insufficiency. Arch Dis Child Fetal Neonatal Ed 1998;79(1):F61–3.
7. Wallace MJ, Probyn ME, Zahra VA, et al. Early biomarkers and potential mediators of ventilation-induced lung injury in very preterm lambs. Respir Res 2009; 10:19.
8. Ratner V, Sosunov SA, Niatsetskaya ZV, et al. Mechanical ventilation causes pulmonary mitochondrial dysfunction and delayed alveolarization in neonatal mice. Am J Respir Cell Mol Biol 2013;49(6):943–50.
9. Brew N, Hooper SB, Allison BJ, et al. Injury and repair in the very immature lung following brief mechanical ventilation. Am J Physiol Lung Cell Mol Physiol 2011; 301(6):L917–26.
10. Allison BJ, Crossley KJ, Flecknoe SJ, et al. Ventilation of the very immature lung in utero induces injury and BPD-like changes in lung structure in fetal sheep. Pediatr Res 2008;64(4):387–92.
11. Hillman NH, Polglase GR, Pillow JJ, et al. Inflammation and lung maturation from stretch injury in preterm fetal sheep. Am J Physiol Lung Cell Mol Physiol 2011; 300(2):L232–41.
12. Donn SM, Sinha SK. Minimising ventilator induced lung injury in preterm infants. Arch Dis Child Fetal Neonatal Ed 2006;91(3):F226–30.
13. Hart SM, McNair M, Gamsu HR, et al. Pulmonary interstitial emphysema in very low birthweight infants. Arch Dis Child 1983;58(8):612–5.
14. Fan E, Villar J, Slutsky AS. Novel approaches to minimize ventilator-induced lung injury. BMC Med 2013;11:85.
15. Ratner I, Whitfield J. Acquired subglottic stenosis in the very-low-birth-weight infant. Am J Dis Child 1983;137(1):40–3.
16. Diblasi RM. Nasal continuous positive airway pressure (CPAP) for the respiratory care of the newborn infant. Respir Care 2009;54(9):1209–35.
17. Schmolzer GM, Kumar M, Pichler G, et al. Non-invasive versus invasive respiratory support in preterm infants at birth: systematic review and meta-analysis. BMJ 2013;347:f5980.
18. Chowdhury O, Wedderburn CJ, Duffy D, et al. CPAP review. Eur J Pediatr 2012; 171(10):1441–8.
19. Finer NN, Carlo WA, Walsh MC, et al. Early CPAP versus surfactant in extremely preterm infants. N Engl J Med 2010;362(21):1970–9.
20. Ammari A, Suri M, Milisavljevic V, et al. Variables associated with the early failure of nasal CPAP in very low birth weight infants. J Pediatr 2005;147(3):341–7.

21. Bhandari V. Nasal intermittent positive pressure ventilation in the newborn: review of literature and evidence-based guidelines. J Perinatol 2010;30(8):505–12.

22. Meneses J, Bhandari V, Alves JG. Nasal intermittent positive-pressure ventilation vs nasal continuous positive airway pressure for preterm infants with respiratory distress syndrome: a systematic review and meta-analysis. Arch Pediatr Adolesc Med 2012;166(4):372–6.

23. Davis PG, Morley CJ, Owen LS. Non-invasive respiratory support of preterm neonates with respiratory distress: continuous positive airway pressure and nasal intermittent positive pressure ventilation. Semin Fetal Neonatal Med 2009;14(1): 14–20.

24. DiBlasi RM. Neonatal noninvasive ventilation techniques: do we really need to intubate? Respir Care 2011;56(9):1273–94 [discussion: 95–7].

25. Moretti C, Giannini L, Fassi C, et al. Nasal flow-synchronized intermittent positive pressure ventilation to facilitate weaning in very low-birthweight infants: unmasked randomized controlled trial. Pediatr Int 2008;50(1):85–91.

26. Tang S, Zhao J, Shen J, et al. Nasal intermittent positive pressure ventilation versus nasal continuous positive airway pressure in neonates: a systematic review and meta-analysis. Indian Pediatr 2013;50(4):371–6.

27. Kirpalani H, Millar D, Lemyre B, et al. A trial comparing noninvasive ventilation strategies in preterm infants. N Engl J Med 2013;369(7):611–20.

28. Stein H, Beck J, Dunn M. Non-invasive ventilation with neurally adjusted ventilatory assist in newborns. Semin Fetal Neonatal Med 2016;21(3):154–61.

29. Carlo WA. Should nasal high-frequency ventilation be used in preterm infants? Acta Paediatr 2008;97(11):1484–5.

30. Avery ME, Tooley WH, Keller JB, et al. Is chronic lung disease in low birth weight infants preventable? A survey of eight centers. Pediatrics 1987;79(1):26–30.

31. Lee KS, Dunn MS, Fenwick M, et al. A comparison of underwater bubble continuous positive airway pressure with ventilator-derived continuous positive airway pressure in premature neonates ready for extubation. Biol Neonate 1998;73(2): 69–75.

32. Morley CJ, Lau R, De Paoli A, et al. Nasal continuous positive airway pressure: does bubbling improve gas exchange? Arch Dis Child Fetal Neonatal Ed 2005; 90(4):F343–4.

33. Liptsen E, Aghai ZH, Pyon KH, et al. Work of breathing during nasal continuous positive airway pressure in preterm infants: a comparison of bubble vs variable-flow devices. J Perinatol 2005;25(7):453–8.

34. Courtney SE, Kahn DJ, Singh R, et al. Bubble and ventilator-derived nasal continuous positive airway pressure in premature infants: work of breathing and gas exchange. J Perinatol 2011;31(1):44–50.

35. Courtney SE, Asselin JM. High-frequency jet and oscillatory ventilation for neonates: which strategy and when? Respir Care Clin N Am 2006;12(3):453–67.

36. Chang HK, Harf A. High-frequency ventilation: a review. Respir Physiol 1984; 57(2):135–52.

37. Pillow JJ. High-frequency oscillatory ventilation: mechanisms of gas exchange and lung mechanics. Crit Care Med 2005;33(Suppl 3):S135–41.

38. Clark RH, Slutsky AS, Gerstmann DR. Lung protective strategies of ventilation in the neonate: what are they? Pediatrics 2000;105(1 Pt 1):112–4.

39. Thompson WK, Marchak BE, Froese AB, et al. High-frequency oscillation compared with standard ventilation in pulmonary injury model. J Appl Physiol Respir Environ Exerc Physiol 1982;52(3):543–8.

40. Hamilton PP, Onayemi A, Smyth JA, et al. Comparison of conventional and high-frequency ventilation: oxygenation and lung pathology. J Appl Physiol Respir Environ Exerc Physiol 1983;55(1 Pt 1):131–8.
41. Truog WE, Standaert TA, Murphy JH, et al. Effects of prolonged high-frequency oscillatory ventilation in premature primates with experimental hyaline membrane disease. Am Rev Respir Dis 1984;130(1):76–80.
42. Bell RE, Kuehl TJ, Coalson JJ, et al. High-frequency ventilation compared to conventional positive-pressure ventilation in the treatment of hyaline membrane disease in primates. Crit Care Med 1984;12(9):764–8.
43. Gerstmann DR, Fouke JM, Winter DC, et al. Proximal, tracheal, and alveolar pressures during high-frequency oscillatory ventilation in a normal rabbit model. Pediatr Res 1990;28(4):367–73.
44. Jackson JC, Truog WE, Standaert TA, et al. Reduction in lung injury after combined surfactant and high-frequency ventilation. Am J Respir Crit Care Med 1994;150(2):534–9.
45. Yoder BA, Siler-Khodr T, Winter VT, et al. High-frequency oscillatory ventilation: effects on lung function, mechanics, and airway cytokines in the immature baboon model for neonatal chronic lung disease. Am J Respir Crit Care Med 2000;162(5):1867–76.
46. Cools F, Askie LM, Offringa M, et al. Elective high-frequency oscillatory versus conventional ventilation in preterm infants: a systematic review and meta-analysis of individual patients' data. Lancet 2010;375(9731):2082–91.
47. Cools F, Offringa M, Askie LM. Elective high frequency oscillatory ventilation versus conventional ventilation for acute pulmonary dysfunction in preterm infants. Cochrane Database Syst Rev 2015;(3):CD000104.
48. Zivanovic S, Peacock J, Alcazar-Paris M, et al. Late outcomes of a randomized trial of high-frequency oscillation in neonates. N Engl J Med 2014;370(12):1121–30.
49. Salvo V, Zimmermann LJ, Gavilanes AW, et al. First intention high-frequency oscillatory and conventional mechanical ventilation in premature infants without antenatal glucocorticoid prophylaxis. Pediatr Crit Care Med 2012;13(1):72–9.
50. Rimensberger PC, Beghetti M, Hanquinet S, et al. First intention high-frequency oscillation with early lung volume optimization improves pulmonary outcome in very low birth weight infants with respiratory distress syndrome. Pediatrics 2000;105(6):1202–8.
51. De Luca D, Carnielli VP, Conti G, et al. Noninvasive high frequency oscillatory ventilation through nasal prongs: bench evaluation of efficacy and mechanics. Intensive Care Med 2010;36(12):2094–100.
52. De Luca D, Piastra M, Pietrini D, et al. Effect of amplitude and inspiratory time in a bench model of non-invasive HFOV through nasal prongs. Pediatr Pulmonol 2012;47(10):1012–8.
53. Mukerji A, Finelli M, Belik J. Nasal high-frequency oscillation for lung carbon dioxide clearance in the newborn. Neonatology 2013;103(3):161–5.
54. Null DM, Alvord J, Leavitt W, et al. High-frequency nasal ventilation for 21 d maintains gas exchange with lower respiratory pressures and promotes alveolarization in preterm lambs. Pediatr Res 2014;75(4):507–16.
55. Rehan VK, Fong J, Lee R, et al. Mechanism of reduced lung injury by high-frequency nasal ventilation in a preterm lamb model of neonatal chronic lung disease. Pediatr Res 2011;70(5):462–6.

56. Hadj-Ahmed MA, Samson N, Nadeau C, et al. Laryngeal muscle activity during nasal high-frequency oscillatory ventilation in nonsedated newborn lambs. Neonatology 2015;107(3):199–205.

57. Hoehn T, Krause MF. Effective elimination of carbon dioxide by nasopharyngeal high-frequency ventilation. Respir Med 2000;94(11):1132–4.

58. Colaizy TT, Younis UM, Bell EF, et al. Nasal high-frequency ventilation for premature infants. Acta Paediatr 2008;97(11):1518–22.

59. Dumas De La Roque E, Bertrand C, Tandonnet O, et al. Nasal high frequency percussive ventilation versus nasal continuous positive airway pressure in transient tachypnea of the newborn: a pilot randomized controlled trial (NCT00556738). Pediatr Pulmonol 2011;46(3):218–23.

60. Czernik C, Schmalisch G, Buhrer C, et al. Weaning of neonates from mechanical ventilation by use of nasopharyngeal high-frequency oscillatory ventilation: a preliminary study. J Matern Fetal Neonatal Med 2012;25(4):374–8.

61. Aktas S, Unal S, Aksu M, et al. Nasal HFOV with binasal cannula appears effective and feasible in ELBW newborns. J Trop Pediatr 2016;62(2):165–8.

62. Mukerji A, Singh B, Helou SE, et al. Use of noninvasive High-frequency ventilation in the neonatal intensive care unit: a retrospective review. Am J Perinatol 2015; 30(2):171–6.

Noninvasive Respiratory Support During Transportation

Donald Null Jr, MD[a],*, Kevin Crezee, BS, RRT-NPS[b],
Tamara Bleak, BSN, RN, MBA[c]

KEYWORDS

- Neonatal • Transport • Noninvasive • CPAP • High-flow nasal cannula
- High-frequency nasal ventilation • Nasal intermittent positive-pressure ventilation

KEY POINTS

- Noninvasive (NIV) techniques of neonatal respiratory support are increasing. Intubating all infants with significant respiratory distress for transport is no longer the only acceptable option.
- Determining the best technique requires more study. It is likely that many neonates can be transported on any of the NIV modes.
- Determining those infants who require a specific NIV mode is challenging.
- All transport teams need to collect and report data relevant to NIV transport experiences to assist in appropriate patient selection and NIV management to improve outcomes.

INTRODUCTION

During the past 10 to 15 years, there has been a steady increase in the use of noninvasive (NIV) respiratory support for all gestational age newborns.[1] This has been accomplished for multiple reasons, including (1) increased use of antenatal steroids; (2) high-risk maternal transfers to level 3 facilities; (3) surfactant replacement therapy[2]; (4) improved resuscitation protocols; and (5) improved knowledge, availability, and use of NIV modes. However, many newborns still require transfer to a higher level of care due to respiratory difficulties. Common reasons include respiratory distress syndrome (RDS), pneumonia, meconium aspiration, barotrauma, persistent pulmonary

[a] Division of Neonatology, Newborn ICU, Neonatal Transport, UC Davis Children's Hospital, 2516 Stockton Boulevard, Sacramento, CA 95817, USA; [b] Department of Medical Affairs, Mallinckrodt Pharmaceuticals, Perryville III Corporate Park, 53 Frontage Road, 3rd Floor, PO Box 9001, Hampton, NJ 08827-9001, USA; [c] Intermountain Life Flight Children's Services, 250 North 2370 West, Salt Lake City, UT 84116, USA
* Corresponding author.
E-mail address: dnull@ucdavis.edu

Clin Perinatol 43 (2016) 741–754
http://dx.doi.org/10.1016/j.clp.2016.07.009
0095-5108/16/© 2016 Elsevier Inc. All rights reserved.

perinatology.theclinics.com

hypertension, and surgical issues. In the past, neonates with respiratory insufficiency who required anything more than oxygen supplementation via a hood or low-flow (<2 liters per minute [Lpm]) nasal cannula were intubated for transport.[3] This article focuses on the modes and approaches to NIV that can be used during transport, as well as the appropriate inclusion and exclusion criteria for these patients.

The use of NIV in transport starts with a recognition of appropriate selection and exclusion criteria for which neonates might be safely and effectively transported, as shown in **Box 1**. Selection criteria are guidelines; one must look carefully at each neonate individually before proceeding with NIV transport. A high success rate with both short-term and long-term neonatal transport can be achieved with appropriate patient selection (see later discussion).

Box 1
Criteria for consideration of neonatal transport via noninvasive respiratory support

Inclusion criteria

1. Acute respiratory distress

2. Chronic lung disease

3. Stable on some form of NIV support for 2 or more hours

4. Chest radiograph for adequate lung expansion

5. Fio_2 50% or less stable or decreasing

6. Arterial P_{aco_2} less than 60 and stable

7. pH greater than 7.3 and stable

8. Transport team comfortable with patient status

Exclusion criteria

1. Pulmonary hypertension unresponsive to nitric oxide

2. Poor lung expansion on upper levels of NIV support
   a. HFNC 6 Lpm or greater
   b. CPAP 8 cm of water (cm H_2O) or greater
   c. NIPPV rate greater than 20 and/or PIP greater than 20 cm H_2O and/or PEEP greater than 7 cm H_2O
   d. HFNV positive airway pressure greater than 8 cm H_2O

3. Persistent apnea

4. Sepsis with poor cardiac output

5. Surgical problems
   a. Diaphragmatic hernia
   b. Tracheoesophageal fistula
   c. Bowel obstruction
   d. Necrotizing enterocolitis
   e. Gastroschisis
   f. Omphalocele

6. Significant acidosis
   a. Respiratory: pH less than 7.25 and/or $Paco_2$ greater than 60 mm Hg
   b. Metabolic: pH less than 7.20 and base deficit greater than −10 mEq/dL

7. Transport team is uncomfortable moving the patient on a NIV technique

Abbreviations: CPAP, continuous positive airway pressure; Fio_2, fraction of inspired oxygen; HFNC, high-flow nasal cannula; HFNV, high-frequency nasal ventilation; NIPPV, nasal intermittent positive pressure ventilation; PEEP, positive end-expiratory pressure; PIP, peak inspiratory pressure.

Before transporting neonates on any NIV mode, a few simple clinical assessments are required to minimize potential failure of NIV during transport and to assess for potential complications en route (**Box 2**). It is important to remember that during transport there is a significant loss of the ability to assess the patient, determine if and what caused any deterioration, as well as to assess the response to any intervention made by the transport team. Intubation before transport is always preferable to during transport.

There are now multiple approaches available for NIV support of the neonate (**Box 3**).

HIGH-FLOW NASAL CANNULA

This technique has gained popularity due to its ease of application, decrease in nasal injury, success in reducing need for invasive ventilation and recently reported comparability to nasal continuous positive airway pressure (CPAP) for postextubation support of neonates[4–7] (**Table 1**). Limited data are available for high-flow nasal cannula (HFNC) support during transport. Two reports have documented the use of HFNC in neonates and infants or pediatric patients. In a brief commentary, Boyle and colleagues[8] reported on the successful interhospital transport of 31 neonates (gestational ages 28–43 weeks) in England. In a larger retrospective study, Schlapbach and colleagues[9] reported on the impact of allowing HFNC during pediatric transport. They reported a 4-fold increase in the use of NIV support (from 7% of patients to 33%) following the incorporation of HFNC as a NIV transport mode. The importance of patient selection was highlighted in that none of the 150 patients transported on HFNC required intubation during transport over distances as long as 465 miles and times as long as 4 hours. Commonly available systems for supporting HFNC in infants and neonates are shown in **Table 1**. For interhospital transport, the authors typically use the Neo-Pod T system coupled with the Lava Bed for humidification (**Fig. 1**).

NASAL CONTINUOUS POSITIVE AIRWAY PRESSURE

CPAP for neonates with RDS was introduced by Gregory and colleagues[10] in 1971. Over the past 1 to 2 decades there has been a marked resurgence in the use of nasal CPAP as a NIV technique of respiratory support in neonates. It is the oldest and best studied of the available NIV modes.[11,12] There are several retrospective reports

---

Box 2
Pretransport assessments to consider before attempted noninvasive respiratory transport of neonates with respiratory insufficiency

Pretransport assessment

1. Breath sounds, breathing rate, depth of respiration, retractions

2. Positions of palpable edge of liver at right costal margin

3. Recovery of oxygen saturation after brief loss of NIV support

4. Stability of patient during repositioning, suctioning, and examining

5. If changing or starting NIV technique
   a. Wait minimum of 30 minutes to access stability
   b. Obtain chest radiograph to assess lung expansion
   c. Measure blood gas before departure

Box 3
Currently available approaches to noninvasive respiratory support that may be applicable to neonatal transport

Techniques of NIV ventilation

1. Oxyhood
2. Oxygen delivered into isolette
3. Nasal cannula less than 2 Lpm
4. Heated humidified high-flow nasal cannula ≥2 Lpm
5. Nasal CPAP
6. Nasal intermittent positive-pressure ventilation
7. High-frequency nasal ventilation

---

regarding neonatal transport with nasal CPAP.[13–16] The 2 largest reports are from Australia and demonstrate increasing successful use of nasal CPAP for the transport of ill neonates, with minimal evidence for intratransport risk with appropriate pretransport assessment.[15,16] Common approaches to nasal CPAP, and potential benefits and risks, are noted in **Table 2**. Of these, interhospital transport is feasible primarily using the transport ventilator. Appropriate sizing of the nasal prongs is necessary to optimize pressure delivery while minimizing injury to the nares (**Table 3**).

NASAL INTERMITTENT POSITIVE PRESSURE VENTILATION

Although controversial, some studies suggest that the addition of intermittent positive-pressure breaths added to nasal CPAP may improve overall ventilation and/or oxygenation, especially in very preterm neonates with apnea.[17–21] It is possible to incorporate NIV during neonatal transport but, to date, there are no published reports describing this approach.

HIGH-FREQUENCY NASAL VENTILATION

High-frequency pulsations with variable rate and amplitude can be delivered nasally. This NIV mode has been described in several clinical reports as a means of improving oxygenation and ventilation in neonates with more severe lung disease and/or with significant apnea.[22–27] Varieties of ventilators are capable of providing high-frequency

---

Table 1
Systems for delivering heated humidified high-flow nasal cannula therapy to infants and neonates

High-Flow Nasal Cannula Delivery Systems				
Devices	Cannula	Flow Rates	Benefits	Risks
Fisher & Paykel Vapotherm Neo Pod T w/Lava Bed	Preterm, neonatal or infant Westmed NC (has pressure relief valve at 21 cm H_2O)	2–8 Lpm	Proper gas humidification Easy to use Well-tolerated Supports gas exchange	May not support significant apnea Pressure related injury with too large nasal cannula

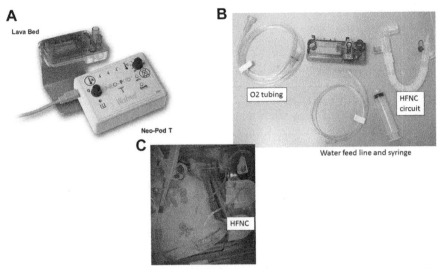

Fig. 1. (*A*) Neo-Pod T power controller with on-off control, temperature setting controller, and alarms silence. The controller provides 12 V power to the Lava Bed for production of heat. The heater adds to the heat that is provided externally by the isolette. The HFNC or high-frequency nasal ventilation circuit is attached to the Lava Bed to allow gas to wick heated moisture from the absorbent material. (*B*) The components of the transport HFNC system. (*C*) The connection of the HFNC to the circuit.

nasal ventilation (HFNV) (**Table 4**). The authors have primarily used the Percussionaire Bronchotron (Percussionaire Inc, Sandy Point, ID, USA) for HFNV during neonatal transport (**Fig. 2**). An integral component to using the Bronchotron for NIV respiratory support is the combination of the Turbohub with the Phasitron (**Fig. 3**). Demographic features of 64 infants transported via Bronchotron HFNV over the past 3 years are shown in **Table 5**. Of note, many of these infants were very preterm and HFNV was safely and effectively provided over long distances and times. The approach to setting up the Bronchotron for neonatal transport to support HFNV is as follows:

HFNV: Bronchotron set-up
  1. Attach circuit to ventilator
     a. White tubing to white port on vent
     b. Red tubing to filter, then to red port on vent (see **Fig. 2**B; **Figs. 4**, and **5A**)
     c. Green tubing to green port if on vent, or to flowmeter at 2 Lpm if not on vent

Table 2			
Commonly used neonatal nasal continuous positive airway pressure delivery systems			
		CPAP	
Device	**Delivery Cannula**	**Benefits**	**Risks**
Flow Driver	Binasal prongs	Measured delivery pressure	Nasal injury
Bubble	RAM cannula	Reduces apnea	Air leak
Ventilator	Nasal mask	Maintains lung volume	
	Single NP/ETT	Reduces need for intubation	

Abbreviations: ETT, endotracheal tube; NP, nasopharyngeal.

Table 3
Binasal Hudson nasal cannula sizing chart

Hudson CPAP Cannula Sizing Chart	
Weight Range	Suggested Cannula Size
<700 g	0
700 to 1250 g	1
1250 to 2000 g	2
2000 to 3000 g	3
Over 3000 g	4
1–2 y of age	5

Nasal prongs: align to fill the nares space. General rule is to use largest prongs size that comfortably fills the nares. If the prong goes all the way in to the nares like a nasal cannula, it is too small.

2. Check Turbohub for red control valve, spring, and white cap (see **Fig. 4**)
   a. Attach white to white
   b. Attach green to green
   c. Attach 2 lengths of corrugated tubing
   d. Attach 500 mL reservoir bag
3. Place Turbohub in bracket and gently secure with clamp (**Fig. 5B**)
4. Assemble infant disposable circuit
5. Attach disposable circuit to Turbohub and heater with circuit provided from Turbohub to humidifier (**Fig. 6**)
6. Attach temperature probes or heated wire cables to circuit
7. Attach other end of green filter to disposable circuit pressure line
8. Measure; select and secure appropriate bonnet on infant head, as needed
9. Select appropriate sized nasal prong interface (eg, Hudson, Drager, RAM)
10. Attach via tapered adaptors to vent circuit
11. Initial ventilator settings (**Fig. 7**)
    a. Working pressure (pounds per square inch) at 40
    b. High flow rate at 350 to 400
    c. Maximize oscillatory CPAP and expiratory time (E-time)
    d. Minimize inspiratory time (I-time) and pulsatile flow

Table 4
High-frequency ventilators with potential for providing noninvasive high-frequency nasal ventilation

High-frequency Nasal Ventilation			
Delivery Device	Cannulas	Benefits	Risks
Bronchotron	Binasal prongs	Supports apneic infants	Potential for air leak
Bunnell Life Pulse Jet	Single NP/ETT	Recruit lung volumes	Potential nasal trauma
SensorMedics 3100A	RAM NC[a,b]	Improve ventilation	Lung overinflation
Drager VN500[a]		Improve oxygenation	
Leoni Plus[a]		Prevents laryngeal	
Stephanie/Sophie[a]		constriction	

Abbreviations: ETT, endotracheal tube; NC, nasal cannula; NP, nasopharyngeal.
[a] Not approved in United States for high-frequency ventilation.
[b] Not approved in United States for nasal CPAP or NIMV.

A   B

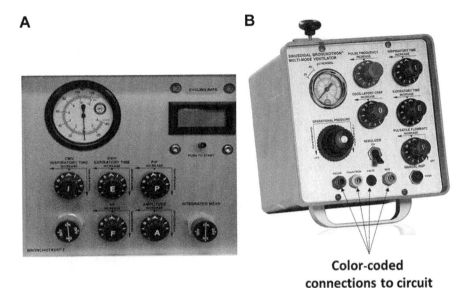

**Color-coded
connections to circuit**

Fig. 2. (*A*) The Bronchotron I that is built in to a transport isolette and provides time-cycled, pressure-limited conventional ventilation or high-frequency ventilation (HFV). The lower level of controls is used for HFNV. Controls from left to right: mode selector for CV or HFV, high frequency (HF) rate controller and amplitude controller used for adjusting CPAP and amplitude for HFNV. (*B*) Sinusoidal Bronchotron (SB) ventilator that can be used for invasive or NIV ventilation. The SB provides HF at 2 pressure levels with 2 different rates similar to NIMV (nasal intermittent mandatory ventilation) with an HFV overlay. The Oscillary CPAP controller is primarily used for controlling CPAP and amplitude during HFNV.

    e. Adjust fraction of inspired oxygen (Fio$_2$) to targeted arterial oxygen saturation (SpO$_2$)

    f. Increase I-time and pulsatile flow, and decrease E-time to achieve target CPAP

    g. Monitor SpO$_2$ and transcutaneous carbon dioxide (TcCO$_2$)

12. Turn on humidifier (allow the humidifier to heat up before placing on patient)
13. Verify CPAP level
14. Place prongs on patient; ensure prongs are correctly fit and positioned
15. Evaluate patient, CPAP level, breath sounds, and chest rise or bounce (not required to be present); increase settings as needed to achieve ordered mean airway pressure or CPAP (see **Fig. 7**)
16. Obtain arterial blood gas (ABG) capillary blood gas (CBG) per transport or unit policy
17. Trend and document patient assessments, TcCO$_2$, SpO$_2$, ventilator settings, and so forth.

PULMONARY HYPERTENSION

Persistent pulmonary hypertension of the newborn (PPHN) is a common problem seen in all gestational age infants with respiratory distress. Echocardiograms are frequently not available for patients being transported. Preductal SpO$_2$ greater than 5% higher than postductal SpO$_2$ suggests probable underlying PPHN. Clinically, a patient who desaturates when being handled and slowly recovers (minute to minutes) may have a component of PPHN. Nitric oxide can be used with any of the NIV techniques

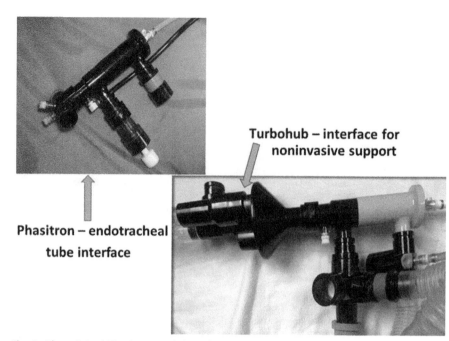

Turbohub – interface for noninvasive support

Phasitron – endotracheal tube interface

Fig. 3. The original Phasitron on left is the basis for the Turbohub Phasitron on the right. The addition of the reversed cone introduces a 1-way valve system that directs the flow from the ventilator in 1 direction out and 1 direction in, allowing use of a humidifier and a regular ventilator type circuit. A small pinhole in the bottom of the cone prevents condensate from building up in the cone and introduces a constant leak to maintain flushing of mixed gas in the cone. The base Phasitron with hub adapters are glued at the factory versus the traditional Phasitron that requires assembly.

previously discussed and most NIV systems have been validated for use with the INO-max DS_{IR} (Mallinckrodt Pharmaceuticals, Derbyshire, UK).

MONITORING DURING TRANSPORT

Due to the ease with which pressure support may be temporarily lost, NIV respiratory support modes are inherently less stable than invasive mechanical ventilation. Thus, the authors recommend aggressive application of appropriate monitoring tools to facilitate the safe transport of these infants (**Box 4**). In particular, the authors strongly recommend the use of both preductal and postductal SpO_2 monitoring for those infants at risk of or diagnosed with pulmonary hypertension, as well as the application of $TcCO_2$ monitoring for all infants.[28] In our experience providing NIV support over long distances and times, the authors have found the $TcCO_2$ monitoring to be very helpful as a tool to minimize problems with hypercapnia or hypocapnia (**Table 6**).

ALTITUDE

During air transport (or ground transport in mountains) adjusting NIV support may be needed due to increases in lung volumes or abdominal gas volumes (**Table 7**). Appropriate adjustments are critical for infants with underlying thoracic or abdominal problems such as diaphragmatic hernia, bowel obstruction or pneumoperitoneum, pneumothorax, or relative increased lung volumes.

Table 5
Patients managed on high-frequency nasal ventilation during transport

Total Number	64
Gestation at birth (wk)	
<28	15
28–35	15
>36	25
Undocumented	9
Birth weight (g)	
<1500	16
1500–1999	3
2000–4800	40
Undocumented	5
Postnatal age	1–160 d
Duration of transport	1->3 h
CPAP pressure (cmH$_2$O) (10%–90%)	4–10 5–8
Lowest SpO$_2$ in transport, noncardiac	86%
Nitric oxide	3
Complications	None
Unable to convert to HFNV	1

Data from Intermountain Health Care neonatal transport service.

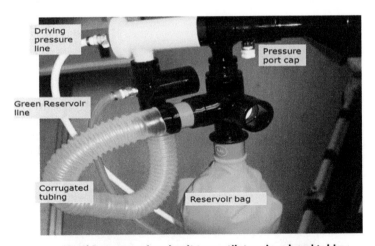

Driving pressure line

Pressure port cap

Green Reservoir line

Corrugated tubing

Reservoir bag

Attaching percussive circuit to ventilator via colored tubing

Fig. 4. The Turbohub Phasitron with attached ventilator connecting lines and spontaneous breathing reservoir system. The high pressure burst is delivered through the white driving pressure line to the sliding Venturi valve. Green gas line provides fresh gas flow to support spontaneous breathing and provides gas mixed at the set oxygen concentration (Fio$_2$) to the sliding Venturi system if entrainment occurs. The reservoir reduces the possibility that the Fio$_2$ delivered to the patient will be diluted with room air.

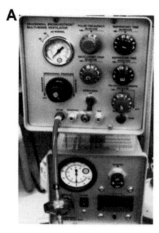

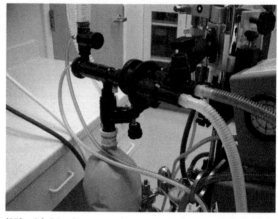

A

B   **Completed ventilator-percussive circuit**

**Red to filter, then to red
pressure gauge on vent**

Fig. 5. (*A*) Sinusoidal Bronchotron (SB) with Monitron monitor mounted to a transport pole. The red line is attached to the hydrophobic filter, then the patient vent circuit pressure line. The pressure is displayed on the monitor below, along with high-frequency rate. A battery-operated disconnect alarm is built in to the monitor. (*B*) Fully assembled Turbohub Phasitron attached to the SB. The blue corrugated vent circuit line is the gas outlet to the humidifier and the white corrugated vent circuit line returns exhaled gas from the patient.

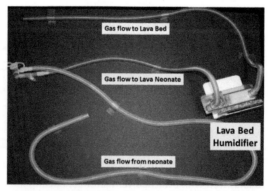

Fig. 6. The transport patient ventilator circuit with a Lava Bed humidifier. Gas is delivered to the patient through the blue tubing and humidifier to the patient wye connector. The wye connector can be removed for NIV and replaced with appropriately sized nasal prongs. Exhaled gas is returned to the Turbohub Phasitron through the white corrugated vent tubing.

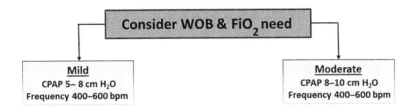

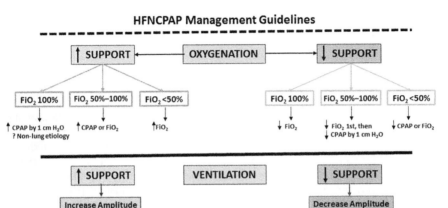

Fig. 7. An example of an HFNV transport management algorithm used with the Bronchron I ventilator where the level of CPAP also determines the level of amplitude provided to the NIV interface. HFNCPAP, high-flow nasal continuous positive airway pressure; WOB, work of breathing.

Box 4
Suggested options for monitoring during transport of neonates supported by noninvasive respiratory techniques

Monitoring During Transport on NIV

1. Preductal and postductal SpO2
2. Invasive blood pressure, except for minimally supported patients
3. TcCO$_2$ monitor
4. Central or 2 peripheral intravenous line preferable
5. Heart rate and respiratory rate
6. Ability to perform laboratory studies, especially blood gas, glucose, and electrolytes
7. Pretransport and intratransport physical examination

Table 6
Paired sample comparison of in transport measurements of transcutaneous and arterial measurements of carbon dioxide

Number Samples = 23	TcO$_2$	Paco$_2$
Mean (all values mm Hg)	51	52
Standard deviation	11	11
Minimum	29	32
Maximum	74	70

Table 7	
Increase in gas volume with change in altitude	
Altitude (feet)	Relative Gas Volume
Sea level	1.00
5000	1.20
8000	1.35
10,000	1.45
20,000	2.20

SUMMARY

NIV ventilation continues to expand as a primary support for neonatal patients with various respiratory disorders during the past 15 years. It has now become necessary for transport teams to be able to move patients on various modes of NIV support. It is important that both inclusion and exclusion criteria are developed to ensure safe as well as effective neonatal transport. Understanding the utility of specific modes of NIV support for various pulmonary pathophysiology is paramount to success during transport. The transport environment is not stable. Infants who do well in a neonatal ICU on NIV may not do as well while being transported. Transport personnel must be trained to determine at the bedside if a neonate can be safely and effectively transported on NIV; they are better suited for this role than the accepting physician. During transport, every issue is more difficult: from physical examination, to intubation, to determining why an infant is not doing well, to deciding if the treatment has actually helped the problem. Appropriate patient management revolves around risks and benefits. Because NIV carries less risk in the neonatal intensive care unit (NICU) does not mean for a given infant it will be less risky in the transport environment. Significant ongoing efforts are needed to safely determine who, how, when, and why any particular infant should be transported with NIV. In the NICU, a single specific approach to NIV does not suit all patients and that will also be true in the transport arena.

Best practices

Current practice

Term, late preterm, and preterm infants with respiratory distress have been transported on all modes of NIV ventilation. These patients tend to be grouped as
1. Newborns with acute respiratory problems
2. Previous preterm infants with chronic lung disease being managed on NIV respiratory support and previous preterm infants being back transported.

Best practice

Proper selection of patients for using an acceptable NIV mode to avoid intubation.

Patients who have not been stable on an NIV mode should be excluded.

If it is necessary to change NIV mode, an observation period to document stability is required.

Transport team must be knowledgeable on the modes of NIV and the risks and benefits of NIV.

Care path objective

To safely and effectively transport neonates with respiratory difficulties, avoiding intubation, invasive ventilation, and complications associated with NIV should reduce the risk of lung injury to such infants. Transport teams need to develop protocols for using NIV during transport and become skilled with the various techniques.

Major recommendation

1. Develop appropriate inclusion and exclusion criteria for transporting patients on NIV.
2. Develop skills with the various NIV techniques, especially their strengths and weaknesses.
3. Have appropriate monitoring techniques in place for these patients.
4. Practice scenarios of how to assess and manage sudden clinical decompensation.

Strength of Evidence

Fair

Summary

NIV techniques of neonatal respiratory support are increasing. Intubating all infants with significant respiratory distress for transport is no longer the only acceptable option. Determining the best technique requires more study. It is likely that many neonates can be transported on any of the NIV modes. Determining those infants that requires a specific NIV mode will be challenging. Clinicians may often learn more from the patient who fails a treatment than those successfully treated. All transport teams need to collect and report data relevant to NIV transport experiences to assist in appropriate patient selection and NIV management to improve outcomes.

Data from Refs.[8,13–16,23]

REFERENCES

1. Schmölzer GM, Kumar M, Pichler G, et al. Non-invasive versus invasive respiratory support in preterm infants at birth: systematic review and meta-analysis. BMJ 2013;347:f5980.
2. Polin RA, Carlo WA. Committee on Fetus and Newborn; American Academy of Pediatrics. Surfactant replacement therapy for preterm and term neonates with respiratory distress. Pediatrics 2014;133(1):156–63.
3. Fenton AC, Leslie A, Skeoch CH. Optimising neonatal transfer. Arch Dis Child Fetal Neonatal Ed 2004;89(3):F215–9.
4. Holleman-Duray D, Kaupie D, Weiss MG. Heated humidified high-flow nasal cannula: use and a neonatal early extubation protocol. J Perinatol 2007;27(12):776–81.
5. Collins CL, Holberton JR, Barfield C, et al. A randomized controlled trial to compare heated humidified high-flow nasal cannulae with nasal continuous positive airway pressure postextubation in premature infants. J Pediatr 2013;162:949–54.
6. Yoder BA, Stoddard RA, Li M, et al. Heated, humidified high-flow nasal cannula versus nasal CPAP for respiratory support in neonates. Pediatrics 2013;131:e1482–90.
7. Manley BJ, Owen LS, Doyle LW, et al. High-flow nasal cannulae in very preterm infants after extubation. N Engl J Med 2013;369:1425–33.
8. Boyle M, Chaudhary R, Kent S, et al. High-flow nasal cannula on transport: moving with the times. Acta Paediatr 2014;103:e181.
9. Schlapbach LJ, Schaefer J, Brady AM, et al. High-flow nasal cannula (HFNC) support in interhospital transport of critically ill children. Intensive Care Med 2014;40(4):592–9.
10. Gregory GA, Kitterman JA, Phibbs RH, et al. Treatment of the idiopathic respiratory-distress syndrome with continuous positive airway pressure. N Engl J Med 1971;284(24):1333–40.

11. Speidel B, Dunn P. Effect of continuous positive airway pressure on breathing pattern of infants with respiratory-distress syndrome. Lancet 1975;305(7902): 302–4.

12. Morley CJ, Davis PG, Doyle LW, et al. Nasal CPAP or intubation at birth for very preterm infants. N Engl J Med 2008;358(7):700–8.

13. Simpson J, Ahmed I, McLaren J, et al. Use of nasal continuous positive airway pressure during neonatal transfer. Arch Dis Child Fetal Neonatal Ed 2004;89(4): F374.

14. Bomont RK, Cheema IU. Use of nasal continuous positive airway pressure during neonatal transfers. Arch Dis Child Fetal Neonatal Ed 2006;91(2):F85–9.

15. Murray PG, Stewart MJ. Use of nasal continuous positive airway pressure during retrieval of neonates with acute respiratory distress. Pediatrics 2008;121(4): e754–8.

16. Resnick S, Sokol J. Impact of introducing binasal continuous positive airway pressure for acute respiratory distress in newborns during retrieval: experience from Western Australia. J Paediatr Child Health 2010;46(12):754–9.

17. Owen LS, Morley CJ, Davis PG. Pressure variation during ventilator generated nasal intermittent positive pressure ventilation in preterm infants. Arch Dis Child Fetal Neonatal Ed 2010;95(5):F359–64.

18. Salvo V, Lista G, Lupo E, et al. Noninvasive ventilation strategies for early treatment of RDS in preterm infants: an RCT. Pediatrics 2015;135(3):444–51.

19. Silveira CST, Leonardi KM, Melo AP, et al. Response of preterm infants to 2 noninvasive ventilatory support systems: nasal CPAP and nasal intermittent positive-pressure ventilation. Respir Care 2015;60(12):1772–6.

20. Owen LS, Manley BJ. Nasal intermittent positive pressure ventilation in preterm infants: equipment, evidence, and synchronization. Semin Fetal Neonatal Med 2016;21(3):146–53.

21. Davis PG, Lemyre B, De Paoli AG. Nasal intermittent positive pressure ventilation (NIPPV) versus nasal continuous positive airway pressure (NCPAP) for preterm neonates after extubation. Cochrane Database Syst Rev 2014;(9):CD003212.

22. Yoder BA, Albertine KH, Null DM. High-frequency ventilation for non-invasive respiratory support of neonates. Semin Fetal Neonatal Med 2016;21(3):162–73.

23. van der Hoeven M, Brouwer E, Blanco CE. Nasal high frequency ventilation in neonates with moderate respiratory insufficiency. Arch Dis Child Fetal Neonatal Ed 1998;79(1):F61–3.

24. Mukerji A, Singh B, Helou SE, et al. Use of noninvasive high-frequency ventilation in the neonatal intensive care unit: a retrospective review. Am J Perinatol 2015; 30(2):171–6.

25. Fischer HS, Bohlin K, Bührer C, et al. Nasal high-frequency oscillation ventilation in neonates: a survey in five European countries. Eur J Pediatr 2015;174(4): 465–71.

26. Hadj-Ahmed MA, Samson N, Nadeau C, et al. Laryngeal muscle activity during nasal high-frequency oscillatory ventilation in nonsedated newborn lambs. Neonatology 2015;107(3):199–205.

27. Null DM, Alvord J, Leavitt W, et al. High-frequency nasal ventilation for 21 d maintains gas exchange with lower respiratory pressures and promotes alveolarization in preterm lambs. Pediatr Res 2013;75(4):507–16.

28. O'Connor TA, Grueber R. Transcutaneous measurement of carbon dioxide tension during long-distance transport of neonates receiving mechanical ventilation. J Perinatol 1997;18(3):189–92.

Minimally Invasive Surfactant Therapy and Noninvasive Respiratory Support

CrossMark

Angela Kribs, MD

KEYWORDS

- Continuous positive airway pressure • Minimally invasive surfactant therapy
- Less invasive surfactant therapy • Respiratory distress syndrome • Preterm infant

KEY POINTS

- CPAP and mechanical ventilation with surfactant application are efficacious therapies of RDS.
- Use of noninvasive modes of respiratory support is recommended as primary therapy in RDS of premature infants.
- Several strategies of minimally invasive surfactant therapy (MIST) to combine the advantages of noninvasive respiratory support and of surfactant therapy have been reported.
- Available data suggest that these strategies may reduce the need for mechanical ventilation and improve outcome of preterm infants under certain conditions.
- Research is still needed to define the conditions for adequate use of MIST.

INTRODUCTION

Respiratory distress syndrome (RDS) caused by surfactant deficiency remains one of the major reasons of neonatal mortality and short- and long-term morbidity in preterm infants. Use of noninvasive modes of respiratory support and intubation, positive pressure ventilation, and surfactant therapy are efficacious therapies of RDS. Continuous positive airway pressure (CPAP) can only be used as primary respiratory support in infants who start spontaneous breathing after birth. When perinatal care of premature infants is optimized by using antenatal steroids and optimizing birth management most preterm infants start spontaneous breathing. In this setting recent studies demonstrate that outcome of preterm infants treated with CPAP alone is at least comparable with that of infants treated with intubation, positive pressure ventilation, and surfactant application.[1–3] Three meta-analyses suggest a superiority of CPAP

No funding was obtained for this review. A. Kribs has received speaking fees and travel grants from Abbott, Chiesi, and Lyomark.
Department of Neonatology and Pediatric Intensive Care, Children's Hospital, University of Cologne, Kerpener Str 62, Cologne 50937, Germany
E-mail address: angela.kribs@uk-koeln.de

regarding the outcome of bronchopulmonary dysplasia (BPD).[4–6] These findings led to the recommendation to use noninvasive modes as primary respiratory support in premature infants by the European Association of Perinatal Medicine and the American Academy of Pediatrics.[7,8]

Nevertheless surfactant, after its introduction at the end of the 1980s, has significantly improved outcome of premature infants. Therefore the combination of noninvasive modes of respiratory support with the administration of surfactant may combine two efficacious principles. The intubation surfactant extubation (INSURE) approach is a well-established strategy to combine both principles. A recent systematic review and meta-analysis pooled nine trials that compared early INSURE with CPAP alone in infants with RDS who had never before been intubated. This revealed no statistically significant differences between INSURE and CPAP alone for BPD and/or death, but the relative risk estimates seemed to favor INSURE.[9] As a consequence further adequately powered trials are needed.

However, although INSURE is well-established and seems to be beneficial it still needs at least a short period of positive pressure ventilation that could induce lung injury. Avoidance of any positive pressure ventilation combined with surfactant may have further benefits. Therefore, some strategies to combine noninvasive modes with surfactant therapy have been reported. These strategies are minimally invasive surfactant therapy or less invasive surfactant application.

DIFFERENT MODES OF MINIMALLY INVASIVE SURFACTANT THERAPY

In a metanarrative review More and coworkers[10] reported the different modes of minimally invasive surfactant therapy. These are surfactant application into the pharynx, surfactant nebulization, surfactant application via a laryngeal mask, and surfactant application via a thin endotracheal catheter. **Box 1** provides an overview of available human data for the different approaches.

Surfactant Application into the Pharynx

Surfactant application into the pharynx is the oldest approach that was tested in a randomized trial.[11] This approach is based on the idea that surfactant spreads at the fluid-air interface when the baby starts breathing. Infants with a gestational age of 27 to 29 weeks were included into the study. Surfactant was given immediately after birth, without noninvasive respiratory support. The study found a decrease in severity of RDS, less mechanical ventilation during the first 10 days, and a lower mortality (19% vs 30%) in the intervention group. However, the interpretation of the study is difficult because many infants also received surfactant via an endotracheal tube after intubation. Surprisingly the method was only evaluated in one further study, where surfactant was given into the nasopharynx immediately after birth of the shoulders.[12] In contrast to the first study in this trial the surfactant application was combined with postnatal respiratory support with CPAP. A total of 13 of 15 infants who were delivered vaginally were weaned quickly to room air, whereas five of eight infants who were delivered by caesarean section had to be intubated soon after birth. Because this approach is really minimally invasive, it warrants further investigation.

Surfactant Nebulization

Nebulization of surfactant is also an old idea. If efficacious it would be an attractive alternative to any other mode of application because it is really noninvasive. Any manipulation of the airways is avoided and the application is independent of the

---

Box 1
Clinical studies on different modes of minimally invasive surfactant application

Administration into the pharynx

Ten Centre Study Group,[11] 1987

Kattwinkel et al,[12] 2004

Nebulization of surfactant

Jorch et al,[14] 1997

Berggren et al,[15] 2000

Finer et al,[16] 2010

Minocchieri et al,[17] 2013

Administration via laryngeal mask

Brimacombe et al,[18] 2004

Trevisanuto et al,[19] 2005

Micaglio et al,[20] 2008

Barbosa et al,[21] 2012

Attridge et al,[22] 2013

Sadeghnia et al,[23] 2014

Pinheiro et al,[24] 2016

Administration via a thin catheter

Verder et al,[25] 1992

Kribs et al,[26] 2007

Kribs et al,[27] 2008

Kribs et al,[28] 2010

Göpel et al,[29] 2011

Dargaville et al,[30] 2011

Mehler et al,[31] 2012

Dargaville et al,[32] 2013

Kanmaz et al,[33] 2013

Klebermass-Schrehof et al,[34] 2013

Heidarzadeh et al,[35] 2013

Aguar et al,[36] 2014

Canals Candela et al,[37] 2016

Kribs et al,[38] 2015

Bao et al,[39] 2015

Mohammadizadeh et al,[40] 2015

Göpel et al,[41] 2015

Krajewski et al,[42] 2015

Boldfaced: Prospective randomized controlled trials.
Normal: Observational studies with or without control group.
Italic: Case reports or case series.

experience of the therapist. But using surfactant as an aerosol has many technical implications: the particle size has to be optimized to 0.5 to 2.0 μm, the substance must be stable during the process of nebulization, and the loss of substance should be minimized to make the therapy inexpensive. Therefore different types of nebulizers have been tested for aerolization of surfactant. Fok and colleagues[13] studied in an animal model nebulization of two different surfactant preparations with a jet nebulizer and an ultrasonic nebulizer. They found a very low pulmonary deposition of the initial dose in all groups and a limited clinical effect even in the group with the highest deposition of 1% of the initial dose. They conclude that the aerosol route with these types of nebulizers is not effective for surfactant treatment.

In the new generation of studies, two feasibility studies and two randomized trials evaluating this are published. One further feasibility study is ongoing (NCT02294630). **Table 1** gives the characteristics of these studies. Results of the existent studies vary. Pillow and Minocchieri[43] have reviewed the available animal and human studies and the technical implications of surfactant nebulization.[44] Many questions remain. These questions concern the ideal nebulizer, the correct positioning of the nebulizer in the circuit, the ideal interface for the noninvasive respiratory support during nebulization, the best surfactant preparation and dosing, and the group of infants who can take benefit of surfactant nebulization. Well-designed and appropriately powered studies are needed. It does seem, however, that surfactant nebulization is the most attractive approach to avoid any manipulation of the airways during surfactant application.

Surfactant Application via Laryngeal Mask

The laryngeal mask is a supraglottic device that is usually used to apply positive pressure ventilation for short periods of time. In 2004 Brimacombe and coworkers[18] described the feasibility of using the laryngeal mask for surfactant application in the report of two cases. This was followed by several case reports and case series.[19–21] The method was subsequently compared with CPAP alone in one randomized controlled trial (RCT) including 26 infants with a birth weight greater than 1200 g.[22] In two further more recent RCTs administration of surfactant via laryngeal mask was compared with the INSURE procedure.[23,24] **Table 2** provides an overview of the studies available.

In summary the studies report some effect on the oxygenation, and one study reports a decreased proportion of newborns who require intubation, as compared with the INSURE method.[2] The authors speculate that this is by avoiding morphine premedication, which is often routine in INSURE. In all studies the placement of the device is described as easy by experienced users. Premedication is not routinely needed.

Nevertheless in one trial coughing, transient bradycardia or apnea, and desaturation were observed during placement of the device and during surfactant instillation. These events were judged to be less than those that commonly occur during intubation and surfactant application.[22]

In the two trials that compared the laryngeal mask approach with the INSURE procedure surfactant reflux and the need of more than one attempt to place the device were reported. But the frequency of these adverse events was similar between the two groups.[23,24]

It should be emphasized that placement of the device requires experience, and that the method is limited to relatively large and mature infants because of technical reasons. The use of premedication to minimize adverse events requires further consideration. Further studies are needed to define an optimal group of infants.

Table 1
Clinical studies on surfactant nebulization: study characteristics and main findings

Reference	Study Type	Number of Patients Included	GA of Included Patients	Rescue/Prophylaxis	Nebulizer	Surfactant Preparation and Dose	Primary and Predefined Secondary Outcome	Main Findings
Jorch et al,[14] 1997	Feasibility	20	28–35	Rescue	Jet	Alveofact, 2 × 150 mg/kg	Feasibility Clinical outcome	Rapid improvement of (A-a)Po$_2$ and dyspnea
Berggren et al,[15] 2000	RCT	34	28–33	Rescue	Jet	Curosurf, 480 mg/kg	Course of (A-a)Po$_2$, respiratory support	No differences in (A-a) Po$_2$, No differences in BPD, IVH, need for mechanical ventilation, duration of CPAP support and supplemental oxygen
Finer et al,[16] 2010	Feasibility, phase II	17	28–32	Prophylactic	Vibrating membrane	Lucinactant, up to 4 × 72 mg during 48 h	Safety and feasibility of nebulization Clinical outcomes for efficacy	Procedure is well tolerated
Minocchieri et al,[17] 2013 ACTRN1261000857000	RCT	—	29–33 and 34–39	Early rescue	—	Curosurf	—	Reduction of need for intubation, no differences in BPD
NCT02294630	RCT Recruiting patients	140	24–36	Early rescue	Two different nebulizers	Survanta, 100 mg/kg or 200 mg/kg	Safety and feasibility, need for intubation during the first 72 h, optimal dose of surfactant	Not yet available

Abbreviations: GA, gestational age; IVH, intraventricular hemorrhage; RCT, randomized controlled trial.

Table 2
Clinical studies on surfactant via laryngeal mask: study characteristics and main findings

Reference	Study Type	Number of Patients Included	Control Intervention	GA of Included Patients (wk)	Birthweight	Surfactant Preparation and Dose	Primary and Predefined Secondary Outcome	Main Findings
Attridge et al,[22] 2013	RCT, single center	26 (13 control, 13 intervention)	Only CPAP	31–35	>1200 g	Infasurf, 105 mg/kg	Feasibility Oxygen requirement	Feasible without problems Marked decrease of oxygen requirement
Sadeghnia et al,[23] 2014	RCT, multicenter	70 (35 control, 35 intervention)	INSURE	Mean GA 35	>2000 g	Survanta, 100 mg/kg	AaPo2, need for repeated surfactant, need for mechanical ventilation, duration of CPAP and hospitalization, pneumothorax	Higher aaPo2 after procedure in the LMA group, no further differences
Pinheiro et al,[24] 2016	RCT, single center	60 (30 control, 3 intervention)	INSURE	29 infants <33, 31 infants ≥33	Mean: 2118 g in intervention group, 1945 g in control group	Infasurf, 105 mg/kg	Failure to avoid mechanical ventilation, early failure (1 h), late failure (>1 h)	Failure rate 77% in control group vs 30% in intervention group, mainly caused by differences in early failure

Abbreviation: GA, gestational age.

Surfactant Application via a Thin Catheter

Surfactant application via a thin catheter is the alternative mode of surfactant application for which most human data are available.

History

Surfactant application via a thin endotracheal catheter was first described by Verder and coworkers,[25] who used it as an equivalent to the INSURE procedure. The intent of his trial was avoidance of intubation and mechanical ventilation in preterm infants who started breathing after birth and who could be stabilized with CPAP. At the time of this study the idea of giving surfactant via a thin catheter during CPAP-supported spontaneous breathing was not widely accepted. Based on the experience with surfactant therapy in ventilated infants most neonatologists were convinced that positive pressure ventilation was necessary to optimize distribution of surfactant. That is why the INSURE approach was more accepted and spread over the world.

During the following years an increasing number of extremely preterm infants who could be stabilized with CPAP in the delivery room were observed. It is possible that this phenomena relies on an optimized perinatal management (including the use of antenatal steroids and a proactive birth management with a high rate of caesarean section). INSURE often fails in infants with an extremely low gestational age and an extremely low birth weight because these infants often do not restart breathing after the short period of ventilation.[44]

Rationale

CPAP failure is related to an increase of adverse outcomes, such as pneumothorax, intraventricular hemorrhage, and even death.[45] It was possible that withholding of surfactant led to CPAP failure. This hypothesis led to the revival of the idea of surfactant application via an endotracheal catheter during CPAP-supported spontaneous breathing.

Human Data

The first feasibility study was performed in Cologne and published in 2007.[26] In summary, a thin catheter is placed into the trachea with aid of a Magill forceps under direct laryngoscopy. In general the procedure is well tolerated without pharmacologic sedation. The procedure is embedded in a whole package of intervention aimed at avoidance of positive pressure ventilation especially during neonatal transition and the first 72 hours of postnatal life.[27,31] This package includes use of antenatal steroids, very early CPAP, and use of early postnatal caffeine. Further observational single and multicenter studies from centers describe outcomes from the Cologne approach.[34,36]

In 2011 the procedure was modified by Dargaville and coworkers[30] for physicians not familiar with the use of a Magill forceps. This uses a more rigid vascular catheter instead of a soft catheter, which can be introduced into the trachea without the use of a Magill forceps. The modified procedure is called the Hobart method. Another difference to the Cologne approach is that during the procedure the infant is not connected to CPAP. The Hobart method was evaluated in two observational studies.[30,32] Importantly, a large RCT (Optimist A trial, NCT02140580) is now being performed now.[46]

The characteristics of the observational studies are shown in **Table 3**. In summary, the observational trials had consistent findings concerning efficacy include decrease of fraction of inspired oxygen and distending pressure after procedure, less need for

Table 3
Nonrandomized studies on surfactant via thin catheter: study characteristics and main findings

	Type of Study	Number of Patients Receiving Intervention	Inclusion Criteria	Control Intervention	Surfactant Preparation and Dose	Main Results
Kribs et al,[26] 2007	Observational single center	29	≤27 wk	Historical control, standard care	Survanta, 100 m/kg	Lower mortality, less IVH >II°, less PIE compared with historical control
Kribs et al,[27] 2008	Observational single center	150	≤1000 g	n.a.	Survanta, 100 m/kg	Less CPAP failure after introduction of the method, lower mortality in infants with CPAP success regardless whether with or without surfactant
Kribs et al,[28] 2010	Observational multicenter	319	<31 wk and ≤1500 g	Any kind of standard care	Curosurf, Survanta, Alveofact, variable doses	Lower prevalence of mechanical ventilation, less BPD compared with standard care
Dargaville et al,[30] 2011	Observational single center	25	≤34 wk	Historical control, CPAP	Curosurf, 100 mg/kg	Increase of Spo_2 after the procedure, reduction of Fio_2 and CPAP pressure
Mehler et al,[31] 2012	Observational single center	164	<26 wk	Historical control, standard care	Survanta, 100 m/kg	Improved survival and reduced morbidity in infants with GA <26 wk after introduction of the procedure
Dargaville et al,[32] 2013	Feasibility, two center	61	25–32 wk	Historical control, CPAP	Curosurf, 100–200 mg/kg	Increase of Spo_2 after the procedure, reduction of Fio_2 and CPAP pressure

Study	Design	N	GA	Control	Surfactant/Dose	Outcome
Klebermass-Schrehof et al,[34] 2013	Observational single center	224	23–27 wk	Historical control, standard care	Curosurf, 200 mg/kg	Lower mortality, especially in infants <26 wk, less IVH, less severe IVH, less cystic PVL, but more ROP and severe ROP, more PDA, less death or BPD
Aguar et al,[36] 2014	Observational single center	44	24–35 wk	Historical control, INSURE	Curosurf, 100 mg/kg	Procedure is feasible without differences in any observed outcome compared with INSURE
Canals Candela et al,[37] 2016	Observational single center	19	25–34 wk	Historical control, CPAP	Curosurf 200 mg/kg	Procedure is feasible without adverse events, less intubation during the first 72 h compared with historical control
Goepel et al,[41] 2015	Matched pairs from German Neonatal Network	1103	<32 wk and ≤1500 g	Matched pairs from the German Neonatal Network	Curosurf, Survanta, Alveofact, variable doses	Lower rates of mechanical ventilation and BPD
Krajewski et al,[42] 2015	Observational single center	26	Mean 29.5 wk	Historical control, MV, surfactant rapid extubation	Curosurf	Procedure is feasible and is associated with less intubation and mechanical ventilation compared with mechanical ventilation with rapid extubation

Abbreviations: FIO$_2$, fraction of inspired oxygen; GA, gestational age; IVH, intraventricular hemorrhage; MV, mechanical ventilation; PDA, persistent arterial duct; PIE, pulmonary interstitial emphysema; PVL, periventricular leukomalacia; ROP, retinopathy of prematurity; SpO$_2$, oxygen saturation as measured by pulse oximetry.

intubation during the first 72 hours compared with historical control subjects, and trend to shorter duration of different kinds of respiratory support. For infants with a gestational age less than 26 weeks there was lower mortality, less severe intraventricular hemorrhage, and less air leak.

In total five published randomized trials have evaluated surfactant application via a small endotracheal catheter. They included different patient populations, had different endpoints, and had different interventions for control. **Table 4** shows the characteristics and the mean results of the studies.

In summary, the RCTs confirmed the findings of the observational studies. All studies showed a trend toward a reduction of adverse pulmonary and nonpulmonary outcomes, but only one study shows a statistically significant reduction of the important outcome of death or BPD. Four further prospective randomized trials are registered (NCT02140580, NCT01848262, NCT02772081, NCT01615016), including Optimist A.[46]

Short-Term Safety Aspects

Every new method raises the question of safety. The reported adverse events during the procedure were very similar in the observational and controlled trials. The following adverse events were observed:

- Need for more than one attempt to be successful (5%–30%)
- Apnea and need for positive pressure ventilation via mask after procedure (12%–44%)
- Bradycardia or desaturation greater than 10 seconds (10%–30%)
- Dislocation (1%)
- Coughing and gagging resulting in surfactant reflux (3%–40%)

However, the incidence of the events differed in the studies according to different characteristics of the included patients and the experience of the persons performing the procedure. Coughing and gagging are more frequent in the more mature infant, whereas apnea occurs more often in the more immature infant. Need for positive pressure ventilation is more frequent after the Horbart method, perhaps because the infants are not on CPAP during the procedure when the method is used.

Catheter application is usually performed without sedation. It is a point of intense discussion whether adequate premedication could be beneficial. Premedication could minimize adverse side effects as surfactant reflux caused by gagging and coughing, but it may increase the rate of failure of the method with need for subsequent intubation. It is also an ethical issue, whether a potentially painful procedure should be done without analgesia. A recent study demonstrated that use of sedation during the procedure increases the comfort of the infants but also the need for positive pressure ventilation and intubation.[47] Research to identify adequate strategies for premedication is urgently needed.

Long-Term Safety Aspects

To date there are only two reports of later follow-up of infants treated with catheter application.[48,49] One of them is the 6-year follow-up of the cohort from the first feasibility study.[48] More patients in the intervention group survived, compared with the surviving infants of the control group. Despite being more immature, infants of the intervention group showed a trend to a higher rate of being without disability. The second report is a 36-month follow-up of a cohort of infants treated with the catheter approach.[49] In this study the catheter-treated infants performed better than a historical control. In the Bayley Scales the MDI (Mental Developmental Index) was 98 versus 89 and the PDI (Psychomotor Developmental Index) 91 versus 83.

DISCUSSION

During the last decades perinatal management of very and extremely preterm birth has improved. This optimization includes the increasing use of antenatal steroids and proactive birth management aimed at avoiding perinatal asphyxia. As a consequence most premature infants start spontaneous breathing after birth, and therefore do not have an obligatory need for intubation and positive pressure ventilation. They are stabilized with noninvasive modes of respiratory support. Such support has been shown to be as efficacious as intubation, positive pressure ventilation, and surfactant application. However, the use of noninvasive modes of respiratory support is related to withholding of surfactant and this remains an issue. Different approaches to overcome this dilemma have been reported.

The INSURE method has been shown to be efficacious in reducing the need for mechanical ventilation. Because it is still related to a short period of positive pressure ventilation it has the risk to induce lung injury. Furthermore this approach has a high failure rate in the most vulnerable infants, the infants with an extremely low gestational age and an extremely low birth weight.[44,45] Therefore, there is an urgent need for further strategies to combine noninvasive modes of respiratory support with surfactant application.

Application of surfactant into the pharynx seems to be an attractive approach because it is possible without any manipulation of the airways. Sparse data prevent its recommendation, but it merits further study.

Nebulization of surfactant also avoids manipulation of the airways. Available human data suggest that it may be efficacious but many technical problems are not yet solved. The approach remains an issue of intense research.

Application of surfactant via a laryngeal mask has technical limitations because of the available sizes of the device. Available data, however, suggest that it might be an alternative to the INSURE procedure. INSURE is usually done after premedication with analgesics and/or sedatives, whereas the laryngeal mask is placed without premedication. A recent study shows a lower incidence of need for intubation after surfactant application via laryngeal mask than after INSURE.[24] This may be an effect of the avoidance of analgesics and sedatives. However, it is not clear whether the avoidance of premedication is a real benefit for the infants. The approach should be further evaluated but it is not yet ready for wide clinical use.

Most clinical data are available for surfactant application via a thin endotracheal catheter. The method is feasible in preterm infants down to a gestational age of 23 completed weeks.[38] Available studies suggest that the method has the potential to improve pulmonary and nonpulmonary outcomes. The catheter application is the sole approach where some long-term data are available.[48,49] These data show no adverse long-term effects of the method and a trend toward a better neurodevelopmental outcome.

However, there remain a lot of questions. The studies were done in different patient groups, with different catheters and different surfactant preparations. It is not clear which is the ideal catheter, the ideal surfactant, and which infants would benefit most from the method. Furthermore, the question of premedication remains unanswered.

In most of the trials the surfactant application via the catheter was embedded in a package of interventions aiming to avoid mechanical ventilation, antenatal steroids, very early CPAP with high pressure levels, and very early use of caffeine. It is not clear to which extent these interventions influence the success of the approach.

Table 4
Randomized studies on surfactant via thin catheter: study characteristics and main findings

	Gestational Age (wk)	Control Group	Number of Included Infants	Number of Patients Receiving Intervention	Surfactant Preparation and Dose	Primary Outcome	Main Results
Göpel et al,[29] 2011	26–28	Any kind of standard care	220	65	Curosurf, Survanta, or Alveofact depending on center-specific standard, 100 mg/kg	Need for any MV or being not ventilated but having a P_{CO_2} >65 mm Hg or a FiO_2 >0.6 or both for more than 2 h between 25 and 72 h of age	Lower rate of primary outcome in the intervention group (28 vs 46%), significantly shorter duration MV and oxygen requirement in the intervention group
Kanmaz et al,[33] 2013	<32	INSURE	200	100	Curosurf, 100 mg/kg	Need for early MV	Lower rate of MV during the first 72 h in the intervention group (30 vs 45%), significantly shorter duration of MV and CPAP in the intervention group, less BPD in the intervention group
Heidarzadeh et al,[35] 2013	≤32	INSURE	80	38	Curosurf, 200 mg/kg	Feasibility, description of outcomes	Lower rate of NEC and shorter duration of CPAP and hospital stay in the intervention group, no further differences

Study	GA	Comparator	N	N	Surfactant	Outcomes	Results
Kribs et al,[38] 2015	23–26	Intubation and mechanical ventilation	211	107	Curosurf, 100 mg/kg	Survival without BPD at 36 wk	No differences in survival without BPD (67% in the intervention group vs 59% in the control group). higher rates of survival without severe morbidity in the intervention group (51% in the intervention group vs 36% in the control group)
Mohammadizadeh et al,[39] 2015	≤34	INSURE	38	19	Curosurf, 200 mg/kg	Need for MV and duration of oxygen therapy	No difference in need for MV, but duration of surfactant therapy significantly shorter in intervention group
Bao et al,[40] 2015	28–32	INSURE	90	47	Curosurf, 200 mg/kg	Feasibility, rate of MV in the first 72 h, duration of MV, CPAP, and oxygen requirement, neonatal morbidities	No differences in rate of MV in the first 72 h, duration of oxygen and neonatal morbidities, duration of MV and CPAP significantly less in the intervention group

Abbreviations: Fio$_2$, fraction of inspired oxygen; GA, gestational age; MV, mechanical ventilation; NEC, necrotizing enterocolitis.

SUMMARY

There is an increasing use of noninvasive modes of respiratory support as primary respiratory therapy in infants with RDS. However, there is an urgent need for strategies to combine them with less invasive surfactant application to enhance success of noninvasive modes. The INSURE method is well-established but may still be too invasive.

There is growing evidence that application via a laryngeal mask or a thin catheter may be an alternative to the INSURE procedure. Catheter application seems safe under conditions described in randomized trials.

Surfactant application into the pharynx and surfactant nebulization are even less invasive but available data do not allow recommendation outside of clinical studies.

Best practices

What is the current practice?

Either noninvasive modes of respiratory support or intubation mechanical ventilation and surfactant application are used as primary respiratory therapy for preterm infants with RDS. Early surfactant therapy is recommended for every extremely preterm infant and for all infants with moderate to severe RDS.

What changes in current practice are likely to improve outcomes?

Perinatal management should aim for the birth of a well-prepared nonasphyxiated infant. This includes particularly the use of antenatal steroids. Postnatal stabilization should aim for the avoidance of positive pressure ventilation. This is reached by early use of CPAP. CPAP and other modes of noninvasive respiratory support should be combined with early rescue surfactant therapy. The INSURE procedure is the best evaluated approach. Surfactant administration via a thin endotracheal catheter during spontaneous breathing with CPAP seems to be safe under certain conditions.

REFERENCES

1. SUPPORT Study Group of the Eunice Kennedy Shriver NICHD Neonatal Research Network, Finer NN, Carlo WA, Walsh MC, et al. Early CPAP versus surfactant in extremely preterm infants. N Engl J Med 2010;362(21):1970–9.
2. Morley CJ, Davis PG, Doyle LW, et al, COIN Trial Investigators. Nasal CPAP or intubation at birth for very preterm infants. N Engl J Med 2008;358(7):700–8.
3. Dunn MS, Kaempf J, de Klerk A, et al, Vermont Oxford Network DRM Study Group. Randomized trial comparing 3 approaches to the initial respiratory management of preterm neonates. Pediatrics 2011;128(5):e1069–76.
4. Schmölzer GM, Kumar M, Pichler G, et al. Non invasive versus invasive respiratory support in preterm infants at birth: systematic review and meta-analysis. BMJ 2013;347:f5980.
5. Rojas-Reyes MX, Morley CJ, Soll R. Prophylactic versus selective use of surfactant in preventing morbidity and mortality in preterm infants. Cochrane Database Syst Rev 2012;(3):CD000510.
6. Fischer HS, Bührer C. Avoiding endotracheal ventilation to prevent bronchopulmonary dysplasia: a meta-analysis. Pediatrics 2013;132(5):e1351–60.
7. Sweet DG, Carnielli V, Greisen G, et al, European Association of Perinatal Medicine. European consensus guidelines on the management of neonatal respiratory distress syndrome in preterm infants—2013 update. Neonatology 2013;103(4): 353–68.

8. Committee on Fetus and Newborn, American Academy of Pediatrics. Respiratory support in preterm infants at birth. Pediatrics 2014;133(1):171–4.

9. Isayama T, Chai-Adisaksopha C, McDonald SD. Noninvasive ventilation with vs without early surfactant to prevent chronic lung disease in preterm infants: a systematic review and meta-analysis. JAMA Pediatr 2015;169(8):731–9.

10. More K, Sakhuja P, Shah PS. Minimally invasive surfactant administration in preterm infants: a meta-narrative review. JAMA Pediatr 2014;168(10):901–8.

11. Ten centre trial of artificial surfactant (artificial lung expanding compound) in very premature babies. Ten Centre Study Group. Br Med J (Clin Res Ed) 1987; 294(6578):991–6.

12. Kattwinkel J, Robinson M, Bloom BT, et al. Technique for intrapartum administration of surfactant without requirement for an endotracheal tube. J Perinatol 2004; 24(6):360–5.

13. Fok TF, al-Essa M, Dolovich M, et al. Nebulisation of surfactants in an animal model of neonatal respiratory distress. Arch Dis Child Fetal Neonatal Ed 1998; 78(1):F3–9.

14. Jorch G, Hartl H, Roth B, et al. Surfactant aerosol treatment of respiratory distress syndrome in spontaneously breathing premature infants. Pediatr Pulmonol 1997; 24(3):222–4.

15. Berggren E, Liljedahl M, Winbladh B, et al. Pilot study of nebulized surfactant therapy for neonatal respiratory distress syndrome. Acta Paediatr 2000;89(4): 460–4.

16. Finer NN, Merritt TA, Bernstein G, et al. An open label, pilot study of Aerosurf combined with nCPAP to prevent RDS in preterm neonates. J Aerosol Med Pulm Drug Deliv 2010;23(5):303–9.

17. Minocchieri S, Berry CA, Pillow J. Nebulized surfactant for treatment of respiratory distress in the first hours of life: the CureNeb study. Abstract presented at: Annual Meeting of the Pediatric Academic Society. Washington, DC; May 6, 2013. Session 3500.

18. Brimacombe J, Gandini D, Keller C. The laryngeal mask airway for administration of surfactant in two neonates with respiratory distress syndrome. Paediatr Anaesth 2004;14(2):188–90.

19. Trevisanuto D, Grazzina N, Ferrarese P, et al. Laryngeal mask airway used as a delivery conduit for the administration of surfactant to preterm infants with respiratory distress syndrome. Biol Neonate 2005;87(4):217–20.

20. Micaglio M, Zanardo V, Ori C, et al. ProSeal LMA for surfactant administration. Paediatr Anaesth 2008;18(1):91–2.

21. Barbosa RF, Marcatto Jde O, Silva AC, et al. ProSealTM laryngeal mask airway for surfactant administration in the treatment of respiratory distress syndrome in a premature infant. Rev Bras Ter Intensiva 2012;24(2):207–10 [in English, Portuguese].

22. Attridge JT, Stewart C, Stukenborg GJ, et al. Administration of rescue surfactant by laryngeal mask airway: lessons from a pilot trial. Am J Perinatol 2013;30(3): 201–6.

23. Sadeghnia A, Tanhaei M, Mohammadizadeh M, et al. A comparison of surfactant administration through i-gel and ET-tube in the treatment of respiratory distress syndrome in newborns weighing more than 2000 grams. Adv Biomed Res 2014;3:160.

24. Pinheiro JM, Santana-Rivas Q, Pezzano C. Randomized trial of laryngeal mask airway versus endotracheal intubation for surfactant delivery. J Perinatol 2016; 36(3):196–201.

25. Verder H, Agertoft L, Albertsen P, et al. Surfactant treatment of newborn infants with respiratory distress syndrome primarily treated with nasal continuous positive air pressure. A pilot study. Ugeskr Laeger 1992;154(31):2136–9 [in Danish].

26. Kribs A, Pillekamp F, Hünseler C, et al. Early administration of surfactant in spontaneous breathing with nCPAP: feasibility and outcome in extremely premature infants (postmenstrual age </=27 weeks). Paediatr Anaesth 2007;17(4):364–9.

27. Kribs A, Vierzig A, Hünseler C, et al. Early surfactant in spontaneously breathing with nCPAP in ELBW infants: a single centre four year experience. Acta Paediatr 2008;97(3):293–8.

28. Kribs A, Härtel C, Kattner E, et al. Surfactant without intubation in preterm infants with respiratory distress: first multi-center data. Klin Padiatr 2010;222(1):13–7.

29. Göpel W, Kribs A, Ziegler A, et al, German Neonatal Network. Avoidance of mechanical ventilation by surfactant treatment of spontaneously breathing preterm infants (AMV): an open-label, randomised, controlled trial. Lancet 2011; 378(9803):1627–34.

30. Dargaville PA, Aiyappan A, Cornelius A, et al. Preliminary evaluation of a new technique of minimally invasive surfactant therapy. Arch Dis Child Fetal Neonatal Ed 2011;96(4):F243–8.

31. Mehler K, Grimme J, Abele J, et al. Outcome of extremely low gestational age newborns after introduction of a revised protocol to assist preterm infants in their transition to extrauterine life. Acta Paediatr 2012;101(12):1232–9.

32. Dargaville PA, Aiyappan A, De Paoli AG, et al. Minimally-invasive surfactant therapy in preterm infants on continuous positive airway pressure. Arch Dis Child Fetal Neonatal Ed 2013;98(2):F122–6.

33. Kanmaz HG, Erdeve O, Canpolat FE, et al. Surfactant administration via thin catheter during spontaneous breathing: randomized controlled trial. Pediatrics 2013; 131(2):e502–9.

34. Klebermass-Schrehof K, Wald M, Schwindt J, et al. Less invasive surfactant administration in extremely preterm infants: impact on mortality and morbidity. Neonatology 2013;103(4):252–8.

35. Heidarzadeh M, Mirnia K, Hoseini MB, et al. Surfactant administration via thin catheter during spontaneous breathing: randomized controlled trial in Alzahra hospital. Iran J Neonatol 2013;4:5–9.

36. Aguar M, Cernada M, Brugada M, et al. Minimally invasive surfactant therapy with a gastric tube is as effective as the intubation, surfactant, and extubation technique in preterm babies. Acta Paediatr 2014;103(6):e229–33.

37. Canals Candela FJ, VizcaínoDíaz C, FerrándezBerenguer MJ, et al. Surfactant replacement therapy with a minimally invasive technique: experience in a tertiary hospital. An Pediatr (Barc) 2016;84(2):79–84 [in Spanish].

38. Kribs A, Roll C, Göpel W, et al, NINSAPP Trial Investigators. Nonintubated surfactant application vs conventional therapy in extremely preterm infants: a randomized clinical trial. JAMA Pediatr 2015;169(8):723–30.

39. Bao Y, Zhang G, Wu M, et al. A pilot study of less invasive surfactant administration in very preterm infants in a Chinese tertiary center. BMC Pediatr 2015; 14(15):21.

40. Mohammadizadeh M, Ardestani AG, Sadeghnia AR. Early administration of surfactant via a thin intratracheal catheter in preterm infants with respiratory distress syndrome: feasibility and outcome. J Res Pharm Pract 2015;4(1):31–6.

41. Göpel W, Kribs A, Härtel C, et al, German Neonatal Network (GNN). Less invasive surfactant administration is associated with improved pulmonary outcomes in spontaneously breathing preterm infants. Acta Paediatr 2015;104(3):241–6.

42. Krajewski P, Chudzik A, Strzałko-Głoskowska B, et al. Surfactant administration without intubation in preterm infants with respiratory distress syndrome: our experiences. J Matern Fetal Neonatal Med 2015;28(10):1161–4.
43. Pillow JJ, Minocchieri S. Innovation in surfactant therapy II: surfactant administration by aerosolization. Neonatology 2012;101(4):337–44.
44. Dani C, Corsini I, Poggi C. Risk factors for intubation-surfactant-extubation (INSURE) failure and multiple INSURE strategy in preterm infants. Early Hum Dev 2012;88(Suppl 1):S3–4.
45. Fuchs H, Lindner W, Leiprecht A, et al. Predictors of early nasal CPAP failure and effects of various intubation criteria on the rate of mechanical ventilation in preterm infants of <29 weeks gestational age. Arch Dis Child Fetal Neonatal Ed 2011;96(5):F343–7.
46. Dargaville PA, Kamlin CO, De Paoli AG, et al. The OPTIMIST-a trial: evaluation of minimally-invasive surfactant therapy in preterm infants 25-28 weeks gestation. BMC Pediatr 2014;14:213.
47. Dekker J, Lopriore E, Rijken M, et al. Sedation during minimal invasive surfactant therapy in preterm infants. Neonatology 2016;109(4):308–13.
48. Porath M, Korp L, Wendrich D, et al. Surfactant in spontaneous breathing with nCPAP: neurodevelopmental outcome at early school age of infants ≤27 weeks. Acta Paediatr 2011;100(3):352–9.
49. Teig N, Weitkämper A, Rothermel J, et al. Observational study on less invasive surfactant administration (LISA) in preterm infants<29 weeks: short and long-term outcomes. Z Geburtshilfe Neonatol 2015;219(6):266–73.

The Role of Caffeine in Noninvasive Respiratory Support

 CrossMark

Nicole R. Dobson, MD[a], Ravi Mangal Patel, MD, MSc[b],*

KEYWORDS

- Caffeine • Apnea • Bronchopulmonary dysplasia • Premature infant
- Noninvasive ventilation

KEY POINTS

- Caffeine is safe, effectively treats apnea, and reduces the risk of bronchopulmonary dysplasia.
- Caffeine facilitates the successful transition from invasive to noninvasive respiratory support and decreases the duration of positive airway pressure support.
- Observational studies suggest early initiation of caffeine within 2 days of birth may have greater benefits compared with later initiation, including fewer days of invasive respiratory support and lower risk of bronchopulmonary dysplasia.
- Additional studies are needed to determine the optimal dose and duration of caffeine therapy and whether prophylactic use of caffeine can prevent the need for rescue interventions among infants receiving early noninvasive respiratory support.

INTRODUCTION

Management of apnea of prematurity plays a critical role in the success of noninvasive ventilation strategies in preterm infants. Methylxanthines have been used in the neonatal intensive care unit for more than 40 years to treat and prevent apnea of prematurity. Among methylxanthines (aminophylline, theophylline, caffeine), caffeine is

Disclaimer and Conflicts of Interest: The views expressed in this article are those of the authors and do not reflect the official policy or position of the United States Army, Department of Defense, the US Government, or the National Institutes of Health. The authors have no relevant conflicts of interest.
This review was supported, in part, by the National Institutes of Health under award numbers KL2 TR000455 and UL1 TR000454 (R.M. Patel).
a Department of Pediatrics, Uniformed Services University of Health Sciences, 4301 Jones Bridge Road, Bethesda, MD 20814, USA; b Division of Neonatal-Perinatal Medicine, Department of Pediatrics, Emory University School of Medicine, Children's Healthcare of Atlanta, 2015 Uppergate Drive Northeast, 3rd Floor, Atlanta, GA 30322, USA
* Corresponding author.
E-mail address: rmpatel@emory.edu

used most commonly because of its wide therapeutic index and longer half-life that allows once-daily administration.[1] Caffeine accounted for 96% of all methylxanthine use in very-low-birth weight (VLBW) infants in 2010.[2] In addition, caffeine is one of the most common medications administered to infants in neonatal intensive care units.[3] Several beneficial effects of caffeine have been well established, whereas other benefits are plausible, and yet others require additional study (**Box 1**). This review focuses on the use of caffeine in preterm infants receiving noninvasive respiratory support with specific emphasis on clinical effects of caffeine, mechanisms of action, timing of initiation, and optimal dose and duration of therapy.

EFFECT OF CAFFEINE ON RESPIRATORY OUTCOMES IN PRETERM INFANTS
Apnea and Intermittent Hypoxia

Despite advances in neonatal care, apnea remains a common and pervasive problem in preterm infants that often leads to failure of noninvasive respiratory support.[4] Apnea can lead to intermittent hypoxia,[5] and intermittent hypoxemic episodes (oxygen saturation <80%) among extremely preterm infants are associated with a higher risk of death or disability at 18 months of age (relative risk 1.53; 95% confidence interval [CI] 1.21–1.94).[6] Caffeine, a trimethylxanthine that primarily exerts its effects by blocking adenosine A1 and A2A receptors, effectively treats apnea[7,8] and reduces intermittent hypoxia.[9] The primary mechanism by which methylxanthines reduce apnea is through antagonism of A2A receptors on GABAergic neurons.[10,11] Caffeine decreases apnea by stimulating the medullary respiratory centers, increasing carbon dioxide sensitivity, and enhancing diaphragmatic function, leading to increased minute

---

Box 1
Known, potential, and uncertain respiratory benefits of caffeine therapy

Known respiratory benefits of caffeine in infants weighing less than 1250 g at birth

- Decreases apnea episodes in preterm infants[7,8]
- Decreases risk of bronchopulmonary dysplasia[20]
- Decreases duration of positive airway pressure support[20]
- Decreases treatment of a patent ductus arteriosus[20]
- Increases successful extubation within 1 week of initiation of treatment[23]

Potential additional respiratory benefits of early initiation of caffeine in VLBW infants

- May further decrease risk of bronchopulmonary dysplasia[2,42–44]
- May further decrease duration of invasive respiratory support[2,42–44]
- May further decrease duration of noninvasive respiratory support[42]
- May further decrease treatment of a patent ductus arteriosus[2,42–44]

Uncertain respiratory benefits of caffeine in VLBW infants

- Does prophylactic caffeine on the day of birth, compared with later initiation, reduce failure of initial noninvasive respiratory support?
- Does prophylactic caffeine on the day of birth, compared with later initiation, reduce the duration of noninvasive respiratory support?
- Does caffeine improve long-term respiratory health into adolescence?
- Is high-dose caffeine, compared with standard-dose caffeine, a safer and more effective alternative to decrease apnea?

ventilation, improved respiratory pattern, and reduced hypoxic respiratory depression.[1,12] As discussed later, these and other physiologic effects of caffeine are likely to mediate many of the respiratory benefits of caffeine observed in clinical studies.

Methylxanthines are effective in reducing the frequency of apneic events and the use of mechanical ventilation in the first week after starting treatment.[7] Higher dosing regimens appear to more effectively treat apnea,[13,14] but a recent pilot study suggests that early high-dose caffeine (80 mg/kg total) given over 36 hours to preterm infants born less than or equal to ≤ 30 weeks' gestation increases the incidence of cerebellar hemorrhage with subsequent alteration in early motor performance.[15] These findings raise concerns about the safety of high-dose caffeine. Although the study found no differences in neurodevelopmental outcomes at 2 years, the findings of increased intracranial hemorrhage parallel nonsignificant trends of increased grade 3 or 4 intraventricular hemorrhage seen in another trial of high-dose caffeine[13] and warrant further study to determine the safety of early high-dose caffeine to decrease apnea.

Studies that have evaluated the efficacy of caffeine as prophylaxis to prevent apnea have not shown definitive benefit, with a systematic review concluding that the available evidence does not support the use of caffeine as prophylaxis to prevent apnea.[16] However, given the favorable safety profile and common occurrence of apnea among extremely preterm infants, the authors think the prophylactic use of caffeine in premature infants to prevent apnea is a reasonable approach among high-risk preterm infants (eg, birth weight <1250 g) who may have cardiorespiratory compromise from apnea. A recent cross-sectional survey of neonatologists in Thailand, Lebanon, Australia, and the United States revealed that prophylactic use of methylxanthines for apnea of prematurity is common, with 62% of those surveyed reporting prophylactic use.[17] Similarly, caffeine was used for apnea prophylaxis in 37% of preterm infants in a multicenter prospective study in Austria, Czech Republic, Greece, Italy, and Spain.[18]

Bronchopulmonary Dysplasia

Among VLBW infants receiving respiratory support, bronchopulmonary dysplasia (BPD) is the most common serious chronic lung disease of infancy and can cause long term respiratory problems including decreased lung function and asthma-like symptoms.[19] The Caffeine for Apnea of Prematurity (CAP) trial, a large, randomized trial conducted from 1999 to 2004, provides the most comprehensive data regarding the effects of caffeine on short- and long-term neonatal outcomes in infants weighing less than 1250 g at birth. Although the trial did not specifically evaluate the effectiveness of caffeine in reduction of apnea of prematurity, the study showed that infants treated with caffeine, compared with placebo, had a lower risk of BPD (adjusted odds ratio [OR] 0.64; 95% CI 0.52–0.78).[20] Other benefits of caffeine demonstrated in the trial included decreased need for treatment of a patent ductus arteriosus, reduced severity of retinopathy of prematurity, and, perhaps most importantly, improved motor function and visual function at 5-year follow-up.[20–22] The CAP trial did not reveal any significant short- and long-term adverse effects of caffeine therapy, supporting the safety of caffeine use in preterm infants. The association of caffeine with improved clinical outcomes combined with its safety profile has led to a consensus that caffeine is the "preferred drug" for treatment of apnea of prematurity.[7]

Facilitation of Transition to Noninvasive Respiratory Support

In preterm infants requiring mechanical ventilation, caffeine therapy facilitates the transition to noninvasive respiratory support. Administration of caffeine around the time of extubation in premature infants results in a significant reduction in the failure of extubation within 1 week (relative risk 0.48; 95% CI 0.32–0.71).[23] In the CAP trial, caffeine-treated infants had younger postmenstrual ages (PMA) at last use of endotracheal intubation (median 29.1 vs 30.0 weeks; $P<.001$).[20] Higher caffeine dosing regimens in the periextubation period may be more effective in preventing apnea and reducing extubation failure rates. A randomized trial of 3 different maintenance dosing regimens of caffeine citrate (3, 15, and 30 mg/kg) for periextubation management of 127 infants born at less than 32 weeks' gestation revealed significantly less apnea in the 2 higher dose groups compared with the lowest dose group, although there was no difference in extubation failure rates between groups.[14] Another trial comparing maintenance dosing regimens of 5 and 20 mg/kg/d of caffeine citrate showed a significant reduction in extubation failure in the high-dose group (relative risk 0.51, 95% CI 0.31–0.85).[13] A more recent trial in preterm infants born less than 32 weeks' gestation comparing high-dose (loading 40 mg/kg/d and maintenance of 20 mg/kg/d) versus low-dose (loading 20 mg/kg/d and maintenance of 10 mg/kg/d) caffeine citrate showed that high-dose caffeine was associated with a significant reduction in extubation failure.[24] However, the potential benefits of high-dose caffeine in reducing extubation failure need to be balanced with safety concerns related to a higher incidence of intracranial hemorrhage among infants receiving high-dose caffeine in the first 36 hours of life,[15] as previously mentioned.

Duration of Respiratory Support

Caffeine therapy reduces the duration of noninvasive respiratory support in preterm infants. In the CAP trial, caffeine-treated infants, compared with placebo-treated infants, had younger PMA at last use of positive pressure ventilation (PPV) (median age of 31 weeks vs 32 weeks; $P<.001$) and oxygen therapy (33.6 weeks vs 35.1 weeks; $P<.001$).[20] An additional post-hoc subgroup analysis of the CAP trial demonstrated that the effects of caffeine on the PMA at last PPV was consistent across infants who received invasive and noninvasive respiratory support as well as those without PPV at time of randomization (test for heterogeneity $P = .80$).[25] Current data suggest that high-dose caffeine (20 mg/kg/d maintenance therapy) does not provide additional benefit over standard dosing (5 mg/kg/d maintenance therapy) on the duration of noninvasive respiratory support after extubation.[24,26]

Reports have suggested that standardizing use of caffeine may reduce the use of invasive respiratory support. A report focusing on noninvasive respiratory support from centers participating in the Vermont Oxford Network–sponsored Neonatal Intensive Care Quality Improvement Collaborative (NIC/Q 2005) showed increases in the routine use of caffeine were temporally associated with fewer days of invasive ventilation but not a lower risk of BPD.[27] In this study of infants less than 30 weeks' gestation, caffeine exposure increased from 47% at baseline to 98% after implementation ($P<.001$), with a decrease in median days of ventilation (8.5 vs 4.0, $P<.001$) and a concomitant increase in days of continuous positive airway pressure (CPAP) use (4.0–8.0, $P<.001$). Although several other practices were changed along with caffeine use limiting any inference of the specific effects of caffeine, these data suggest that standardizing caffeine use is one important component of efforts to improve postnatal respiratory care of preterm infants.

PHYSIOLOGIC EFFECTS OF CAFFEINE ON PULMONARY FUNCTION

Studies in both humans and animals have shown that caffeine has multiple effects on pulmonary function and respiratory health (**Fig. 1**). These effects include improving lung compliance and airway resistance,[28,29] increasing minute ventilation,[28,30]

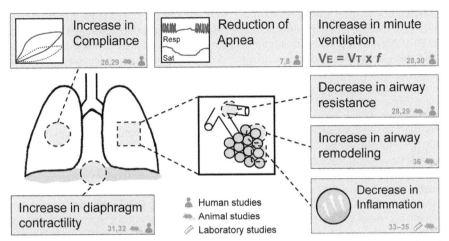

Fig. 1. Effects of caffeine on neonatal respiratory health: potential mechanisms. Study references are noted in the bottom right of each box. f, respiratory frequency; Resp, respiration; Sat, oxygen saturation; VE, minute ventilation; VT, tidal volume.

increasing diaphragm muscle contractility,[31,32] decreasing lung inflammation,[33–35] and improving airway remodeling.[36] Although it is unclear which of these potential mechanisms are responsible for the clinical benefits of caffeine observed in large clinical trials, it is likely that multiple mechanisms, beyond a reduction in apnea, are responsible for the benefits of caffeine on pulmonary health. The potential effects of caffeine on improving lung compliance and respiratory muscle function are likely to be important in ensuring infants on noninvasive respiratory support maintain effective ventilation. However, additional investigation is needed to translate the study of effects of caffeine observed in animal studies to preterm infants.

MECHANISMS OF FAILURE OF NONINVASIVE RESPIRATORY SUPPORT

Noninvasive respiratory support is commonly initiated in the delivery room. However, many VLBW infants will need additional "rescue" therapy with surfactant or mechanical ventilation. Data from randomized controlled trials report incidences of CPAP failure needing "rescue" between 22% and 36% for VLBW infants[37–39] and 46% and 66% for extremely preterm infants.[40,41] Those infants who fail CPAP therapy are at higher risk of adverse outcomes, including death or BPD.[38] Because some infants will have an interval of several hours or days between initial noninvasive respiratory support therapy and failure, early caffeine therapy has the potential to decrease failure rates. However, limited studies have evaluated the effect of early caffeine initiation on the risk of initial noninvasive respiratory support failure. Additional prospective studies are needed to determine if prophylactic use of caffeine on the day of birth can improve the success of initial noninvasive respiratory support therapy, especially in extremely preterm infants.

TIMING OF CAFFEINE INITIATION IN INFANTS RECEIVING NONINVASIVE RESPIRATORY SUPPORT

Several studies have demonstrated an association with earlier initiation of caffeine in the first few days of life, compared with later initiation, and improved respiratory outcomes in preterm infants, including a reduced risk of BPD[2,42–44] and shorter duration of respiratory support with ventilation or CPAP therapy.[2,25,43] In a post-hoc subgroup analysis of the CAP trial, the effect of caffeine, compared with placebo, on the PMA at last PPV appeared greater for infants initiating caffeine within the first 3 days of age compared with later initiation (mean difference: early, −1.35 days vs late −0.55 days, test for heterogeneity adjusted $P = .03$).[25]

In an initial study reporting the comparative effectiveness of early (initiation < 3 days of life) versus late (initiation at or after 3 days of life) caffeine therapy at a single center, early caffeine therapy was associated with a lower risk of BPD (adjusted OR 0.26, 95% CI 0.09–0.70; $P<.01$) and shorter duration of invasive ventilation (median 6 vs 22 days, $P<.01$).[43] Subsequently, 3 large multicenter cohort studies in the United States and Canada have confirmed these findings.[2,42,44] In a multicenter cohort study of 62,056 VLBW infants who were propensity matched to reduce confounding, early caffeine initiation was associated with a lower risk of BPD (OR 0.68; 95% CI 0.69–0.08) and a shorter duration of mechanical ventilation (median 3 vs 6 days, $P<.001$) compared with infants receiving late caffeine.[2] In a large multicenter cohort study in Canada of infants born before 31 weeks' gestation, infants receiving early caffeine in the first 2 days of life, compared with later caffeine, had a shorter duration of invasive mechanical ventilation and a shorter duration of noninvasive respiratory support.[42] Early caffeine use in this study was also associated with a decreased risk of BPD (adjusted OR 0.79; 95% CI 0.64–0.96) and surgical treatment of a patent ductus arteriosus (adjusted OR 0.58; 95% CI 0.42–0.80). Similar findings of a decrease in the risk of BPD associated with early caffeine (0–2 days of age), compared with later initiation (3–10 days) were reported in a study of 2951 infants weighing less than or equal to 1250 g at birth (adjusted OR 0.69; 95% CI 0.58–0.82).[44] However, this study reported an increased risk of necrotizing enterocolitis (NEC) among infants receiving early caffeine (adjusted OR 1.41; 95% CI 1.04–1.91).[44] By contrast, none of the other studies evaluating the effects of early initiation of caffeine, compared with later initiation, found an association between early caffeine exposure and NEC.[2,42,43]

A recent pilot randomized trial evaluated the use of early prophylactic caffeine very soon after birth.[45] In this study, infants less than 29 weeks' gestation were randomized to early prophylactic use of caffeine before 2 hours of age or caffeine initiation at 12 hours of age. The study reported fewer infants in the early caffeine treatment arm required intubation by 12 hours of age, compared with those receiving caffeine at 12 hours of age, although this was not a statistically significant difference (27% vs 70%, $P = .08$). By contrast, there was no reduction in days of mechanical ventilation between infants receiving caffeine before 2 hours versus 12 hours of age (mean 6 days vs 3 days; $P = .40$). Additional studies are necessary to determine if prophylactic caffeine can successfully prevent the need for intubation among preterm infants initially supported with noninvasive respiratory modalities.

DOSE AND DURATION OF CAFFEINE THERAPY

Pharmacodynamic studies investigating the relationship between caffeine dose, plasma concentrations, and ventilatory responses show a rapid increase in minute ventilation followed by a plateau in response with increasing doses of caffeine.[46] These observations resulted in the widely used regimens of a loading dose followed by daily maintenance therapy. Approval of caffeine citrate by the US Food and Drug Administration for the treatment of apnea of prematurity was based on the standard dosing regimen of a loading dose of 20 mg/kg (10 mg/kg of caffeine base) followed by a daily maintenance dose of 5 mg/kg.[8] This dosing regimen usually achieves plasma caffeine concentrations of 8 to 20 mg/L in infants less than 32 weeks PMA.

After 32 weeks PMA, and particularly after 36 weeks PMA, caffeine metabolism increases and the standard dosing regimen may result in subtherapeutic levels.[47] Higher doses may be required beyond 36 weeks PMA to maintain therapeutic effects.

As discussed previously, some studies have reported that higher doses of caffeine may be more efficacious in facilitating extubation and reducing the frequency of apnea.[13,14,24,26,48] In the United States, most neonatal centers currently use a maintenance dose of 5 to 10 mg/kg/d of caffeine citrate for routine therapy. However, some international centers have reported use of maintenance doses of up to 20 mg/kg/d.[13,24] Maintenance doses up to 30 mg/kg/d have been reported without significant adverse effects, and preterm infants have been shown to safely tolerate caffeine concentrations as high as 50 to 84 mg/L.[13,14,26] However, safety concerns still exist with the use of early high-dose caffeine, particularly with the recent report of increased rates of cerebellar hemorrhage in infants exposed to early high-dose caffeine,[15] and further study is warranted.

Studies suggest that measurement of serum caffeine concentration is not routinely needed, because most preterm infants, including those with hepatic and renal impairment, attain goal plasma levels with current dosing regimens.[49,50] A recent retrospective study associated higher average caffeine concentrations in infants less than 30 weeks' gestation with improved outcomes, including a decreased duration of ventilation, lower incidence of BPD, and shorter duration of supplemental oxygen use.[51] Confirmation of these findings in a prospective study may guide additional studies to identify the optimal dosing and therapeutic levels of caffeine.

Caffeine treatment is usually terminated at 33 to 35 weeks PMA following resolution of clinically apparent apnea.[1] In the CAP trial, the median PMA at discontinuation of caffeine was 34 weeks.[20] Extended caffeine therapy in preterm infants nearing initial hospital discharge has been shown to reduce intermittent hypoxia, especially in infants at 35 and 36 weeks PMA.[9] However, the routine practice of extended caffeine therapy cannot be recommended at this time because it is unknown whether intermittent hypoxia adversely affects outcomes in preterm infants nearing term-equivalent age.

SUMMARY

Caffeine has an important role in noninvasive respiratory support by facilitating transition from invasive to noninvasive support, reducing the duration of positive airway pressure support, and decreasing the risk of BPD. Multiple mechanisms of action beyond a reduction in apnea are likely to mediate the beneficial effects of caffeine. Additional studies are necessary to guide optimal use of caffeine, including treatment decisions on the dose, duration, and timing of therapy.

REFERENCES

1. Dobson NR, Hunt CE. Pharmacology review: caffeine use in neonates: indications, pharmacokinetics, clinical effects, outcomes. Neoreviews 2003;14: e540–50.

2. Dobson NR, Patel RM, Smith PB, et al. Trends in caffeine use and association between clinical outcomes and timing of therapy in very low birth weight infants. J Pediatr 2014;164(5):992–8.e3.

3. Clark RH, Bloom BT, Spitzer AR, et al. Reported medication use in the neonatal intensive care unit: data from a large national data set. Pediatrics 2006;117(6): 1979–87.

4. Abu-Shaweesh JM, Martin RJ. Neonatal apnea: what's new? Pediatr Pulmonol 2008;43(10):937–44.

5. Martin RJ, Di Fiore JM, Macfarlane PM, et al. Physiologic basis for intermittent hypoxic episodes in preterm infants. Adv Exp Med Biol 2012;758:351–8.

6. Poets CF, Roberts RS, Schmidt B, et al. Association between intermittent hypoxemia or bradycardia and late death or disability in extremely preterm infants. JAMA 2015;314(6):595–603.

7. Henderson-Smart DJ, De Paoli AG. Methylxanthine treatment for apnoea in preterm infants. Cochrane Database Syst Rev 2010;(12):CD000140. [denotes systematic reviews and meta-analyses].

8. Erenberg A, Leff RD, Haack DG, et al. Caffeine citrate for the treatment of apnea of prematurity: a double-blind, placebo-controlled study. Pharmacotherapy 2000; 20(6):644–52.

9. Rhein LM, Dobson NR, Darnall RA, et al. Effects of caffeine on intermittent hypoxia in infants born prematurely: a randomized clinical trial. JAMA Pediatr 2014;168(3):250–7.

10. Mayer CA, Haxhiu MA, Martin RJ, et al. Adenosine A2A receptors mediate GABAergic inhibition of respiration in immature rats. J Appl Physiol (1985) 2006;100(1):91–7.

11. Wilson CG, Martin RJ, Jaber M, et al. Adenosine A2A receptors interact with GABAergic pathways to modulate respiration in neonatal piglets. Respir Physiol Neurobiol 2004;141(2):201–11.

12. Bhatt-Mehta V, Schumacher RE. Treatment of apnea of prematurity. Paediatr Drugs 2003;5(3):195–210.

13. Steer P, Flenady V, Shearman A, et al. High dose caffeine citrate for extubation of preterm infants: a randomised controlled trial. Arch Dis Child Fetal Neonatal Ed 2004;89(6):F499–503.

14. Steer PA, Flenady VJ, Shearman A, et al. Periextubation caffeine in preterm neonates: a randomized dose response trial. J Paediatr Child Health 2003;39(7): 511–5.

15. McPherson C, Neil JJ, Tjoeng TH, et al. A pilot randomized trial of high-dose caffeine therapy in preterm infants. Pediatr Res 2015;78(2):198–204.

16. Henderson-Smart DJ, De Paoli AG. Prophylactic methylxanthine for prevention of apnoea in preterm infants. Cochrane Database Syst Rev 2010;(12):CD000432. [denotes systematic reviews and meta-analyses].

17. Abu Jawdeh EG, O'Riordan M, Limrungsikul A, et al. Methylxanthine use for apnea of prematurity among an international cohort of neonatologists. J Neonatal Perinatal Med 2013;6(3):251–6.

18. Lista G, Fabbri L, Polackova R, et al. The real-world routine use of caffeine citrate in preterm infants: a European Postauthorization Safety Study. Neonatology 2016; 109(3):221–7.

19. Baraldi E, Filippone M. Chronic lung disease after premature birth. N Engl J Med 2007;357(19):1946–55.

20. Schmidt B, Roberts RS, Davis P, et al. Caffeine therapy for apnea of prematurity. N Engl J Med 2006;354(20):2112–21.

21. Schmidt B, Roberts RS, Davis P, et al. Long-term effects of caffeine therapy for apnea of prematurity. N Engl J Med 2007;357(19):1893–902.

22. Schmidt B, Anderson PJ, Doyle LW, et al. Survival without disability to age 5 years after neonatal caffeine therapy for apnea of prematurity. JAMA 2012;307(3): 275–82.

23. Henderson-Smart DJ, Davis PG. Prophylactic methylxanthines for endotracheal extubation in preterm infants. Cochrane Database Syst Rev 2010;(12):CD000139. [denotes systematic reviews and meta-analyses].

24. Mohammed S, Nour I, Shabaan AE, et al. High versus low-dose caffeine for apnea of prematurity: a randomized controlled trial. Eur J Pediatr 2015;174(7): 949–56.

25. Davis PG, Schmidt B, Roberts RS, et al. Caffeine for Apnea of Prematurity trial: benefits may vary in subgroups. J Pediatr 2010;156(3):382–7.

26. Gray PH, Flenady VJ, Charles BG, et al. Caffeine Collaborative Study G. Caffeine citrate for very preterm infants: effects on development, temperament and behaviour. J Paediatr Child Health 2011;47(4):167–72.

27. Mola SJ, Annibale DJ, Wagner CL, et al. NICU bedside caregivers sustain process improvement and decrease incidence of bronchopulmonary dysplasia in infants < 30 weeks gestation. Respir Care 2015;60(3):309–20.

28. Davis JM, Bhutani VK, Stefano JL, et al. Changes in pulmonary mechanics following caffeine administration in infants with bronchopulmonary dysplasia. Pediatr Pulmonol 1989;6(1):49–52.

29. Yoder B, Thomson M, Coalson J. Lung function in immature baboons with respiratory distress syndrome receiving early caffeine therapy: a pilot study. Acta Paediatr 2005;94(1):92–8.

30. Aranda JV, Turmen T, Davis J, et al. Effect of caffeine on control of breathing in infantile apnea. J Pediatr 1983;103(6):975–8.

31. Supinski GS, Deal EC Jr, Kelsen SG. The effects of caffeine and theophylline on diaphragm contractility. Am Rev Respir Dis 1984;130(3):429–33.

32. Kassim Z, Greenough A, Rafferty GF. Effect of caffeine on respiratory muscle strength and lung function in prematurely born, ventilated infants. Eur J Pediatr 2009;168(12):1491–5.

33. Weichelt U, Cay R, Schmitz T, et al. Prevention of hyperoxia-mediated pulmonary inflammation in neonatal rats by caffeine. Eur Respir J 2013;41(4):966–73.

34. Nagatomo T, Jimenez J, Richter J, et al. Caffeine prevents hyperoxia-induced functional and structural lung damage in preterm rabbits. Neonatology 2016; 109(4):274–81.

35. Koroglu OA, MacFarlane PM, Balan KV, et al. Anti-inflammatory effect of caffeine is associated with improved lung function after lipopolysaccharide-induced amnionitis. Neonatology 2014;106(3):235–40.

36. Fehrholz M, Speer CP, Kunzmann S. Caffeine and rolipram affect Smad signalling and TGF-β1 stimulated CTGF and transgelin expression in lung epithelial cells. PLoS One 2014;9(5):e97357.

37. Aly H, Massaro AN, Patel K, et al. Is it safer to intubate premature infants in the delivery room? Pediatrics 2005;115(6):1660–5.

38. Dargaville PA, Aiyappan A, De Paoli AG, et al. Continuous positive airway pressure failure in preterm infants: incidence, predictors and consequences. Neonatology 2013;104(1):8–14.

39. Ammari A, Suri M, Milisavljevic V, et al. Variables associated with the early failure of nasal CPAP in very low birth weight infants. J Pediatr 2005;147(3):341–7.

40. Finer NN, Carlo WA, Walsh MC, et al. Early CPAP versus surfactant in extremely preterm infants. N Engl J Med 2010;362(21):1970–9.

41. Morley CJ, Davis PG, Doyle LW, et al. Nasal CPAP or intubation at birth for very preterm infants. N Engl J Med 2008;358(7):700–8.

42. Lodha A, Seshia M, McMillan DD, et al. Association of early caffeine administration and neonatal outcomes in very preterm neonates. JAMA Pediatr 2015;169(1): 33–8.

43. Patel RM, Leong T, Carlton DP, et al. Early caffeine therapy and clinical outcomes in extremely preterm infants. J Perinatol 2013;33(2):134–40.

44. Taha D, Kirkby S, Nawab U, et al. Early caffeine therapy for prevention of bronchopulmonary dysplasia in preterm infants. J Matern Fetal Neonatal Med 2014; 27(16):1698–702.

45. Katheria AC, Sauberan JB, Akotia D, et al. A pilot randomized controlled trial of early versus routine caffeine in extremely premature infants. Am J Perinatol 2015;32(9):879–86.

46. Turmen T, Davis J, Aranda JV. Relationship of dose and plasma concentrations of caffeine and ventilation in neonatal apnea. Semin Perinatol 1981;5(4):326–31.

47. Charles BG, Townsend SR, Steer PA, et al. Caffeine citrate treatment for extremely premature infants with apnea: population pharmacokinetics, absolute bioavailability, and implications for therapeutic drug monitoring. Ther Drug Monit 2008; 30(6):709–16.

48. Scanlon JE, Chin KC, Morgan ME, et al. Caffeine or theophylline for neonatal apnoea? Arch Dis Child 1992;67(4 Spec No):425–8.

49. Natarajan G, Botica ML, Thomas R, et al. Therapeutic drug monitoring for caffeine in preterm neonates: an unnecessary exercise? Pediatrics 2007;119(5):936–40.

50. Leon AE, Michienzi K, Ma CX, et al. Serum caffeine concentrations in preterm neonates. Am J Perinatol 2007;24(1):39–47.

51. Alur P, Bollampalli V, Bell T, et al. Serum caffeine concentrations and short-term outcomes in premature infants of 29 weeks of gestation. J Perinatol 2015;35(6): 434–8.

Noninvasive Support

Does It Really Decrease Bronchopulmonary Dysplasia?

 CrossMark

Clyde J. Wright, MD[a],*, Richard A. Polin, MD[b]

KEYWORDS

- CPAP (continuous positive airway pressure) • nCPAP (nasal CPAP)
- BPD (bronchopulmonary dysplasia) • Ventilatory-induced lung injury
- SLI (sustained lung inflation) • INSURE (INtubate, SURfactant, Extubate)
- Mechanical ventilation • High frequency ventilation

KEY POINTS

- The incidence of bronchopulmonary dysplasia (BPD) and death or BPD is decreased with early initiation of nasal continuous positive airway pressure (CPAP).
- There is no benefit on the incidence of BPD to using prophylactic or "early" administration of surfactant.
- The optimal way to administer CPAP is unknown; however, there may be considerable differences in the efficacy of various CPAP devices.
- Sustained lung inflation may increase the rate of CPAP success, but may not decrease the incidence of BPD if positive pressure ventilation is needed.
- The benefits of administering surfactant through a thin plastic catheter requires further investigation.

INTRODUCTION

Bronchopulmonary dysplasia (BPD) is the most serious and common complication of mechanical ventilation in the neonate, resulting in increased morbidity and mortality. The first description of BPD by Northway and colleagues[1] identified oxygen and

Conflict of Interest: C.J. Wright is a past recipient of a Young Investigator Award from Actelion Pharmaceuticals (2014–15). The research funded by that grant was unrelated to the topic discussed here, and none of the current submission was supported by the grant. R.A. Polin is a consultant for Discovery Labs and Fisher Paykel and has a grant from Fisher Paykel.
[a] Section of Neonatology, Department of Pediatrics, Perinatal Research Center, Children's Hospital Colorado, University of Colorado School of Medicine, Mail Stop F441, 13243 East 23rd Avenue, Aurora, CO 80045, USA; [b] Department of Pediatrics, Morgan Stanley Children's Hospital, 3959 Broadway, New York, NY 10032, USA
* Corresponding author.
E-mail address: clyde.wright@ucdenver.edu

Clin Perinatol 43 (2016) 783–798
http://dx.doi.org/10.1016/j.clp.2016.07.012
0095-5108/16/© 2016 Elsevier Inc. All rights reserved.

prolonged mechanical ventilation of preterm infants with respiratory distress syndrome (RDS) as the main etiologic factors. In 1987, Avery and colleagues[2] surveyed 8 hospitals with significant inborn populations weighing between 700 to 1500 g to compare respiratory outcomes. BPD was defined as the need for supplemental oxygen at 28 days of life. Columbia University (Babies Hospital) had the lowest percentage of infants needing oxygen at 28 days and 3 months of life that was not explained by other variables. The conclusion of that observational study was that early intervention with continuous distending pressure, reduced dependence on mechanical ventilation, and lack of use of muscle relaxants with mechanical ventilation were practices that seemed to improve outcomes. In the intervening years, a number of interventions have been studied and used clinically in an attempt to decrease the risk of BPD. These include vitamin A,[3] postnatal and antenatal steroids,[4] and caffeine.[5] Probably as a result, the incidence of the severe form of BPD has decreased, although the overall incidence of BPD has remained relatively stable.[6,7] Given the early observations of Avery and colleagues,[2] and the unchanging incidence of BPD,[6] it is somewhat surprising that the use of CPAP has not become more widespread. This qualitative review summarizes the evidence supporting the use of noninvasive ventilation to decrease the incidence of BPD and defines best practices for increasing the successful use of CPAP.

DOES MECHANICAL VENTILATION CONTRIBUTE TO BRONCHOPULMONARY DYSPLASIA?

The association of mechanical ventilation, pulmonary inflammation, and severe chronic lung disease has been known since the 1970s.[8,9] Studies in experimental animals revealed a strong association of positive pressure ventilation with lung injury.[10,11] The effect of CPAP on lung inflammation and injury has been studied in preterm sheep.[12] Compared with preterm sheep that were ventilated, lambs placed on CPAP had fewer neutrophils and less hydrogen peroxide in alveolar washes, both suggesting that lung injury was reduced. However, if lipopolysaccharide was instilled into the trachea as an inflammatory stimulus before CPAP or ventilation, lambs placed on CPAP demonstrated no benefit in either the cytokine markers of lung injury or the systemic response to intratracheal lipopolysaccharide.[13] More recently, Wu and colleagues[14] demonstrated that rats with ventilator-induced lung injury randomized to bubble CPAP (vs spontaneous breathing) had decreased alveolar protein levels and lung injury scores.

Randomized clinical trials in preterm infants receiving other modes of mechanical ventilation (high-frequency jet ventilation[15] or high-frequency oscillatory ventilation)[16] have demonstrated a significant reduction in BPD; however, a recent metaanalysis revealed only a small benefit on the incidence of chronic lung disease.[17] Other ventilation strategies, including synchronized mechanical ventilation[18] and volume-targeted ventilation,[19] are promising, but await further large clinical trials. Additionally, no benefit on the incidence of BPD has been demonstrated using a permissive hypercapnea strategy.[20]

ADVENT OF NONINVASIVE VENTILATION

In 1971, Gregory and associates[21] reported the use of CPAP delivered via endotracheal tube or head box to treat 20 spontaneously breathing neonates with RDS. Application of a continuous distending pressure of 6 to 12 mm Hg increased survival from an expected 25% to a remarkable 80%. Given the earlier observations of Northway and colleagues[1] on the importance of oxygen toxicity in the pathogenesis of BPD, the authors focused on the ability of CPAP to facilitate delivery of the "lowest concentration of oxygen compatible with adequate arterial oxygenation." Over the ensuing years, CPAP was extensively studied, using a variety of interfaces to provide positive airway pressure[4–6] (nasal prongs, head box, and face mask). Randomized trials showed that CPAP improved oxygenation and work of breathing, and improved survival, especially in babies greater than 1.5 kg.[22] Despite this evidence, worry over the complications associated with CPAP (eg, pneumothorax), high rates of failure (approximately 60%) in the smallest babies, and an inability to effectively treat apnea, invasive ventilation replaced routine use of CPAP for treatment of RDS in many centers.[22,23] However, experience with CPAP in the neonatal intensive care unit grew, and it was suggested that it was a powerful tool in preventing extubation failure.[24] Although data from randomized controlled trials were lacking, observational studies suggested that avoiding intubation decreased the risk of developing BPD.[25,26]

Between 1970 and 1990, respiratory care for the preterm neonate evolved quickly. Evidence mounted that routine use of antenatal corticosteroids decreased the incidence of RDS and decreased mortality.[27] The National Institutes of Health recommended it as the standard of care for anticipated delivery between 24 and 34 weeks in 1994.[28] Multiple trials supported that early (vs delayed) administration of surfactant for treatment of RDS improved survival and decreased the incidence of air leak.[29] Furthermore, prophylactic use of surfactant in babies at highest risk of developing RDS improved survival.[30] Based on these trials, prophylactic surfactant became the standard of care babies at high risk of developing RDS and lung injury.[31,32] Unfortunately, neither antenatal corticosteroids nor surfactant have significantly decreased the incidence of BPD.[28–30] Additionally, only 3 pharmacologic interventions—caffeine, vitamin A, and dexamethasone—have been shown to prevent the development of BPD in at-risk infants.[33,34] Postnatal dexamethasone, used early and without consideration of the baseline risk of developing BPD, has been demonstrated to increase the risk of cerebral palsy, and its use was discouraged by the American Academy of Pediatrics in 2002.[35–37] Thus, despite the introduction of interventions that improved the survival in preterm infants, BPD remained a problem without effective preventive therapies.

Thus, lack of preventive therapies, combined with the increasing survival of vulnerable preterm neonates, has resulted in a relatively stable—or even increasing—incidence of BPD. Data collected by the Neonatal Research Network recently on more than 34,000 infants born at 22 to 28 weeks gestation between 1993 and 2012 showed that the incidence of BPD increased over this interval from 32% to 47%, disproportionally affecting those born at the earliest gestational ages (<26 weeks' gestational age).[7] These data necessitate a thoughtful reevaluation of respiratory care practices. Of note, more than 85% of the infants in the Neonatal Research Network cohort were exposed to mechanical ventilation during their stay in the neonatal intensive care unit.[7] As stated, routine intubation and prophylactic surfactant for the highest risk neonates was accepted as the standard of care at many centers. However, studies that informed this practice included very few extremely preterm infants and were performed in a time when many babies did not receive antenatal steroids.[30,38] Furthermore, "control" infants were mechanically ventilated without surfactant, leaving the effectiveness of noninvasive support understudied. Therefore, as antenatal corticosteroid use increased and smaller babies survived, it remained unknown whether prophylactic surfactant, compared with noninvasive support, provided the same benefits to infants less than 1000 g. Alternatively stated, during the time when care for the smallest babies became more invasive, rates of BPD remained stagnant or increased. Would a less invasive approach yield similar results?

TRIALS EVALUATING WHETHER NONINVASIVE VENTILATION PREVENTS BRONCHOPULMONARY DYSPLASIA

Until recently, there were no randomized trials demonstrating a beneficial effect of CPAP on the incidence of BPD. However, beginning in 2008, 5 randomized clinical trials were published comparing nasal CPAP with intubation and surfactant.[39–43] Although the studies had similar primary endpoints, the criteria used to define CPAP failure and the devices used to provide CPAP were different. Almost all study infants weighed less than 1500 g and most were born at less than 28 weeks gestation. The COIN (CPAP or Intubation) trial compared the effectiveness of nasal CPAP (nCPAP) with mechanical ventilation.[42] There was a trend toward a lower rate of death or BPD (oxygen need at 36 weeks gestation) in the CPAP group (odds ratio [OR], 0.80; 95% confidence interval [CI], 0.58–1.12). However, the incidence of pneumothoraces was significantly greater in the CPAP group (9% vs 3%; $P<.001$). Of the CPAP cohort, 46% required mechanical ventilation and 50% of those infants received surfactant. Therefore, the comparison was actually between early CPAP (with 50% of the infants receiving surfactant) and intubation/ventilation with most infants receiving surfactant. In a subsequent subgroup analysis, infants randomized to nCPAP demonstrated significantly lower respiratory rates, better respiratory compliance and improved elastic work of breathing at 2 months postterm age.[44]

SUPPORT (Surfactant Positive Pressure and Oximetry Randomized Trial) randomized 1310 infants to early CPAP or intubation and surfactant.[41] The rate of death or BPD was not different in the CPAP group versus the intubation/surfactant group (OR, 0.91; 95% CI, 0.83–1.01 $P = .07$). Two-thirds of the infants in the nCPAP group ultimately received surfactant. At 18 to 22 months of age, the incidence of wheezing without a cold was 28.9% in the nCPAP group and 36.5% in the ventilation/surfactant group ($P<.05$). In addition, the number of respiratory illnesses diagnosed by a doctor and physician or emergency room visits were significantly less in the nCPAP group.[45]

The VON-DRM (Vermont Oxford Network Delivery Room Management Trial) randomized 647 infants to nCPAP, prophylactic surfactant followed by rapid extubation (INSURE [INtubate, SURfactant, Extubate]) or prophylactic surfactant with stabilization on mechanical ventilation for at least 6 hours.[40] There were no differences in outcomes between the groups. However, compared with the group stabilized on mechanical ventilation, the relative risk (RR) of death or BPD was 0.83 (95% CI, 0.64–1.09) in the CPAP group and 0.78 (95% CI, 0.59–1.03) in the INSURE group.

The CURPAP (An International, Open, Randomized, Controlled Study to Evaluate the Efficacy of Combining Prophylactic Curosurf® With Early Nasal CPAP Versus Early Nasal CPAP Alone in Very Preterm Infants at Risk of Respiratory Distress Syndrome) trial randomized 208 infants to prophylactic surfactant or CPAP within 30 minutes of birth.[43] Rescue surfactant was given to infants failing CPAP followed by an attempt at extubation within 1 hour. The primary endpoint was a need for mechanical ventilation in the first 5 days of life, There were no significant differences in the rates of death or oxygen need at 36 weeks gestation. In the NEOCOSUR study conducted by 12 centers in South America, 256 infants were randomized to CPAP and selective use of INSURE or oxygen followed by selective use of mechanical ventilation.[39] Infants with an of FiO_2 greater than 0.35 received surfactant. The primary endpoint in this study was subsequent need for mechanical ventilation at any time before discharge. The need for mechanical ventilation was reduced in the CPAP/INSURE group ($P = .001$). There was no significant difference in the rate of death or BPD.

There have been 3 recent metaanalyses of these trials.[46–48] The authors of these metaanalyses papers chose slightly different papers to include in their respective reviews. Importantly, only 2 trials, SUPPORT and the Vermont Oxford DRM Study Group trial, have directly compared routine CPAP with routine prophylactic surfactant.[40,41] The COIN trial did not compare routine CPAP with prophylactic surfactant because babies randomized to intubation did not routinely receive surfactant.[42] The CURPAP study randomized infants to prophylactic surfactant followed by rapid extubation to CPAP (if possible) with CPAP alone. This approach, often referred to as INSURE, is arguably different than routine intubation and prophylactic surfactant administration, where the duration of intubation is invariably longer. Speaking to this important difference, the Vermont Oxford DRM Study Group trial showed that in the first hour following intubation and surfactant, approximately 85% of babies (180/216) randomized to INSURE were extubated compared with only 1 of 209 babies randomized to prophylactic surfactant.[40] Thus, considering only the direct comparison of CPAP to prophylactic surfactant (SUPPORT and VON-DRM trials), routine use of CPAP decreases the incidence of death or BPD, with a number needed to treat of 17.7 (**Fig. 1**).[46] The systematic review of Schmolzer and colleagues[47] combined 4 trials (SUPPORT, VON-DRM, CURPAP, and COIN; 2780 infants) and concluded that the combined outcome of death or BPD was significantly lower in babies treated with nCPAP (RR, 0.91; 95% CI, 0.84–0.99; number needed to treat, 25; **Fig. 2**). Finally, the metaanalysis of Fischer and Buhrer included trials comparing CPAP to mechanical ventilation with or without prophylactic surfactant,[40–42] trials comparing CPAP with INSURE,[43,49] as well as trials evaluating less invasive methods of administering surfactant.[50,51] This analysis is the largest and most inclusive (7 trials with 3289 infants), and compared the interventions aimed at "avoiding intubation" to "control." The authors reached a reached a similar conclusion; the OR for death or BPD was 0.83 (95% CI, 0.71–0.96) with an number needed to treat of 35 favoring strategies aimed at avoiding intubation (**Fig. 3**).[48]

Many centers are routinely using the INSURE approach in preterm infants with RDS. A Cochrane systematic review published in 2007 demonstrated that the INSURE approach versus selective surfactant administration and continued ventilation reduced the incidence of BPD at 28 days, but not at 36 weeks gestation.[52] However, the incidence of air leak and mechanical ventilation were significantly reduced. In a recent metaanalysis comparing early CPAP (alone) with INSURE,[53] there were no differences in the rates of chronic lung disease (defined as oxygen need and/or respiratory support) at 36 weeks gestation and/or death, but there was a 12% RR reduction in death or chronic lung disease (RR, 0.88; 95% CI, 0.76–1.02) and a 14% decrease in chronic lung disease (RR, 0.86; 95% CI, 0.71–1.03) in infants randomized to INSURE. The authors concluded that currently no evidence suggests that early INSURE or nCPAP alone is superior to the other.

Given the concerns about surfactant administration through an endotracheal tube, there has been recent interest in administering surfactant through a thin plastic catheter. The less invasive methods have been variably described as "Take care" or "Less invasive surfactant administration." **Table 1** summarizes the results of 5 clinical studies.[50,51,54–56] In 2 of the randomized trials, the incidence of death or BPD was reduced compared with surfactant administration using an endotracheal tube.[50,51] More studies are needed to determine if that approach is efficacious.

WHY DOES IT NOT WORK BETTER? FAILURE OF CONTINUOUS POSITIVE AIRWAY PRESSURE

Unfortunately, routine use of CPAP in the babies at highest risk of lung injury is associated with high rates of failure. In the randomized clinical trials comparing nCPAP with

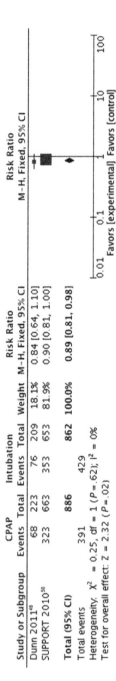

Fig. 1. Effect of routine continuous positive airway pressure (CPAP) versus prophylactic surfactant on death or bronchopulmonary dysplasia. (*From* Wright CJ, Polin RA, Kirpalani H. Continuous positive airway pressure to prevent neonatal lung injury: how did we get here, and how do we improve? J Pediatr 2016;173:17–24.e2; with permission.)

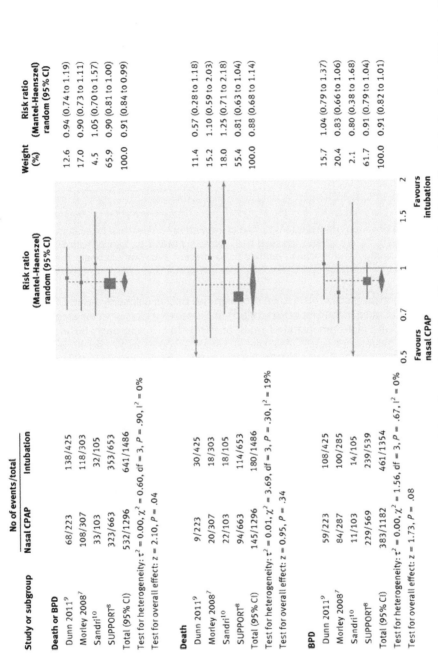

Fig. 2. Effect of routine continuous positive airway pressure (CPAP) versus intubation with or without surfactant/prophylactic surfactant INtubate, SURfactant, Extubate, Extubate/(INSURE)/on death or bronchopulmonary dysplasia. CI, confidence interval. (*From* Schmolzer GM, Kumar M, Pichler G, et al. Non-invasive versus invasive respiratory support in preterm infants at birth: systematic review and meta-analysis. BMJ 2013;347:f5980.)

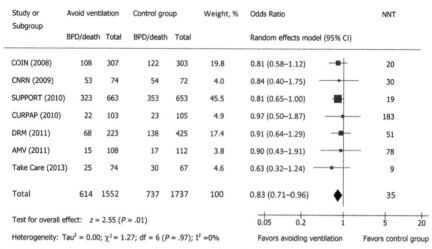

Study or Subgroup	Avoid ventilation		Control group		Weight, %	Odds Ratio		NNT
	BPD/death	Total	BPD/death	Total		Random effects model (95% CI)		
COIN (2008)	108	307	122	303	19.8	0.81 (0.58–1.12)		20
CNRN (2009)	53	74	54	72	4.0	0.84 (0.40–1.75)		30
SUPPORT (2010)	323	663	353	653	45.5	0.81 (0.65–1.00)		19
CURPAP (2010)	22	103	23	105	4.9	0.97 (0.50–1.87)		183
DRM (2011)	68	223	138	425	17.4	0.91 (0.64–1.29)		51
AMV (2011)	15	108	17	112	3.8	0.90 (0.43–1.91)		78
Take Care (2013)	25	74	30	67	4.6	0.63 (0.32–1.24)		9
Total	614	1552	737	1737	100	0.83 (0.71–0.96)		35

Test for overall effect: $z = 2.55$ ($P = .01$)

Heterogeneity: $Tau^2 = 0.00$; $\chi^2 = 1.27$; df = 6 ($P = .97$); $I^2 = 0\%$

0.05   0.2   1   5   20

Favors avoiding ventilation   Favors control group

Fig. 3. Effect of various interventions to "avoid intubation" on death or bronchopulmonary dysplasia (BPD). CI, confidence interval; NNT, number needed to treat. (*From* Fischer HS, Buhrer C. Avoiding endotracheal ventilation to prevent bronchopulmonary dysplasia: a meta-analysis. Pediatrics 2013;132(5):e1355; with permission.)

intubation and surfactant, 45% to 50% of high-risk babies ultimately failed CPAP and required intubation in the first week of life.[40–42] Rates were highest in the smallest babies: the COIN trial demonstrated rates of CPAP failure approach 60% at 25 to 26 weeks' gestational age.[42] This rate is similar to other published observational data.[57–59] Given the high rate of CPAP failure in this group of patients, efforts to optimize CPAP success are necessary to ensure any lung protective effect.

Table 1
Clinical trials evaluating surfactant administration using a thin catheter

Study, Year	Number	Entry Criteria	Need for MV (Catheter/ Endotracheal Tube)	BPD (Catheter/ Endotracheal Tube)
Gopel,[48] 2011	220 26–28 wk	Fio₂ >0.3 and CPAP for the catheter group	33%/73% P<.0001	36 wk PMA 8%/13% P = .268
Kanmaz,[49] 2013	200 <32 wk	Fio₂ ≥0.4 and CPAP	40%/49% P = NS	Moderate to severe 10.3.%/20.2% P = .009
Kribs,[53] 2015	211 23.0–26.8 wk	Fio₂ ≥0.3 and CPAP in the first 2 h	74.8%/99% P<.001	Survival without BPD 67.3%/58.7% NS
Mohammadizadeh,[52] 2015	n = 38 <34 wk	CPAP and need for surfactant	15.8%/10.5% P = NS	NS
Gopel,[54] 2015	2206 26–28 wk	Cohort study Not specified	41%/62% P<.001	36 wk PMA 12%/18% P = .001

Abbreviations: BPD, bronchopulmonary dysplasia; CPAP, continuous positive airway pressure; MV, mechanical ventilation; NS, not significant.

Defining Failure of Continuous Positive Airway Pressure

Randomized controlled trials performed in the 1980s and 1990s conclusively showed that surfactant treatment decreased mortality and air leak in intubated babies with RDS.[60] However, the babies enrolled in these studies were very different from the babies enrolled in the most recent randomized clinical trials that sought to answer whether or not CPAP can prevent BPD. These early trials evaluated surfactant in relatively large (>28 weeks' gestational age) infants, who often did not routinely receive antenatal corticosteroids. In general, the surfactant trials required that, before randomization, babies were intubated and had to demonstrate evidence of RDS most frequently quantified as oxygen requirement (approximately 40% Fio_2).[60] It is likely that many clinicians still use these criteria—an oxygen requirement of approximately 40%, with a mean airway pressure of 6 to 7 cm H_2O- to define CPAP failure and trigger surfactant therapy. Whether these limits are appropriate for babies less than 28 weeks' gestational age on CPAP who have benefited from antenatal steroids is unclear.

Importantly, the definition of CPAP failure that triggered intubation in recent randomized trials was more lax.[40–43,49–51,55,61] In these trials, published between 2008 and 2015, a higher Fio_2 requirement (range 40%–75%) and Pco_2 range (60–70 mm Hg) was allowed (**Table 2**). Furthermore, initial CPAP settings ranged from 5 to 8 cm H_2O, and a maximum level of CPAP (7 cm H_2O) was stipulated in only 2 trials.[40,51] These trials suggest that the keys to improving CPAP success are (1) giving every baby an opportunity to succeed on CPAP, starting in the delivery room, (2) using a more "liberal" definition of CPAP failure than derived from the surfactant trials, and (3) delivering a safe, appropriate level of noninvasive support.

Optimizing Delivery of Continuous Positive Airway Pressure

Ultimately, CPAP success relies on effective delivery of distending pressure to the lung. To date, there are no data to suggest that 1 mode of CPAP delivery (bubble vs variable flow vs continuous flow CPAP) is better than any other. One small randomized controlled trial showed no difference between variable and continuous flow CPAP in preventing CPAP failure in infants with RDS.[62] Similarly, significant differences between modalities of CPAP delivery in preventing postextubation failure in preterm infants with RDS have not been established.[63–65] However, Gupta and colleagues[64] showed in a post hoc analysis, that the subgroup of preterm neonates intubated for less than 14 days, bubble CPAP was more effective than variable flow CPAP for preventing extubation failure. These clinical data are consistent with laboratory studies that signal that there may be a beneficial effect of using bubble CPAP to deliver distending pressure.[66,67]

It may be that optimizing CPAP success relies on multiple, small additional interventions that make up a "best practices" approach. Using a T-piece device during resuscitation, rather than a self-inflating bag, seems to decrease intubation rates in the delivery room.[68] When compared with supine positioning, the left lateral and prone positioning decreases work of breathing of infants on CPAP and is a simple way to improve lung mechanics.[69] Routine use of caffeine in premature infants (500–1250 g) limits exposure to mechanical ventilation, and protects against the development of BPD specifically in infants treated with noninvasive ventilation, and is a useful, evidence-based adjunct.[70–72]

Nonetheless, some babies at high risk of developing BPD will, despite best practice, fail CPAP and require intubation. Retrospective data show that even in experienced centers, approximately two-thirds of the smallest infants (<700 g) require intubation.[59]

Table 2
Definition of CPAP failure and CPAP settings in RCTs

Trial, Year	Fio$_2$ and Sat Goals	CPAP Failure Apnea	Apnea
CPAP versus intubation			
COIN,[40] 2008	>60%	>6 needing stimulation in 6 h or >1 needing BMV	>60 and pH <7.25
SUPPORT,[39] 2010	>50% to maintain 88%	Not included	>65
Dunn,[38] 2011	Mandatory: >60% to maintain 86%–94% discretionary: 40%–60% to maintain 86%–94%	>12 needing stimulation in 6 h or >1 needing BMV	>65
CPAP versus surfactant/extubation			
Gopel,[48] 2011	30%–60%	Not included	>60–70 7.15–7.2
Rojas,[47] 2009	>75%	Not included	>65 and pH <7.22
Sandri,[41] 2010	>40% to maintain 85%–92%	>4/h or >2 needing BMV	>65 and pH <7.2
Less invasive surfactant administration techniques			
Kanmaz,[49] 2013	>40%–60% to maintain 85%–92%	Apnea requiring repeated episodes of PPV	>60, pH <7.2,
Dargaville,[59] 2013	>50% to maintain 88%	Apnea	"Respiratory acidosis"
Kribs,[53] 2015	>45% to maintain a Po$_2$ of 45 mm Hg	Severe apnea despite respiratory analeptic therapy	Respiratory acidosis with pH <7.15

Abbreviations: BMV, bag mask ventilation; CPAP, continuous positive airway pressure; PPV, positive pressure ventilation; RCT, randomized controlled trial.

However, the percentage falls to less than 50% when considering only the babies not requiring intubation in the delivery room.[59] One potential way to optimize CPAP success in these babies is to develop clinical screening tools that successfully predict failure, which might allow earlier intervention (increasing CPAP, administering surfactant, etc). The benefit of this approach would be to allow the babies with the highest likelihood of succeeding on CPAP to remain on CPAP, while providing the benefit of surfactant to those infants who are likely to be ventilated. Observational data demonstrate that CPAP failure is most frequently marked by increasing oxygen and CPAP requirements; these events occur early in the postnatal course. Data from randomized controlled trials support these findings. Most babies failing CPAP (approximately 50%) in the CURPAP and COIN trials were intubated for increasing oxygen requirements within the first 8 hours of life.[42,43] However, because an increasing Fio$_2$ is frequently included in the criteria defining "CPAP failure," this association is necessarily confounded, and other markers are needed. Interestingly, lack of receipt of antenatal corticosteroids has not been associated with an increased risk of CPAP failure.[57,58,73–75] Receiving PPV in the delivery room and a chest radiograph consistent with severe RDS are associated with CPAP failure, but without great (approximately

50%) positive predictive value.[59] Other groups have demonstrated consistently that male infants fail CPAP more often than female infants.[57,73,74] The ability of more sophisticated measures of pulmonary function, including tidal volume breaths and peak inspiratory flows immediately after delivery to predict CPAP failure deserves further study.[76] The stable microbubble test was developed to predict which babies would develop RDS.[77,78] It has recently been shown to perform well in babies receiving noninvasive ventilation, and may help to guide selective surfactant therapy.[79,80]

Other potentially helpful adjuncts await further study. It has been proposed that providing positive pressure at 20 to 25 cm H_2O for 5 to 20 seconds shortly after birth via a nasopharyngeal tube or facemask will help to establish functional reserve capacity and prevent CPAP failure in preterm infants.[81,82] However, in experimental animals, sustained lung inflation followed by mechanical ventilation did not reduce the inflammatory response in the lung.[83,84] Results from an ongoing clinical trial will tell us whether sustained lung inflation reduces the combined outcome of BPD or death in babies born at 23 to 26 weeks' GA.[85]

Studies have demonstrated that, when compared with CPAP alone, surfactant plus CPAP and the INSURE protocol decreases the need for mechanical ventilation, but does not decrease the incidence of death or BPD.[40,43,46,49,50,86] An attempt to minimize or completely avoid exposure to mechanical ventilation by using less invasive methods to deliver surfactant to spontaneously breathing babies is important. A large randomized trial directly comparing Minimally Invasive Surfactant Therapy (MIST) to CPAP will be completed in 2019 (NCT02140580).[87]

SUMMARY

Initiation of noninvasive respiratory support using nasal prongs (nCPAP) is replacing intubation and surfactant as the first line of therapy for many preterm infants with RDS. However, the criteria used to define CPAP failure, the selection of infants who are likely to succeed on CPAP, and the optimal way to administer CPAP are unknown. Strategies that are likely to enhance the success of nCPAP (eg, sustained lung inflation or minimally invasive surfactant therapy) need further study.

REFERENCES

1. Northway WH Jr, Rosan RC, Porter DY. Pulmonary disease following respirator therapy of hyaline-membrane disease. Bronchopulmonary dysplasia. N Engl J Med 1967;276(7):357–68.

2. Avery ME, Tooley WH, Keller JB, et al. Is chronic lung disease in low birth weight infants preventable? A survey of eight centers. Pediatrics 1987;79:26–30.

3. Tyson JE, Wright LL, Oh W, et al. Vitamin a supplementation for extremely-low-birth-weight infants. National Institute of Child Health and Human Development Neonatal Research Network. N Engl J Med 1999;340(25):1962–8.

4. Doyle LW, Ehrenkranz RA, Halliday HL. Late (> 7 days) postnatal corticosteroids for chronic lung disease in preterm infants. Cochrane Database Syst Rev 2014;(5):CD001145.

5. Schmidt B, Roberts RS, Davis P, et al. Caffeine therapy for apnea of prematurity. N Engl J Med 2006;354(20):2112–21.

6. Ancel PY, Goffinet F, Group E-W, et al. Survival and morbidity of preterm children born at 22 through 34 weeks' gestation in France in 2011: results of the EPIPAGE-2 cohort study. JAMA Pediatr 2015;169(3):230–8.

7. Stoll BJ, Hansen NI, Bell EF, et al. Trends in care practices, morbidity, and mortality of extremely preterm neonates, 1993-2012. JAMA 2015;314(10):1039–51.
8. Rhodes PG, Hall RT, Leonidas JC. Chronic pulmonary disease in neonates with assisted ventilation. Pediatrics 1975;55(6):788–96.
9. Taghizadeh A, Reynolds EO. Pathogenesis of bronchopulmonary dysplasia following hyaline membrane disease. Am J Pathol 1976;82(2):241–64.
10. Gerstmann DR, deLemos RA, Coalson JJ, et al. Influence of ventilatory technique on pulmonary baroinjury in baboons with hyaline membrane disease. Pediatr Pulmonol 1988;5(2):82–91.
11. Yoder BA, Coalson JJ. Animal models of bronchopulmonary dysplasia. The preterm baboon models. Am J Physiol Lung Cell Mol Physiol 2014;307(12):L970–7.
12. Jobe AH, Kramer BW, Moss TJ, et al. Decreased indicators of lung injury with continuous positive expiratory pressure in preterm lambs. Pediatr Res 2002; 52(3):387–92.
13. Polglase GR, Hillman NH, Ball MK, et al. Lung and systemic inflammation in preterm lambs on continuous positive airway pressure or conventional ventilation. Pediatr Res 2009;65(1):67–71.
14. Wu CS, Chou HC, Huang LT, et al. Bubble CPAP support after discontinuation of mechanical ventilation protects rat lungs with ventilator-induced lung injury. Respiration 2016;91(2):171–9.
15. Keszler M, Modanlou HD, Brudno DS, et al. Multicenter controlled clinical trial of high-frequency jet ventilation in preterm infants with uncomplicated respiratory distress syndrome. Pediatrics 1997;100(4):593–9.
16. Sun H, Cheng R, Kang W, et al. High-frequency oscillatory ventilation versus synchronized intermittent mandatory ventilation plus pressure support in preterm infants with severe respiratory distress syndrome. Respir Care 2014;59(2):159–69.
17. Cools F, Offringa M, Askie LM. Elective high frequency oscillatory ventilation versus conventional ventilation for acute pulmonary dysfunction in preterm infants. Cochrane Database Syst Rev 2015;(3):CD000104.
18. Greenough A, Dimitriou G, Prendergast M, et al. Synchronized mechanical ventilation for respiratory support in newborn infants. Cochrane Database Syst Rev 2008;(1):CD000456.
19. Peng W, Zhu H, Shi H, et al. Volume-targeted ventilation is more suitable than pressure-limited ventilation for preterm infants: a systematic review and meta-analysis. Arch Dis Child Fetal Neonatal Ed 2014;99(2):F158–65.
20. Thome UH, Genzel-Boroviczeny O, Bohnhorst B, et al. Permissive hypercapnia in extremely low birthweight infants (PHELBI): a randomised controlled multicentre trial. Lancet Respir Med 2015;3(7):534–43.
21. Gregory GA, Kitterman JA, Phibbs RH, et al. Treatment of the idiopathic respiratory-distress syndrome with continuous positive airway pressure. N Engl J Med 1971;284(24):1333–40.
22. Roberton NR. Management of hyaline membrane disease. Arch Dis Child 1979; 54(11):838–44.
23. Diblasi RM. Nasal continuous positive airway pressure (CPAP) for the respiratory care of the newborn infant. Respir Care 2009;54(9):1209–35.
24. Morley C. Continuous distending pressure. Arch Dis Child Fetal Neonatal Ed 1999;81(2):F152–6.
25. Van Marter LJ, Allred EN, Pagano M, et al. Do clinical markers of barotrauma and oxygen toxicity explain interhospital variation in rates of chronic lung disease? The Neonatology Committee for the Developmental Network. Pediatrics 2000; 105(6):1194–201.

26. Gittermann MK, Fusch C, Gittermann AR, et al. Early nasal continuous positive airway pressure treatment reduces the need for intubation in very low birth weight infants. Eur J Pediatr 1997;156(5):384–8.

27. Crowley PA. Antenatal corticosteroid therapy: a meta-analysis of the randomized trials, 1972 to 1994. Am J Obstet Gynecol 1995;173(1):322–35.

28. Effect of corticosteroids for fetal maturation on perinatal outcomes. NIH Consens Statement 1994;12(2):1–24.

29. Yost CC, Soll RF. Early versus delayed selective surfactant treatment for neonatal respiratory distress syndrome. Cochrane Database Syst Rev 2000;(2):CD001456.

30. Rojas-Reyes MX, Morley CJ, Soll R. Prophylactic versus selective use of surfactant in preventing morbidity and mortality in preterm infants. Cochrane Database Syst Rev 2012;(3):CD000510.

31. Horbar JD, Carpenter JH, Buzas J, et al. Timing of initial surfactant treatment for infants 23 to 29 weeks' gestation: is routine practice evidence based? Pediatrics 2004;113(6):1593–602.

32. Horbar JD, Rogowski J, Plsek PE, et al. Collaborative quality improvement for neonatal intensive care. NIC/Q Project Investigators of the Vermont Oxford Network. Pediatrics 2001;107(1):14–22.

33. Tin W, Wiswell TE. Drug therapies in bronchopulmonary dysplasia: debunking the myths. Semin Fetal Neonatal Med 2009;14(6):383–90.

34. Schmidt B, Roberts R, Millar D, et al. Evidence-based neonatal drug therapy for prevention of bronchopulmonary dysplasia in very-low-birth-weight infants. Neonatology 2008;93(4):284–7.

35. Doyle LW, Halliday HL, Ehrenkranz RA, et al. An update on the impact of postnatal systemic corticosteroids on mortality and cerebral palsy in preterm infants: effect modification by risk of bronchopulmonary dysplasia. J Pediatr 2014;165(6):1258–60.

36. Demauro SB, Dysart K, Kirpalani H. Stopping the swinging pendulum of postnatal corticosteroid use. J Pediatr 2014;164(1):9–11.

37. Committee on Fetus and Newborn. Postnatal corticosteroids to treat or prevent chronic lung disease in preterm infants. Pediatrics 2002;109(2):330–8.

38. Carlo WA. Gentle ventilation: the new evidence from the support, COIN, VON, CURPAP, Colombian Network, and Neocosur Network trials. Early Hum Dev 2012;88(Suppl 2):S81–3.

39. Tapia JL, Urzua S, Bancalari A, et al. Randomized trial of early bubble continuous positive airway pressure for very low birth weight infants. J Pediatr 2012;161(1):75–80.e71.

40. Dunn MS, Kaempf J, de Klerk A, et al. Randomized trial comparing 3 approaches to the initial respiratory management of preterm neonates. Pediatrics 2011;128(5):e1069–76.

41. Finer NN, Carlo WA, Walsh MC, et al. Early CPAP versus surfactant in extremely preterm infants. N Engl J Med 2010;362(21):1970–9.

42. Morley CJ, Davis PG, Doyle LW, et al. Nasal CPAP or intubation at birth for very preterm infants. N Engl J Med 2008;358(7):700–8.

43. Sandri F, Plavka R, Ancora G, et al. Prophylactic or early selective surfactant combined with nCPAP in very preterm infants. Pediatrics 2010;125(6):e1402–9.

44. Roehr CC, Proquitte H, Hammer H, et al. Positive effects of early continuous positive airway pressure on pulmonary function in extremely premature infants: results of a subgroup analysis of the COIN trial. Arch Dis Child Fetal Neonatal Ed 2011;96(5):F371–3.

45. Stevens TP, Finer NN, Carlo WA, et al. Respiratory outcomes of the Surfactant Positive Pressure and Oximetry Randomized Trial (SUPPORT). J Pediatr 2014; 165(2):240–9.e4.

46. Wright CJ, Polin RA, Kirpalani H. Continuous positive airway pressure to prevent neonatal lung injury: how did we get here, and how do we improve? J Pediatr 2016;173:17–24.e2.

47. Schmolzer GM, Kumar M, Pichler G, et al. Non-invasive versus invasive respiratory support in preterm infants at birth: systematic review and meta-analysis. BMJ 2013;347:f5980.

48. Fischer HS, Buhrer C. Avoiding endotracheal ventilation to prevent bronchopulmonary dysplasia: a meta-analysis. Pediatrics 2013;132(5):e1351–60.

49. Rojas MA, Lozano JM, Rojas MX, et al. Very early surfactant without mandatory ventilation in premature infants treated with early continuous positive airway pressure: a randomized, controlled trial. Pediatrics 2009;123(1):137–42.

50. Gopel W, Kribs A, Ziegler A, et al. Avoidance of mechanical ventilation by surfactant treatment of spontaneously breathing preterm infants (AMV): an open-label, randomised, controlled trial. Lancet 2011;378(9803):1627–34.

51. Kanmaz HG, Erdeve O, Canpolat FE, et al. Surfactant administration via thin catheter during spontaneous breathing: randomized controlled trial. Pediatrics 2013; 131(2):e502–9.

52. Stevens TP, Harrington EW, Blennow M, et al. Early surfactant administration with brief ventilation vs. selective surfactant and continued mechanical ventilation for preterm infants with or at risk for respiratory distress syndrome. Cochrane Database Syst Rev 2007;(4):CD003063.

53. Isayama T, Chai-Adisaksopha C, McDonald SD. Noninvasive ventilation with vs without early surfactant to prevent chronic lung disease in preterm infants: a systematic review and meta-analysis. JAMA Pediatr 2015;169(8):731–9.

54. Mohammadizadeh M, Ardestani AG, Sadeghnia AR. Early administration of surfactant via a thin intratracheal catheter in preterm infants with respiratory distress syndrome: feasibility and outcome. J Res Pharm Pract 2015;4(1):31–6.

55. Kribs A, Roll C, Gopel W, et al. Nonintubated surfactant application vs conventional therapy in extremely preterm infants: a randomized clinical trial. JAMA Pediatr 2015;169(8):723–30.

56. Gopel W, Kribs A, Hartel C, et al. Less invasive surfactant administration is associated with improved pulmonary outcomes in spontaneously breathing preterm infants. Acta Paediatr 2015;104(3):241–6.

57. Dargaville PA, Aiyappan A, De Paoli AG, et al. Continuous positive airway pressure failure in preterm infants: incidence, predictors and consequences. Neonatology 2013;104(1):8–14.

58. Fuchs H, Lindner W, Leiprecht A, et al. Predictors of early nasal CPAP failure and effects of various intubation criteria on the rate of mechanical ventilation in preterm infants of <29 weeks gestational age. Arch Dis Child Fetal Neonatal Ed 2011;96(5):F343–7.

59. Ammari A, Suri M, Milisavljevic V, et al. Variables associated with the early failure of nasal CPAP in very low birth weight infants. J Pediatr 2005;147(3):341–7.

60. Seger N, Soll R. Animal derived surfactant extract for treatment of respiratory distress syndrome. Cochrane Database Syst Rev 2009;(2):CD007836.

61. Dargaville PA, Aiyappan A, De Paoli AG, et al. Minimally-invasive surfactant therapy in preterm infants on continuous positive airway pressure. Arch Dis Child Fetal Neonatal Ed 2013;98(2):F122–6.

62. Bober K, Swietlinski J, Zejda J, et al. A multicenter randomized controlled trial comparing effectiveness of two nasal continuous positive airway pressure devices in very-low-birth-weight infants. Pediatr Crit Care Med 2012;13(2):191–6.

63. Yadav S, Thukral A, Sankar MJ, et al. Bubble vs conventional continuous positive airway pressure for prevention of extubation failure in preterm very low birth weight infants: a pilot study. Indian J Pediatr 2012;79(9):1163–8.

64. Gupta S, Sinha SK, Tin W, et al. A randomized controlled trial of post-extubation bubble continuous positive airway pressure versus Infant Flow Driver continuous positive airway pressure in preterm infants with respiratory distress syndrome. J Pediatr 2009;154(5):645–50.

65. Stefanescu BM, Murphy WP, Hansell BJ, et al. A randomized, controlled trial comparing two different continuous positive airway pressure systems for the successful extubation of extremely low birth weight infants. Pediatrics 2003;112(5):1031–8.

66. Pillow JJ, Hillman N, Moss TJ, et al. Bubble continuous positive airway pressure enhances lung volume and gas exchange in preterm lambs. Am J Respir Crit Care Med 2007;176(1):63–9.

67. Pillow JJ, Travadi JN. Bubble CPAP: is the noise important? an in vitro study. Pediatr Res 2005;57(6):826–30.

68. Szyld E, Aguilar A, Musante GA, et al. Comparison of devices for newborn ventilation in the delivery room. J Pediatr 2014;165(2):234–9.e3.

69. Gouna G, Rakza T, Kuissi E, et al. Positioning effects on lung function and breathing pattern in premature newborns. J Pediatr 2013;162(6):1133–7, 1137.e1.

70. Dobson NR, Patel RM, Smith PB, et al. Trends in caffeine use and association between clinical outcomes and timing of therapy in very low birth weight infants. J Pediatr 2014;164(5):992–8.e3.

71. Davis PG, Schmidt B, Roberts RS, et al. Caffeine for Apnea of Prematurity trial: benefits may vary in subgroups. J Pediatr 2010;156(3):382–7.

72. Schmidt B, Roberts RS, Davis P, et al. Long-term effects of caffeine therapy for apnea of prematurity. N Engl J Med 2007;357(19):1893–902.

73. De Jaegere AP, van der Lee JH, Cante C, et al. Early prediction of nasal continuous positive airway pressure failure in preterm infants less than 30 weeks gestation. Acta Paediatr 2012;101(4):374–9.

74. Rocha G, Flor-de-Lima F, Proenca E, et al. Failure of early nasal continuous positive airway pressure in preterm infants of 26 to 30 weeks gestation. J Perinatol 2013;33(4):297–301.

75. Pillai MS, Sankar MJ, Mani K, et al. Clinical prediction score for nasal CPAP failure in pre-term VLBW neonates with early onset respiratory distress. J Trop Pediatr 2011;57(4):274–9.

76. Siew ML, van Vonderen JJ, Hooper SB, et al. Very preterm infants failing CPAP show signs of fatigue immediately after birth. PLoS One 2015;10(6):e0129592.

77. Chida S, Fujiwara T. Stable microbubble test for predicting the risk of respiratory distress syndrome: I. Comparisons with other predictors of fetal lung maturity in amniotic fluid. Eur J Pediatr 1993;152(2):148–51.

78. Chida S, Fujiwara T, Takahashi A, et al. Precision and reliability of stable microbubble test as a predictor of respiratory distress syndrome. Acta Paediatr Jpn 1991;33(1):15–9.

79. Bhatia R, Morley CJ, Argus B, et al. The stable microbubble test for determining continuous positive airway pressure (CPAP) success in very preterm infants receiving nasal CPAP from birth. Neonatology 2013;104(3):188–93.

80. Fiori HH, Fritscher CC, Fiori RM. Selective surfactant prophylaxis in preterm infants born at < or =31 weeks' gestation using the stable microbubble test in gastric aspirates. J Perinat Med 2006;34(1):66–70.
81. Lista G, Castoldi F, Cavigioli F, et al. Alveolar recruitment in the delivery room. J Matern Fetal Neonatal Med 2012;25(Suppl 1):39–40.
82. Vyas H, Field D, Milner AD, et al. Determinants of the first inspiratory volume and functional residual capacity at birth. Pediatr Pulmonol 1986;2(4):189–93.
83. Hillman NH, Kemp MW, Miura Y, et al. Sustained inflation at birth did not alter lung injury from mechanical ventilation in surfactant-treated fetal lambs. PLoS One 2014;9(11):e113473.
84. Hillman NH, Kemp MW, Noble PB, et al. Sustained inflation at birth did not protect preterm fetal sheep from lung injury. Am J Physiol Lung Cell Mol Physiol 2013; 305(6):L446–53.
85. Foglia EE, Owen LS, Thio M, et al. Sustained Aeration of Infant Lungs (SAIL) trial: study protocol for a randomized controlled trial. Trials 2015;16:95.
86. Verder H, Albertsen P, Ebbesen F, et al. Nasal continuous positive airway pressure and early surfactant therapy for respiratory distress syndrome in newborns of less than 30 weeks' gestation. Pediatrics 1999;103(2):E24.
87. ClinicalTrials.gov. OPTIMIST-A Trials: Minimally-invasive Surfactant Therapy in Preterm Infants 25-28 Weeks Gestation on CPAP, NCT02140580. Available at: https://clinicaltrials.gov/ct2/show/NCT02140580. Accessed August 24, 2016.

Nasal Intermittent Positive Pressure Ventilation for Preterm Neonates: Synchronized or Not?

Markus Waitz, MD[a],*, Lars Mense, MD[a],
Haresh Kirpalani, BM, MSc, FRCPC[b], Brigitte Lemyre, MD, FRCPC[a]

KEYWORDS

• Synchronization • NIPPV • Bilevel • BPD • Noninvasive ventilation • Preterm infant

KEY POINTS

- Nasal intermittent positive pressure ventilation (NIPPV) is a strategy that provides positive pressure above the positive end-expiratory pressure level.
- Bilevel NIPPV and conventional mechanical ventilator-driven NIPPV differ substantially in pressures and cycling times; both methods can be used in a nonsynchronized or synchronized mode.
- Results of a metaanalysis suggest beneficial effects of synchronized CMV NIPPV in preterm infants with regard to extubation failure when compared with continuous positive airway pressure support.
- Little evidence exists on the efficacy of synchronization during CMV NIPPV and bilevel NIPPV and the impact on important outcomes such as bronchopulmonary dysplasia and mortality.

INTRODUCTION

In the last decade, the early use of nasal continuous positive airway pressure (CPAP) has become a cornerstone in the treatment of respiratory distress syndrome in infants born very prematurely.[1] However, CPAP failure occurs in up to 50% of extremely low birth weight infants.[1–4] Apnea of prematurity and progressive respiratory acidosis are the most common reasons for CPAP failure.[5] Nasal intermittent positive pressure ventilation (NIPPV) has become increasingly popular in neonatology, with the goal to avoid intubation and invasive ventilation. NIPPV is defined as any mode of assisted ventilation that delivers pressure throughout the respiratory cycle with additional phasic increase in airway pressure without the presence of an endotracheal tube;

Disclosures: None.
a Department of Pediatrics, University of Ottawa, 401 Smyth Road, Ottawa, ON K1H 8L1, Canada;
b Division of Neonatology, Children's Hospital of Philadelphia, 3401 Civic Center Boulevard, Philadelphia, PA 19104, USA
* Corresponding author.
E-mail address: markus.waitz@paediat.med.uni-giessen.de

NIPPV therefore augments CPAP with superimposed inflations to a set peak pressure.[6] The devices used for this purpose can be broadly classified into 2 categories: bilevel positive airway pressure (bilevel NIPPV) and conventional mechanical ventilator-driven (CMV) NIPPV. They differ substantially in maximal peak inspiratory pressures (PIP) and cycling times.[7] In a large pragmatic randomized controlled trial (RCT), the use of NIPPV did not reduce the rate of death or BPD in extremely low birth weight infants, as compared with CPAP.[8] In this trial, both bilevel NIPPV and CMV NIPPV were used, because of the variability between different NIPPV devices used in clinical practice. Interpretation of results of all studies is complicated by the different devices used to provide NIPPV, the multiple clinical indications, different patient populations, duration and settings of respiratory support (ie, inspiration time, PIP), weaning processes and the use of synchronization during NIPPV.[9] This review focuses on the different NIPPV strategies, indications and reviews current techniques and evidence with regard to synchronization.

RATIONALE FOR THE USE OF NASAL INTERMITTENT POSITIVE PRESSURE VENTILATION

Attention to several perinatal therapies, such as antenatal corticosteroids, surfactant replacement, early CPAP, and the increased use of noninvasive ventilation strategies have improved respiratory outcomes in very preterm infants.[10–12] Nonetheless, prolonged intubation and mechanical ventilation, barotrauma and volutrauma as well as oxygen toxicity are associated with the development of bronchopulmonary dysplasia (BPD).[13] In addition, respiratory instability, including apnea of prematurity and frequent fluctuations in oxygen saturation, may contribute to a poor neurodevelopmental outcome and may increase morbidity as well.[14–17] Although CPAP stabilizes lung volume and improves apnea and upper airway obstruction, it does not effectively improve ventilation and has limited benefits in infants with poor respiratory efforts.[18] Therefore, NIPPV as a mode of noninvasive ventilation has been proposed to avoid mechanical ventilation and stabilize respiration in preterm infants. The mechanisms of action of NIPPV are not yet fully understood. In surfactant-deficient newborn piglets, NIPPV reduced the pulmonary inflammatory response compared with invasive ventilation.[19] Several investigators have shown that NIPPV, especially when used in the synchronized mode, reduces the work of breathing (WOB) and chest wall distortion, and improves gas exchange.[20–23] It is postulated that the intermittent distending pressure above positive end-expiratory pressure (PEEP) level increases the mean airway pressure, which more efficiently recruits the lung and improves functional residual capacity.[24–26]

MODALITIES OF NASAL INTERMITTENT POSITIVE PRESSURE VENTILATION SUPPORT
Differences Between Bilevel Nasal Intermittent Positive Pressure Ventilation and Conventional Mechanical Ventilator-Driven Nasal Intermittent Positive Pressure Ventilation

Devices used to provide bilevel NIPPV mostly deliver a variable flow and aim to provide 2 alternate PEEP levels (high and low). The inspiration times on the bilevel NIPPV are much longer and the respiratory rates are typically lower than those set during CMV NIPPV, to allow spontaneous breathing on both levels of PEEP. The PIP generated by bilevel systems are generally between 9 and 11 cm H_2O.[7] With variable flow systems, the flow toward the baby increases during inspiration and decreases during expiration. Variable flow therefore has been shown to reduce WOB in preterm infants.[27]

CMV NIPPV, in contrast, is delivered by a conventional ventilator and provides a constant flow. Higher PIP are delivered with inspiration times that are comparable with those used during invasive mechanical ventilation (**Fig. 1**). With constant flow

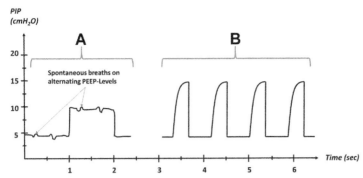

Fig. 1. Differences in pressure wave patterns during (A) bilevel nasal intermittent positive pressure ventilation (NIPPV) and (B) conventional mechanical ventilator-driven NIPPV. PEEP, positive end-expiratory pressure; PIP, peak inspiratory pressure.

systems, inspiratory efforts by the baby typically result in a pressure drop, and a pressure increase occurs during the expiration phase given the constant flow in the respiratory circuit. Those pressure fluctuations in the respiratory circuit may increase WOB.

DO CURRENT METHODS ALLOW EFFECTIVE SYNCHRONIZATION AND WHAT EFFECTS DOES SYNCHRONIZATION HAVE ON RESPIRATORY PARAMETERS?

One of the early NIPPV trials observed that NIPPV was associated with an increased rate of gastrointestinal perforations in neonates.[28] This discouraged further investigations until NIPPV re-emerged with the option of "*synchronization*" using a pneumatic capsule that detects inspiratory efforts based on abdominal wall movements.[9] Subsequent trials confirmed the efficacy of this new trigger technique without gastrointestinal complications.[29,30] Currently, 2 methods are mainly employed to trigger increases in peak pressures, in trials and in clinical practice: (1) a pneumatic capsule (Graseby capsule) detects abdominal wall movements as trigger signal and (2) flow sensors at the airway opening that utilize flow signals to trigger spontaneous breaths. Characteristics and response times of the 2 currently available trigger devices are summarized in **Table 1**. One further method, a pressure trigger, was described in one trial, but trigger effectiveness or response times were not assessed.[31]

Several studies have evaluated physiologic effects such as WOB, accuracy and efficacy of synchronization, gas exchange, tidal volumes and pressure transmission (ie, physiologic studies); they are summarized in **Table 2**. Two studies have shown that tidal volumes in non-synchronized NIPPV only increase when the PIP occurs during spontaneous inspiration; and that synchronized NIPPV (sNIPPV) is associated with increased tidal volumes, minute ventilation, and decreased WOB when compared with CPAP support only.[32,33] The majority of physiologic studies on sNIPPV show decreased WOB, but conflicting results with regard to changes in tidal volumes and gas exchange.[20–22,32] Improvement in tidal volumes were noted in 1 study and increased minute ventilation was reported during synchronized CMV NIPPV along with decreased transcutaneous CO_2 values in another study.[21,32] A post hoc analysis from 1 study revealed enhanced minute ventilation only in infants where higher P_{CO_2} values at baseline ($\geq$55 mm Hg) indicated a more severe lung disease state.[21] The only physiologic study to show a significant improvement in tidal volumes during sNIPPV used very low PEEP levels (ie, 3 cm H_2O).[32]

Table 1
Characteristics of trigger devices used in neonates

Detector	Signal	Response Time (ms)	Advantages	Disadvantages
Air- and sponge-filled abdominal capsule (Graseby capsule)[33,34]	Minimal changes in pressure on capsule surface owing to abdominal wall movements produce mechanical signal processed into electrical signal	53 ± 13	• Easy use • Highly sensitive • Signal not affected by leaks around the interface or water in circuit • Fast response time	• Requires paradoxic abdominal movements • Considerable skills required for placement • No tidal volume measurement
Differential pressure flow transducer[34] or hot wire anemometer[35]	Sensor connected between NIPPV-interface and ventilatory circuit. Flow or volume signal detects spontaneous breathing efforts	25–50 65 ± 12	• Easy placement • Highly sensitive • Fast response time	• Large/variable leaks affect trigger signal • Increased death space • Autotriggering with secretions/water

Abbreviations: NIPPV, noninvasive positive pressure ventilation.

Hence, it remains unclear if improved respiratory parameters were because of inadequate lung recruitment in the CPAP control group, and in contrast the potentially higher mean airway pressure delivered during NIPPV and thus improved functional residual capacity, rather than any effect from synchronization per se. A recent observational study using bilevel NIPPV showed no improvement in tidal volumes, independent of whether the bilevel cycle was triggered or not.[36] This could be related to the relatively small delta pressure of 3 cm H_2O set in that study. The same study detected an overall trigger rate of spontaneous breaths of 82%; and the trigger response time occurred within 50 ms in 83% of all triggered breaths.

In summary, the currently available trigger devices can effectively synchronize spontaneous breaths during both modes of NIPPV (bilevel NIPPV and CMV NIPPV).[23,32,36] Available data from physiologic studies indicate some benefits with regard to WOB and pulmonary mechanics. ,However most of these studies, independent of the device used, suggest that sNIPPV may not be effective to treat severe respiratory failure with hypercarbia. In this condition, inspiratory pressures do not seem to be sufficiently delivered to the alveolar space, especially at very high set PIP levels (ie, >20 cm H_2O).[37] Overall convincing data with regard to improvement in tidal volume or minute ventilation are lacking.[20–23,32,37]

CLINICAL APPLICATION OF SYNCHRONIZED NASAL INTERMITTENT POSITIVE PRESSURE VENTILATION

NIPPV can be used as a "primary mode" of noninvasive respiratory support soon after birth, which may or may not include a brief course of mechanical ventilation, invasive and/or noninvasive surfactant administration. Because there is no clear consensus in

Table 2
Physiologic studies on sNIPPV

Study	Patients	Ventilator/NIPPV Mode/Trigger/Settings	Intervention	Outcome/Results
Aghai et al,[20] 2006	n = 15 BW = 1367 ± 325 g (mean ± SD) GA = 29 ± 2.4 wk (mean ± SD)	• InfantStar ventilator/CMV NIPPV/ Graseby-capsule • CMV NIPPV (ACPC-mode) settings: PEEP 5 cm H_2O, 3 PIP levels were studied (10, 12, 14 cm H_2O), Ti 0.35 sec • CPAP settings: PEEP 5 cm H_2O	• CPAP vs CMV NIPPV • Cross-over design	• sNIPPV reduced inspiratory WOB at all PIP levels with largest reduction at PIP 14 cm H_2O compared with CPAP • Resistive WOB during sNIPPV was significantly lower at PIP levels of 12 and 14 cm H_2O compared with CPAP • Elastic WOB with sNIPPV was only reduced during PIP 14 cm H_2O • No difference in tidal volumes, minute ventilation between sNIPPV and CPAP
Ali et al,[21] 2007	n = 15 BW = 808 ± 201 g (mean ± SD) GA = 25 ± 1.8 wk (mean ± SD)	• Sechrist IV-200 SAVI ventilator/ CMV NIPPV/Inductance plethysmography • CMV NIPPV (PSV-mode) settings: PEEP 5 cm H_2O, pressure support 100%–150% of spontaneous respiratory effort (7.9 ± 1.3 cm H_2O above PEEP), max. Ti 0.45 s • CPAP settings: PEEP 5 cm H_2O	• CPAP vs CMV NIPPV • Cross-over design (2-h each period)	• Lower esophageal pressure during sNIPPV indicates reduced WOB compared with CPAP • No difference in tidal volumes or minute ventilation between CPAP and sNIPPV • Increased minute ventilation during sNIPPV in infants with transcutaneous Pco_2 ≥55 mm Hg (post hoc analysis) • Improved chest wall distortion indicated effective unloading during sNIPPV

(continued on next page)

Table 2
(continued)

Study	Patients	Ventilator/NIPPV Mode/Trigger/Settings	Intervention	Outcome/Results
Chang et al,[22] 2011	n = 16 BW = 993 ± 248 g (mean ± SD) GA = 27.6 ± 2.3 wk (mean ± SD)	• InfantStar ventilator/CMV NIPPV/Graseby-capsule • CMV NIPPV (IMV-mode) settings: no fixed PEEP, PIP 10 cm H_2O above set PEEP, Ti 0.3 s, each mode synchronized nonsynchronized CMV NIPPV studied at respiratory rate 20/min and 40/min • CPAP settings: PEEP set at level before study entry	• CPAP vs synchronized CMV NIPPV vs nonsynchronized CMV NIPPV • Cross-over design (1 h each period)	• No significant differences in gas exchange parameters • Inspiratory WOB was reduced during sNIPPV compared with CPAP or non-sNIPPV at rate 20/min and reduction in WOB was more striking at higher synchronized rates (40/min) • No difference in WOB parameters between non-sNIPPV and CPAP • Non-sNIPPV cycles during exhalation produced increased respiratory effort • 56% of non-sNIPPV ventilator cycles were delivered during exhalation compared with 5% during sNIPPV
Moretti et al,[32] 1999	n = 11 BW = 1141 ± 53 g (mean ± SD) GA = 28.1 ± 0.5 wk (mean ± SD)	• MOG 2000 ventilator/CMV NIPPV/Hot wire flow sensor • CMV NIPPV (SIMV or ACPC mode) settings: PEEP 3 cm H_2O, PIP 12 ± 0.2, Ti 0.36 ± 0.02 s, respiratory rate 38/min (mean) • CPAP-settings: PEEP 3 cm H_2O	• CPAP vs CMV NIPPV • Cross-over design (1-h each period) • Immediately after extubation from RDS treatment	• Lung volumes, tidal volumes, and minute ventilation were significantly greater during sNIPPV • Lower esophageal pressure during synchronized breaths indicated reduced WOB during sNIPPV • Successful trigger rate of 91.2% with a mean trigger response time 65 ± 12 ms (mean ± SD)

Study	Population	Intervention/Settings	Study design	Results

Huang et al,[23] 2015	n = 14
	BW = 928 g (475–1310) Median (range)
	GA = 26.3 ± 2.3 wk
		• Sophie Ventilator/CMV NIPPV/Graseby-capsule
		• CMV NIPPV (SIMV or IMV mode) settings (calculated)
		  ○ SIMV: PEEP 5.6 cm H_2O, PIP 15.0 ± 2.0 cm H_2O, respiratory rate 38 ± 15/min
		  ○ IMV: PEEP 5.6 cm H_2O, PIP 15.1 ± 2.3 cm H_2O, respiratory rate 40 ± 12/min
			• Synchronized CMV NIPPV vs non-sNIPPV
			• Cross-over design (2 h each period)
			• Immediately after extubation from RDS treatment
				• Reduced spontaneous respiratory rate and decreased WOB during sNIPPV
				• Synchrony rate during sNIPPV was 82% (59–97) compared with 26.5% (18–33), median (range), during non-sNIPPV
				• Significantly lower transcutaneous Pco_2 during sNIPPV
				• No significant difference in mean SpO_2, cerebral tissue oxygenation, hypoxemic episodes, or bradycardia between groups

Owen et al,[36] 2015	n = 10
	BW = 776 g (709–816) median (range)
	GA = 26 ± 0 wk (25 ± 5 to 26 ± 2) median (range)
		• Infant flow nCPAP/bilevel NIPPV/Graseby-capsule
		• bilevel-NIPPV settings:
		  ○ Pressure "low" 7 cm H_2O
		  ○ Pressure "high" 10 cm H_2O
		  ○ Ti 0.3 s
		  ○ Apnea time 10 s
		  ○ Backup rate 30/min
			Observational study	• Overall trigger rate was 82%
				• 83% occurred within 50 ms and 9% within 150 ms
				• Synchrony rate was affected by spontaneous respiratory rate
				  ○ With respiratory rate <55/min 89% of spontaneous breaths triggered a bilevel cycle
				  ○ With respiratory rate >55/min 75% of spontaneous breaths triggered a bilevel cycle
				• No changes in tidal volumes during synchronized BIPAP cycles
				• Backup cycle did not deliver measurable tidal volumes

Abbreviations: ACPC, assist control, pressure control; BIPAP, biphasic positive airway pressure; BW, body weight; CMV, conventional mechanical ventilator-driven; CPAP, continuous positive airway pressure; GA, gestational age; IMV, intermittent mechanical ventilation; NIPPV, nasal intermittent positive pressure ventilation; PEEP, positive end-expiratory pressure; PIP, peak inspiratory pressure; RDS, respiratory distress syndrome; SIMV, synchronized intermittent mechanical ventilation; sNIPPV, synchronized nasal intermittent positive pressure ventilation; Ti, inspiratory time; WOB, work of breathing.

the literature on the duration of mechanical ventilation to consider NIPPV being the "primary mode," we define this as mechanical ventilation for less than 24 hours. Therefore, the "secondary mode" refers to its use after a prolonged period of intubation and mechanical ventilation (ie, >24 hours). Additionally, NIPPV can be used to treat symptoms of apnea of prematurity.

Studies Using Synchronized Nasal Intermittent Positive Pressure Ventilation as Primary Mode of Ventilation

There are in total 3 observational and retrospective studies to date in this category (**Table 3**). A prospective observational study by Santin and colleagues[38] compared early synchronized CMV NIPPV following intubation surfactant extubation (INSURE) versus continued mechanical ventilation and later extubation to synchronized CMV NIPPV. Early synchronized CMV NIPPV was associated with significantly less exposure to mechanical ventilation, less supplemental oxygen requirements, and a shorter duration of stay. Gizzi and colleagues[39] conducted a retrospective study that compared the use of CPAP versus synchronized CMV NIPPV following INSURE. Significantly less infants were reintubated within the first 72 hours in the sNIPPV group, the incidence of BPD was lower, and infants needed less surfactant and less methylxanthine compared with the CPAP group. Another retrospective study assessed the use of nonsynchronized bilevel NIPPV versus synchronized CMV NIPPV as either primary mode with or without INSURE in very low birth weight infants and clinical signs of respiratory distress.[40] The investigators did not find a significant difference in the duration or failure of noninvasive respiratory support between the groups.

To date, 3 RCTs have assessed the effect of synchronization during NIPPV in preterm neonates as a primary mode of ventilation (see **Table 3**). In 1 trial, early extubation of preterm infants (n = 41) to synchronized CMV NIPPV resulted in a significantly lower rate of BPD/death when compared with continued mechanical ventilation and later extubation.[41] Kugelman and colleagues[31] randomized 84 infants with clinical signs of respiratory distress syndrome to early CPAP or synchronized CMV NIPPV without foregoing mechanical ventilation or surfactant administration. In this study, infants assigned to early synchronized CMV NIPPV were significantly less likely to be intubated and had a lower incidence of BPD when compared with the early CPAP group. Few infants weighing less than 1000 g were included in this trial. A more recent RCT comparing synchronized CMV NIPPV with unsynchronized bilevel NIPPV (n = 124) did not show a difference in the primary outcomes (failure of or duration of noninvasive respiratory support) between the 2 groups.[42] A potential confounder in this trial is the use of sustained inflation maneuver in the delivery room for all included subjects. This procedure itself has been shown to reduce the need for mechanical ventilation within 72 hours after birth owing to effective lung recruitment and establishment of functional residual capacity.[43] Among all the studies on sNIPPV as primary mode, there was no difference in necrotizing enterocolitis, intraventricular hemorrhage, air leak syndromes, or retinopathy of prematurity.

Studies Using Synchronized Nasal Intermittent Positive Pressure Ventilation as Secondary Mode of Ventilation

Five RCT compared synchronized CMV NIPPV with nasal CPAP as a secondary mode of noninvasive ventilation (**Table 4**).[25,29,30,44,45] In 1 RCT (n = 41), failure of noninvasive respiratory support within the first 48 hours after extubation was significantly lower in the synchronized CMV NIPPV compared with the CPAP group. Notably, 6 infants who met failure criteria in the CPAP group were rescued with synchronized CMV NIPPV.[25] In a trial including 54 infants, Barrington and colleagues[30] demonstrated a significant

Table 3
Studies using sNIPPV as "primary mode"

Study	Intervention/Comparison/Study Type/Outcome	Inclusion Criteria	Ventilator/NIPPV Mode/Trigger/Settings	Outcome/Results
Santin et al,[38] 2004	• Prospective observational • CMV vs early synchronized CMV NIPPV • Primary endpoint: duration of stay	• 28–34 wk GA • RDS with need for surfactant and CMV • n = 59	• InfantStar Ventilator/CMV NIPPV/Graseby-capsule • Settings synchronized CMV NIPPV: ○ PEEP ≤5cm H_2O, PIP 2–4 cm H_2O above preextubation level, flow 8–10 L/min	• sNIPPV group had shorter duration of mechanical ventilation (2.4 ± 0.4 vs 0.3 ± 0.0 d; $P = .001$), less need for additional O_2 requirements (15 ± 3.2 vs 8.2 ± 3.3 d; $P = .04$), fewer days on parenteral nutrition, fewer in-hospital days (37.5 ± 3.0 vs 29.1 ± 3.3 d; $P = .04$) • No difference in IVH, BPD, PVL, NEC, PDA, ROP, or air leak syndromes
Bhandari et al,[41] 2007	• 2-center RCT • CMV vs early synchronized CMV NIPPV • Primary endpoint: combined outcome death or BPD	• 28–34 wk GA • RDS with need for surfactant and CMV • n = 41	• InfantStar Ventilator/CMV NIPPV/Graseby-capsule • Settings synchronized CMV NIPPV: PEEP ≤5 cm H_2O, PIP 2–4 cm H_2O above preextubation level, flow 8–10 L/min	• Significantly lower rate of BPD or death (20% vs 52%; $P = .03$) with sNIPPV • No significant difference in IVH, PVL, NEC, PDA, ROP, air leak syndromes, or neurodevelopmental outcome

(continued on next page)

Table 3 (continued)				
Study	**Intervention/Comparison/Study Type/Outcome**	**Inclusion Criteria**	**Ventilator/NIPPV Mode/Trigger/ Settings**	**Outcome/Results**
Gizzi et al,[39] 2012	• Retrospective analysis • Early CPAP vs early synchronized CMV NIPPV • Primary endpoint: need for mechanical ventilation within 72 h after INSURE	• ≤32 wk GA • RDS treated with INSURE procedure • n = 64	• Giulia Neonatal Ventilator/CMV NIPPV/Hot wire flow sensor • Settings synchronized CMV NIPPV: PEEP 5.5 ± 0.5 cm H_2O, PIP 15 ± 2 cm H_2O, Ti 0.32 ± 0.02, Backup rate 35/min, flow 8.0 ± 0.5 L/min • CPAP settings: PEEP 5–6 cm H_2O, flow 8.0 ± 0.5 L/min	• sNIPPV was associated with less reintubations within 72 h (35.5% vs 6.1%; $P = .004$), less surfactant, less methylxanthine treatment. and lower rate of BPD (12.9% vs 0%; $P = .05$) • No difference in IVH, PVL, NEC, ROP, or air leak syndromes • Higher rate of PDA in CMV NIPPV group
Ricotti et al,[40] 2013	• Retrospective analysis • Early nonsynchronized bilevel NIPPV vs early synchronized CMV NIPPV • Primary endpoint: duration and failure of noninvasive respiratory support	• <32 wk GA and <1500 g BW • RDS with the need of either noninvasive respiratory support and/or INSURE-procedure • n = 78	• Giulia Neonatal Ventilator/CMV NIPPV/Hot wire flow sensor or InfantFlow System for bilevel NIPPV support • Settings synchronized CMV NIPPV: PEEP 4–6 cm H_2O, PIP 15–20 cm H_2O, Ti 0.3–0.4, rate 40–60/min • Bilevel NIPPV-settings: PEEP$_{low}$ 4–6 cm H_2O, PEEP$_{high}$ 8–9 cm H_2O, Ti 0.6–0.7, flow 7–10 L/min	• No significant difference in the duration or failure of noninvasive respiratory support between groups • No difference in IVH, PVL, NEC, ROP, or air leak syndromes, surfactant dose or duration of stay

| Kugelmann et al,[31] 2007 | • RCT
• Early CPAP vs synchronized CMV NIPPV
• Primary endpoint: failure of noninvasive respiratory support | • <35 wk GA
• RDS with need of noninvasive respiratory support
• n = 84 | • SLE 2000 Ventilator/CMV NIPPV/ Pressure trigger
• Settings synchronized CMV NIPPV: PEEP 6–7 cm H_2O, PIP 14–22 cm H_2O, Ti 0.3, Rate 12–30/min
• CPAP-settings: PEEP 6–7 cm H_2O | • Significantly less failure during sNIPPV compared with the CPAP group (49% vs 25%; $P = .04$)
• Infants in sNIPPV-group had significant less incidence of BPD (17% vs 2%; $P = .03$)
• No difference in duration of stay, IVH, or time to reach full feeds |
| Salvo et al,[42] 2015 | • RCT
• Early nonsynchronized bilevel NIPPV vs early synchronized CMV NIPPV
• Primary endpoint: duration and failure of noninvasive respiratory support | • <32 wk GA and BW <1500 g
• RDS with the need of either noninvasive respiratory support and/or INSURE-procedure
• n = 124 | • Giulia Neonatal Ventilator/CMV NIPPV/hot wire flow sensor or InfantFlow System for bilevel NIPPV support
• Settings synchronized CMV NIPPV: PEEP 4–6 cm H_2O, PIP 15–20 cm H_2O, Ti 0.3–0.4, rate 40/min, flow 6–10 L/min
• Bilevel-NIPPV-settings: $PEEP_{low}$ 4–6 cm H_2O, $PEEP_{high}$ 8–9 cm H_2O, Ti 1.0, flow 7–10 L/min | • No difference between groups in failure or duration of noninvasive respiratory support
• No difference in IVH, PVL, NEC, ROP, air leak syndromes, duration of stay, or BPD |

Abbreviations: BPD, bronchopulmonary dysplasia; BW, body weight; CMV, conventional mechanical ventilator-driven; CPAP, continuous positive airway pressure; GA, gestational age; INSURE, intubation surfactant extubation; IVH, intraventricular hemorrhage; NEC, necrotizing enterocolitis; NIPPV, nasal intermittent positive pressure ventilation; PDA, persistent ductus arteriosus; PEEP, positive end-expiratory pressure; PIP, peak inspiratory pressure; PVL, periventricular leukomalacia; RCT, randomized controlled trial; RDS, respiratory distress syndrome; ROP, retinopathy of prematurity; sNIPPV, synchronized nasal intermittent positive pressure ventilation; Ti, inspiratory time.

Table 4
Studies using sNIPPV as "secondary mode"

Study	Intervention/Comparison/Study Type/Outcome	Inclusion Criteria	Ventilator/NIPPV Mode/Trigger/Settings	Outcome/Results
Friedlich et al,[25] 1999	• RCT • CPAP vs synchronized CMV NIPPV • Primary endpoint: failure of noninvasive respiratory support	• BW 500–1500 g • Need for mechanical ventilation • n = 41	• InfantStar Ventilator/CMV NIPPV/Graseby-capsule • Settings synchronized CMV NIPPV: PEEP ≤5 cm H_2O, PIP set at preextubation level, Rate 10/min, Ti 0.6 s • CPAP settings: PEEP set at discretion of clinician	• More infants in CPAP group met criteria for noninvasive respiratory failure compared with sNIPPV (37% vs 5%, $P = .016$) • 6 of 7 infants who failed on CPAP mode were rescued with sNIPPV
Barrington et al,[30] 2001	• RCT • CPAP vs synchronized CMV NIPPV • Primary endpoint: failure of noninvasive respiratory support within 72 h of extubation	• BW <1251 g • Extubation before 6 wk of life • n = 54	• InfantStar Ventilator/CMV NIPPV/Graseby-capsule • Settings synchronized CMV NIPPV: PEEP 6 cm H_2O, PIP 16 cm H_2O, rate 12/min, no Ti reported • CPAP-settings: PEEP 6 cm H_2O	• Lesser incidence of respiratory failure in sNIPPV group compared with CPAP group (14.0% vs 44.4%; $P<.05$) • No difference in NEC, gastrointestinal perforation, BPD, feeding intolerance, or duration of stay • Fewer apneic spells in sNIPPV group (5.1 ± 4.4 vs 8.2 ± 12, mean ± SD)
Gao et al,[45] 2010	• RCT • CPAP vs synchronized CMV NIPPV • Primary endpoint: failure of noninvasive respiratory support after extubation	• <36 wk and/or BW <2 kg • RDS with need for mechanical ventilation within 6 h after birth	• Newport, Teama, Stephan or Millennium ventilators/CMV NIPPV/unspecified synchronization method • Settings synchronized CMV NIPPV: PEEP 5 cm H_2O, PIP 20 cm H_2O, Rate 40/min, no Ti reported • CPAP-settings: PEEP 4–8 cm H_2O, flow 8–10 L/min	• More infants in CPAP group met criteria for reintubation compared with sNIPPV (60% vs 24%; $P<.05$) • Reduction of hypercapnic and hypoxemic episodes during sNIPPV was noted • No difference in air leaks between the 2 groups

Study	Design	Ventilator and Settings	Outcomes
Khalaf et al,[29] 2001	• RCT • CPAP vs synchronized CMV NIPPV • Primary endpoint: failure of noninvasive respiratory support after extubation	• ≤34 wk GA • RDS with need for mechanical ventilation • n = 64	• InfantStar Ventilator/CMV NIPPV/no report on trigger mode • Settings synchronized CMV NIPPV: PEEP ≤5 cm H_2O, PIP 2–4 cm H_2O above preextubation level, rate set at preextubation rate (max. 25/min), • CPAP-settings: PEEP 4–6 cm H_2O	• Need for reintubation within 72 h was lower in sNIPPV group compared with CPAP- group (6% vs 40%; P<.01) • No difference in mortality, NEC, ROP, BPD, duration of stay, sepsis, air leak syndromes or IVH between groups • No difference in apneic spells between the 2 groups
Morettiet al,[44] 2008	• RCT • CPAP vs synchronized CMV NIPPV • Primary endpoint: failure of noninvasive respiratory support within 72 h of extubation	• BW <1251 g • RDS and need for mechanical ventilation within 48 h of life and extubation by day of life 14 • n = 63	• Giulia Neonatal Ventilator/CMV NIPPV/Hot wire flow sensor • Settings synchronized CMV NIPPV: PEEP 3–5 cm H_2O, PIP 10–20 cm H_2O, rate not reported, flow 6–10 L/min, no Ti reported • CPAP-settings: PEEP 3–5 cm H_2O, flow 6–10 L/min	• Failure of noninvasive ventilation was lower in sNIPPV group compared with CPAP group (6% vs 39%;, P = .005) • No difference in secondary outcome: BPD, air leak syndromes, PDA, ROP, IVH, PVL, sepsis, feeding intolerance, or mortality

Abbreviations: BPD, bronchopulmonary dysplasia; BW, body weight; CMV, conventional mechanical ventilator-driven; CPAP, continuous positive airway pressure; GA, gestational age; IVH, intraventricular hemorrhage; NEC, necrotizing enterocolitis; NIPPV, nasal intermittent positive pressure ventilation; PDA, persistent ductus arteriosus; PEEP, positive end-expiratory pressure; PIP, peak inspiratory pressure; PVL, periventricular leukomalacia; RCT, randomized controlled trial; RDS, respiratory distress syndrome; ROP, retinopathy of prematurity; sNIPPV, synchronized nasal intermittent positive pressure ventilation.

reduction in the rate of extubation failure with the use of synchronized CMV NIPPV. A reduction in the number of apneic spells per 24 hours in the CMV NIPPV group was also noted in this trial. In a trial by Khalaf and colleagues,[29] which included 64 patients, significantly fewer infants assigned to synchronized CMV NIPPV met extubation failure criteria, compared with the CPAP group, 72 hours after extubation. Moretti and colleagues[44] evaluated the use of synchronized CMV NIPPV in 63 preterm infants. They found a significantly lower rate of reintubation in the synchronized CMV NIPPV group, compared with CPAP. Gao and colleagues[45] (n = 50) found a significant reduction in the need for reintubation in infants treated with synchronized CMV NIPPV after extubation, compared with CPAP. They also noted a reduced number of hypercapnic and hypoxemic events during synchronized CMV NIPPV. None of the RCT using CMV NIPPV as secondary mode of noninvasive respiratory support reported adverse side effects. In addition, no differences were noted with regard to other important short-term morbidity parameters.

The largest pragmatic RCT conducted by Kirpalani and colleagues[8] compared the use of NIPPV (either bilevel or CMV) versus CPAP as primary or secondary mode in a high-risk population of preterm infants (birth weight <1000 g and gestational age <30 weeks). The study protocol allowed synchronization during both modes of NIPPV, but the trial was not designed to compare sNIPPV versus non-sNIPPV. A secondary analysis of the data for the infants randomized to the NIPPV arm of the trial compared outcomes between infants who received mostly CMV NIPPV and those who received mostly bilevel NIPPV.[46] No difference in the combined outcome of death/BPD (adjusted odds ratio [OR], 0.88; 95% confidence interval [CI], 0.57–1.35; P = .56) was observed. More deaths before 36 weeks gestational age occurred in the bilevel NIPPV group (9.4% vs 2.3%;adjusted OR, 5.01; 95% CI,1.74–14.4; P = .0028) with no difference in the rate of BPD between the 2 groups (30.3% bilevel NIPPV vs 37.1% CMV NIPPV; adjusted OR, 0.64; 95% CI, 0.41–1.02; P = .061). The number of reintubations within the first week of extubation was lower in the bilevel NIPPV group compared with CMV NIPPV group (31.8% vs 39.8%; adjusted OR, 0.69; 95% CI, 0.46–1.06; P = .088). The investigators of this trial point out an important issue with regard to synchronization during NIPPV. With the phasing out of the InfantStar ventilator in the United States and North America, no Food and Drug Administration–approved devices for synchronization during NIPPV are currently available. Only one study compared synchronized versus nonsynchronized CMV NIPPV, used either as primary or secondary mode. In this retrospective analysis (n = 410), Dumpa and colleagues[47] found no difference in the combined outcome of BPD/death after adjustment for significant confounders (adjusted OR, 0.74; 95% CI, 0.42–1.3).

Since the reemergence of NIPPV in clinical practice, several metaanalyses on NIPPV have been published. A recent metaanalysis included 8 trials and compared the impact of NIPPV versus nasal CPAP after extubation.[48] Five of these trials used the synchronized mode of CMV NIPPV by means of a Graseby capsule or a flow sensor. Overall, NIPPV significantly reduced the risk of meeting predefined extubation criteria (relative risk, 0.71; 95% CI, 0.6–0.82). The effect was most marked in studies using sNIPPV (n = 272 infants; relative risk, 0.25; 95% CI, 0.15–0.41). No difference was noted in the rate of BPD between the NIPPV and CPAP trials (relative risk, 0.97; 95% CI, 0.83–1.14).

Synchronized Nasal Intermittent Positive Pressure Ventilation for Treatment of Apnea of Prematurity

Two RCT using synchronized CMV NIPPV compared with nasal CPAP reported on differences in apneic episodes as a secondary outcome.[29,30] Barrington and colleagues[30] noted a significant reduction of apneic episodes during the study period, whereas Khalaf and colleagues[29] did not. An RCT has been recently conducted by Gizzi and colleagues.[49] These investigators assessed the effect of different noninvasive ventilation strategies on symptoms of apnea of prematurity. Nineteen infants were enrolled in this study (median gestational age of 27 weeks and median birth weight of 800 g) and were allocated randomly to flow-synchronized CMV NIPPV, nonsynchronized CMV NIPPV, and CPAP in a cross-over design (4 hours each period). The median event rate of desaturations and/or bradycardia per hour (SpO_2 $\leq$80% >1 sec and HR $\leq$80/min for >1 beat) was 2.9 (range, 0.75–6.8) during sNIPPV, 6.1 (range, 3.1–9.4) during non-sNIPPV, and 5.9 (range, 2–10.3) during CPAP (P<.001 and P<.009, compared with sNIPPV). The median central apnea rate per hour were 2.4 (range, 1–3.6) during sNIPPV, 6.3 (range, 2.8–17) during non-sNIPPV, and 5.4 (range, 3.1–12) during CPAP (P = .001, for both compared with sNIPPV). PEEP and PIP levels during both modes of NIPPV were set at the same level and a back-up rate of 20/min was provided during apneic episodes on synchronized mode (rate nonsynchronized was 20/min as well).

SUMMARY

Results from physiologic studies have shown some advantages with regard to WOB and pulmonary mechanics, whereas conflicting results were reported with regard to the effectiveness of ventilation in infants undergoing NIPPV. There are currently 2 trigger devices clinically available but not Food and Drug Administration approved, both of which have shown to effectively synchronize spontaneous breaths during CMV NIPPV and bilevel NIPPV. Physiologic studies tend to enroll infants that are considered to be stable in terms of their respiratory and cardiovascular status. Thus, it is unclear whether these findings can be translated to preterm infants with active respiratory issues (ie, active respiratory distress syndrome) and this needs further evaluation.

Short-term benefits have been observed for synchronized CMV NIPPV, either as primary or secondary mode, with regard to extubation failure within the first week when compared with CPAP. Nevertheless, none of the currently available modes of NIPPV was able to improve important outcome measures such as BPD or mortality. A recent and well-conceptualized RCT study comparing bilevel NIPPV with synchronized CMV NIPPV as a primary mode of noninvasive ventilation did not show an advantage of 1 of the 2 modes.[42] Attenuation of symptoms of apnea of prematurity have been observed in infants undergoing sNIPPV, in small clinical trials.[30,49]

Given the recent interests in oxygen saturation targeting, influence of hypoxemic events on short and long term morbidities,[4,50] as well as the fact that hypoxemic events mainly occur with advanced gestational age,[16] it would be of interest to assess the effect of prolonged NIPPV support on long-term pulmonary and neurodevelopmental outcomes. The limited availability of devices capable to synchronize makes future trials difficult to facilitate.

REFERENCES

1. Morley CJ, Davis PG, Doyle LW, et al, COIN Trial Investigators. Nasal CPAP or intubation at birth for very preterm infants. N Engl J Med 2008;14:700–8.
2. Ammari A, Suri M, Musavlievic V, et al. Variables associated with the early failure of nasal CPAP in very low birth weight infants. J Pediatr 2005;147:341–7.
3. Aly H, Massaro AN, Patel K, et al. Is it safer to intubate premature infants in the delivery room? Pediatrics 2005;115:1660–5.

4. SUPPORT Study Group of the Eunice Kennedy Shriver NICHD Neonatal Research Network. Early CPAP versus surfactant in extremely preterm infants. N Engl J Med 2010;362:1970–9.
5. Stefanescu MB, Murphy WP, Hansell BJ, et al. A randomized, controlled trial comparing two different continuous positive airway pressure systems for the successful extubation of extremely low birth weight infants. Pediatrics 2003;112: 1031–8.
6. Courtney SE, Barrington KJ. Continuous positive airway pressure and noninvasive ventilation. Clin Perinatol 2007;34:73–92.
7. Roberts CT, Davis PG, Owen LS. Neonatal non-invasive respiratory support: synchronised NIPPV, non-synchronised NIPPV or bi-level CPAP: what is the evidence in 2013? Neonatology 2013;104:203–9.
8. Kirpalani H, Millar D, Lemyre B, et al. A trial comparing noninvasive ventilation strategies in preterm infants. N Engl J Med 2013;369:611–20.
9. John J, Björklund LJ, Svenningsen NW, et al. Airway and body surface sensors for triggering in neonatal ventilation. Acta Paediatr 1994;83:903–9.
10. Crowley P, Chalmers I, Keirse MJNC. The effects of corticosteroid administration before preterm delivery: an overview of the evidence from controlled trials. Br J Obstet Gynaecol 1990;97:11–25.
11. Committee on Fetus and Newborn, American Academy of Pediatrics. Respiratory support in preterm infants at birth. Pediatrics 2014;133:171–4.
12. Stevens TP, Harrington EW, Blennow M, et al. Early surfactant administration with brief ventilation vs. selective surfactant and continued mechanical ventilation for preterm infants with or at risk for respiratory distress syndrome. Cochrane Database Syst Rev 2007;(17):CD003063.
13. Speer CP. Inflammation and bronchopulmonary dysplasia: a continuing story. Semin Fetal Neonatal Med 2006;11:354–62.
14. Di Fiore JM, Bloom JN, Orge F, et al. A higher incidence of intermittent hypoxemic episodes is associated with severe retinopathy of prematurity. J Pediatr 2010; 157:69–73.
15. Hibbs AM, Johnson NL, Rosen CL, et al. Prenatal and neonatal risk factors for sleep disordered breathing in school-aged children born preterm. J Pediatr 2008;153:176–82.
16. Martin RJ, Wang K, Köroğlu O, et al. Intermittent hypoxic episodes in preterm infants: do they matter? Neonatology 2011;100:303–10.
17. Schmidt B, Roberts RS, Davis P, et al. Long-term effects of caffeine therapy for apnea of prematurity. N Engl J Med 2007;357:1893–902.
18. Gregory GA, Kitterman JA, Phibbs RH, et al. Treatment of the idiopathic respiratory-distress syndrome with continuous positive airway pressure. N Engl J Med 1971;284:1333–40.
19. Lampland AL, Meyers PA, Worwa CT, et al. Gas exchange and lung inflammation using nasal intermittent positive-pressure ventilation versus synchronized intermittent mandatory ventilation in piglets with saline lavage-induced lung injury: an observational study. Crit Care Med 2008;36:183–7.
20. Aghai ZH, Saslow JG, Nakhla T, et al. Synchronized nasal intermittent positive pressure ventilation (SNIPPV) decreases work of breathing (WOB) in premature infants with respiratory distress syndrome (RDS) compared to nasal continuous positive airway pressure (NCPAP). Pediatr Pulmonol 2006;41:875–81.
21. Ali N, Claure N, Alegria X, et al. Effects of non-invasive pressure support ventilation (NI-PSV) on ventilation and respiratory effort in very low birth weight infants. Pediatr Pulmonol 2007;42:704–10.

22. Chang HY, Claure N, D'Ugard C, et al. Effects of synchronization during nasal ventilation in clinically stable preterm infants. Pediatr Res 2011;69:84–9.

23. Huang L, Mendler MR, Waitz M, et al. Effects of synchronization during noninvasive intermittent mandatory ventilation in preterm infants with respiratory distress syndrome immediately after extubation. Neonatology 2015;108(2):108–14.

24. Jackson JK, Vellucci J, Johnson P, et al. Evidence-based approach to change in clinical practice: introduction of expanded nasal continuous positive airway pressure use in an intensive care nursery. Pediatrics 2003;111:542–7.

25. Friedlich P, Lecart C, Posen R, et al. A randomized trial of nasopharyngeal synchronized intermittent mandatory ventilation versus nasopharyngeal continuous positive airway pressure in very low birth weight infants after extubation. J Perinatol 1999;19:413–8.

26. Bhandari V. Nasal intermittent positive pressure ventilation in the newborn: review of literature and evidence-based guidelines. J Perinatol 2010;30:505–12.

27. Pandit PB, Courtney SE, Pyon KH, et al. Work of breathing during constant- and variable-flow nasal continuous positive airway pressure in preterm neonates. Pediatrics 2001;108:682–5.

28. Garland JS, Nelson DB, Rice T, et al. Increased risk of gastrointestinal perforations in neonates mechanically ventilated with either face mask or nasal prongs. Pediatrics 1985;76:406–10.

29. Khalaf MN, Brodsky N, Hurley J, et al. A prospective randomized, controlled trial comparing synchronized nasal intermittent positive pressure ventilation versus nasal continuous positive airway pressure as modes of extubation. Pediatrics 2001;108:13–7.

30. Barrington KJ, Bull D, Finer NN. Randomized trial of nasal synchronized intermittent mandatory ventilation compared with continuous positive airway pressure after extubation of very low birth weight infants. Pediatrics 2001;107:638–41.

31. Kugelman A, Feferkorn I, Riskin A, et al. Nasal intermittent mandatory ventilation versus nasal continuous positive airway pressure for respiratory distress syndrome: a randomized, controlled, prospective study. J Pediatr 2007;150:521–6.

32. Moretti C, Gizzi C, Papoff P, et al. Comparing the effects of nasal synchronized intermittent positive pressure ventilation (nSIPPV) and nasal continuous positive airway pressure (nCPAP) after extubation in very low birth weight infants. Early Hum Dev 1999;56:167–77.

33. Owen LS, Morley CJ, Dawson JA, et al. Effects of non-synchronised nasal intermittent positive pressure ventilation on spontaneous breathing in preterm infants. Arch Dis Child Fetal Neonatal Ed 2011;96:422–8.

34. Bernstein G, Cleary JP, Heldt GP, et al. Response time and reliability of three neonatal patient-triggered ventilators. Am Rev Respir Dis 1993;148:358–64.

35. Bernstein G. Patient triggered ventilation using cutaneous sensors. Semin Neonatol 1997;2:89–97.

36. Owen LS, Morley CJ, Davis PG. Effects of synchronisation during SiPAP-generated nasal intermittent positive pressure ventilation (NIPPV) in preterm infants. Arch Dis Child Fetal Neonatal Ed 2015;100:24–30.

37. Owen LS, Morley CJ, Davis PG. Pressure variation during ventilator generated nasal intermittent positive pressure ventilation in preterm infants. Arch Dis Child Fetal Neonatal Ed 2010;95:359–64.

38. Santin R, Brodsky N, Bhandari V. A prospective observational pilot study of synchronized nasal intermittent positive pressure ventilation (SNIPPV) as a primary mode of ventilation in infants > or = 28 weeks with respiratory distress syndrome (RDS). J Perinatol 2004;24:487–93.

39. Gizzi C, Papoff P, Giordano I, et al. Flow-synchronized nasal intermittent positive pressure ventilation for infants <32 weeks' gestation with respiratory distress syndrome. Crit Care Res Pract 2012;2012:301818.

40. Ricotti A, Salvo V, Zimmermann LJ, et al. N-SIPPV versus bi-level N-CPAP for early treatment of respiratory distress syndrome in preterm infants. J Matern Fetal Neonatal Med 2013;26:1346–51.

41. Bhandari V, Gavino RG, Nedrelow JH, et al. A randomized controlled trial of synchronized nasal intermittent positive pressure ventilation in RDS. J Perinatol 2007; 27:697–703.

42. Salvo V, Lista G, Lupo E, et al. Noninvasive ventilation strategies for early treatment of RDS in preterm infants: an RCT. Pediatrics 2015;135:444–51.

43. Schmölzer GM, Kumar M, Aziz K, et al. Sustained inflation versus positive pressure ventilation at birth: a systematic review and meta-analysis. Arch Dis Child Fetal Neonatal Ed 2015;100:361–8.

44. Moretti C, Giannini L, Fassi C, et al. Nasal flow-synchronized intermittent positive pressure ventilation to facilitate weaning in very low-birthweight infants: unmasked randomized controlled trial. Pediatr Int 2008;50:85–91.

45. Gao WW, Tan SZ, Chen YB, et al. Randomized trial of nasal synchronized intermittent mandatory ventilation compared with nasal continuous positive airway pressure in preterm infants with respiratory distress syndrome. Zhongguo Dang Dai Er Ke Za Zhi 2010;12:524–6.

46. Millar D, Lemyre B, Kirpalani H, et al. A comparison of bilevel and ventilator-delivered non-invasive respiratory support. Arch Dis Child Fetal Neonatal Ed 2016;101:21–5.

47. Dumpa V, Katz K, Northrup V, et al. SNIPPV vs NIPPV: does synchronization matter? J Perinatol 2012;32:438–42.

48. Lemyre B, Davis PG, De Paoli AG, et al. Nasal intermittent positive pressure ventilation (NIPPV) versus nasal continuous positive airway pressure (NCPAP) for preterm neonates after extubation. Cochrane Database Syst Rev 2014;(9):CD003212.

49. Gizzi C, Montecchia F, Panetta V, et al. Is synchronised NIPPV more effective than NIPPV and NCPAP in treating apnoea of prematurity (AOP)? A randomised crossover trial. Arch Dis Child Fetal Neonatal Ed 2015;100:17–23.

50. Poets CF, Roberts RS, Schmidt B, et al. Canadian oxygen trial investigators. Association between intermittent hypoxemia or bradycardia and late death or disability in extremely preterm infants. JAMA 2015;11:595–603.

Index

Note: Page numbers of article titles are in **boldface** type.

A

Alveolar development, high-frequency ventilation effects on, 729–731
Apnea, caffeine for, 773–775

B

Babylog 8000, 731, 735
Bilevel nasal intermittent positive pressure ventilation, 800–813
Breathing, physiology of, 621–624
Bronchopulmonary dysplasia, **783–798**
    after nasal high-flow therapy, 686, 688
    caffeine for, 775
    description of, 783–784
    mechanical ventilation association with, 784
    prevention of, noninvasive ventilation for, 784–793
Bubble continuous airway pressure, **647–659, 661–671,** 728
    after extubation, 655–656
    check of, 652
    clinical trials of, 654–656
    device comparisons of, 654–655
    factors affecting, 651–654
    failure of, 653–654
    high amplitude, 665–669
    history of, 662–663
    monitoring of, 651
    nasal interface selection and fixation of, 651
    optimizing delivery, 652
    physiologic basis of, 648–651
    physiology of, 663–665
    weaning from, 652–653
Bunnel Life Pulse ventilator, 727

C

Caffeine therapy, **773–782**
    action of, 622–623
    dose of, 778–779
    duration of, 778–779
    for transition to noninvasive respiratory support, 775–776
    initiation of, 777–778
    physiologic effects of, 776–777
    respiratory benefits of, 774–776

Clin Perinatol 43 (2016) 817–821
http://dx.doi.org/10.1016/S0095-5108(16)30092-6
0095-5108/16

UNITED STATES POSTAL SERVICE ®

Statement of Ownership, Management, and Circulation
(All Periodicals Publications Except Requester Publications)

1. Publication Title	2. Publication Number	3. Filing Date
CLINICS IN PERINATOLOGY	001 – 744	9/18/2016

4. Issue Frequency	5. Number of Issues Published Annually	6. Annual Subscription Price
MAR, JUN, SEP, DEC	4	$273.00

7. Complete Mailing Address of Known Office of Publication (Not printer) (Street, city, county, state, and ZIP+4®)

ELSEVIER INC.
360 PARK AVENUE SOUTH
NEW YORK, NY 10010-1710

Contact Person
STEPHEN R. BUSHING
Telephone (Include area code)
215-239-3688

8. Complete Mailing Address of Headquarters or General Business Office of Publisher (Not printer)

ELSEVIER INC.
360 PARK AVENUE SOUTH
NEW YORK, NY 10010-1710

9. Full Names and Complete Mailing Addresses of Publisher, Editor, and Managing Editor (Do not leave blank)

Publisher (Name and complete mailing address)

ADRIANNE BRIGIDO, ELSEVIER INC.
1600 JOHN F KENNEDY BLVD. SUITE 1800
PHILADELPHIA, PA 19103-2899

Editor (Name and complete mailing address)

KERRY HOLLAND, ELSEVIER INC.
1600 JOHN F KENNEDY BLVD. SUITE 1800
PHILADELPHIA, PA 19103-2899

Managing Editor (Name and complete mailing address)

PATRICK MANLEY, ELSEVIER INC.
1600 JOHN F KENNEDY BLVD. SUITE 1800
PHILADELPHIA, PA 19103-2899

10. Owner (Do not leave blank. If the publication is owned by a corporation, give the name and address of the corporation immediately followed by the names and addresses of all stockholders owning or holding 1 percent or more of the total amount of stock. If not owned by a corporation, give the names and addresses of the individual owners. If owned by a partnership or other unincorporated firm, give its name and address as well as those of each individual owner. If the publication is published by a nonprofit organization, give its name and address.)

Full Name	Complete Mailing Address
WHOLLY OWNED SUBSIDIARY OF REED/ELSEVIER, US HOLDINGS	1600 JOHN F KENNEDY BLVD. SUITE 1800 PHILADELPHIA, PA 19103-2899

11. Known Bondholders, Mortgagees, and Other Security Holders Owning or Holding 1 Percent or More of Total Amount of Bonds, Mortgages, or Other Securities. If none, check box ▶ ☐ None

Full Name	Complete Mailing Address
N/A	

12. Tax Status (For completion by nonprofit organizations authorized to mail at nonprofit rates) (Check one)
The purpose, function, and nonprofit status of this organization and the exempt status for federal income tax purposes:
☐ Has Not Changed During Preceding 12 Months
☐ Has Changed During Preceding 12 Months (Publisher must submit explanation of change with this statement)

13. Publication Title	14. Issue Date for Circulation Data Below
CLINICS IN PERINATOLOGY	JUNE 2016

15. Extent and Nature of Circulation			Average No. Copies Each Issue During Preceding 12 Months	No. Copies of Single Issue Published Nearest to Filing Date
a. Total Number of Copies (Net press run)			1009	1098
b. Paid Circulation (By Mail and Outside the Mail)	(1)	Mailed Outside-County Paid Subscriptions Stated on PS Form 3541 (Include paid distribution above nominal rate, advertiser's proof copies, and exchange copies)	568	678
	(2)	Mailed In-County Paid Subscriptions Stated on PS Form 3541 (Include paid distribution above nominal rate, advertiser's proof copies, and exchange copies)	0	0
	(3)	Paid Distribution Outside the Mails Including Sales Through Dealers and Carriers, Street Vendors, Counter Sales, and Other Paid Distribution Outside USPS®	166	188
	(4)	Paid Distribution by Other Classes of Mail Through the USPS (e.g., First-Class Mail®)	0	0
c. Total Paid Distribution (Sum of 15b (1), (2), (3), and (4))		▶	734	865
d. Free or Nominal Rate Distribution (By Mail and Outside the Mail)	(1)	Free or Nominal Rate Outside-County Copies included on PS Form 3541	56	72
	(2)	Free or Nominal Rate In-County Copies Included on PS Form 3541	0	0
	(3)	Free or Nominal Rate Copies Mailed at Other Classes Through the USPS (e.g., First-Class Mail)	0	0
	(4)	Free or Nominal Rate Distribution Outside the Mail (Carriers or other means)	0	0
e. Total Free or Nominal Rate Distribution (Sum of 15d (1), (2), (3) and (4))		▶	56	72
f. Total Distribution (Sum of 15c and 15e)		▶	790	938
g. Copies not Distributed (See Instructions to Publishers #4 (page #3))		▶	219	160
h. Total (Sum of 15f and g)		▶	1009	1098
i. Percent Paid (15c divided by 15f times 100)		▶	93%	92%

* If you are claiming electronic copies, go to line 16 on page 3. If you are not claiming electronic copies, skip to line 17 on page 3.

PS Form **3526**, July 2014 (Page 2 of 4)

16. Electronic Copy Circulation		Average No. Copies Each Issue During Preceding 12 Months	No. Copies of Single Issue Published Nearest to Filing Date
a. Paid Electronic Copies	▲	0	0
b. Total Paid Print Copies (Line 15c) + Paid Electronic Copies (Line 16a)	▲	734	865
c. Total Print Distribution (Line 15f) + Paid Electronic Copies (Line 16a)	▲	790	938
d. Percent Paid (Both Print & Electronic Copies) (16b divided by 16c × 100)	▲	93%	92%

☒ I certify that 50% of all my distributed copies (electronic and print) are paid above a nominal price.

17. Publication of Statement of Ownership
☒ If the publication is a general publication, publication of this statement is required. Will be printed in the DECEMBER 2016 issue of this publication.

☐ Publication not required.

18. Signature and Title of Editor, Publisher, Business Manager, or Owner

Stephen R. Bushing Date 9/18/2016

STEPHEN R. BUSHING - INVENTORY DISTRIBUTION CONTROL MANAGER

I certify that all information furnished on this form is true and complete. I understand that anyone who furnishes false or misleading information on this form or who omits material or information requested on the form may be subject to criminal sanctions (including fines and imprisonment) and/or civil sanctions (including civil penalties).

PS Form **3526**, July 2014 (Page 2 of 4)

PS Form **3526**, July 2014 (Page 1 of 4 (see instructions page 4)) PSN: 7530-01-000-9931   PRIVACY NOTICE: See our privacy policy on www.usps.com

Moving?

Make sure your subscription moves with you!

To notify us of your new address, find your **Clinics Account Number** (located on your mailing label above your name), and contact customer service at:

Email: journalscustomerservice-usa@elsevier.com

800-654-2452 (subscribers in the U.S. & Canada)
314-447-8871 (subscribers outside of the U.S. & Canada)

Fax number: 314-447-8029

Elsevier Health Sciences Division
Subscription Customer Service
3251 Riverport Lane
Maryland Heights, MO 63043

*To ensure uninterrupted delivery of your subscription, please notify us at least 4 weeks in advance of move.